# Supramolecular Systems for Gene and Drug Delivery, 2nd Edition

# Supramolecular Systems for Gene and Drug Delivery, 2nd Edition


Guest Editors

**Francisco José Ostos**
**José Antonio Lebrón**
**Pilar López-Cornejo**



MDPI

Basel • Beijing • Wuhan • Barcelona • Belgrade • Novi Sad • Cluj • Manchester

*Guest Editors*
Francisco José Ostos
Department of Physical Chemistry
University of Seville
Seville
Spain

José Antonio Lebrón
Department of Physical Chemistry
University of Seville
Seville
Spain

Pilar López-Cornejo
Department of Physical Chemistry
University of Seville
Seville
Spain

*Editorial Office*
MDPI AG
Grosspeteranlage 5
4052 Basel, Switzerland

This is a reprint of the Special Issue, published open access by the journal *Pharmaceutics* (ISSN 1999-4923), freely accessible at: https://www.mdpi.com/journal/pharmaceutics/special_issues/supra_gene_drug_volume_II.

For citation purposes, cite each article independently as indicated on the article page online and as indicated below:

| Lastname, A.A.; Lastname, B.B. Article Title. *Journal Name* **Year**, *Volume Number*, Page Range. |
|---|

**ISBN 978-3-7258-7472-9 (Hbk)**
**ISBN 978-3-7258-7473-6 (PDF)**
**https://doi.org/10.3390/books978-3-7258-7473-6**

# Contents

# About the Editors

**Francisco José Ostos**

Francisco José Ostos is an Assistant Professor in the Department of Physical Chemistry at the University of Seville. His research interests lie at the interface of physical chemistry and biomedicine, specifically focusing on supramolecular and nanostructured systems, including calixarenes, micelles, liposomes, polymeric nanoparticles, and carbon and titanium nanotubes for drug and gene delivery, as well as the development of hydrogels for tissue regeneration. He is currently an emerging Principal Investigator in a regional project (PI-0170-2024). His career is marked by participation in 14 research projects and the awarding of prestigious fellowships, such as the "Sara Borrell" and PAIDI 2020. Among his academic achievements, he obtained his PhD in Chemistry with International Mention (2020, *excellent cum laude*), complemented by strategic research stays at the University of East Anglia (UK) and the University of Pisa (Italy). His impressive scientific track record includes 31 research articles (mostly in Q1/D1 journals), 3 books, and 2 book chapters, accumulating over 650 citations with an h-index of 16. He has presented 58 communications in international meetings, including 5 keynote talks, and serves as a Guest Editor for *Pharmaceutics* and *Discovery Pharmaceutical Sciences*. Beyond his research, he has been recognized with the XIV *Arquímedes* University Prize. He is also highly active in mentorship, supervising numerous BSc and MSc students, as well as a predoctoral candidate. His extensive network of international collaborations includes institutions such as the Institute of Technology Tallaght, the European Molecular Biology Laboratory (Hamburg, Germany), and the National Academy of Sciences of Ukraine.

**José Antonio Lebrón**

José Antonio Lebrón is an Assistant Professor in the Department of Physical Chemistry at the University of Seville. His research focuses on the design and development of advanced nanostructured systems for biomedical and pharmaceutical applications, particularly in drug and gene delivery. His work includes the use of liposomes, polymeric nanoparticles, micelles, aminoclays, and carbon nanotubes as nanocarriers, as well as the study of antimicrobial peptides for applications in biomedicine and aquaculture. He obtained his PhD in Chemistry from the University of Seville in 2019 with the highest distinction (*cum laude*). His academic career has been closely linked to this institution, where he has held predoctoral and postdoctoral positions before his current role. He also completed a postdoctoral research stay at the RENSMA Centre at the University of Huelva.

He has participated in more than 10 competitive research projects and has served as Principal Investigator in a project funded by Fundación ONCE focused on metal–organic frameworks to eradicate HIV reservoirs. His scientific output includes 27 peer-reviewed articles in JCR-indexed journals, mostly in Q1, as well as books, book chapters, and a patent. His work has received over 430 citations, with an h-index of 12. He has presented over 40 contributions at national and international conferences, including invited talks, and serves as reviewer for international journals and Guest Editor for *Pharmaceutics* and *Discovery Pharmaceutical Sciences*. His research has been recognized with several awards, including the XIV *Arquímedes* University Prize. He maintains active collaborations with national and international institutions.

**Pilar López-Cornejo**

Pilar López-Cornejo is a Full Professor in Physical Chemistry at the University of Seville. She is recognized for her extensive contributions to supramolecular chemistry, colloid and interface science, and the physicochemical characterization of complex systems. Her research career encompasses significant advances in electron transfer kinetics, micellar and microemulsion effects, host–guest chemistry, and biomolecular interactions, with pioneering applications of the Pseudophase Model in heterogeneous media. She has authored more than one hundred peer reviewed publications in leading international journals, including *Pharmaceutics*, *J. Mat. Chem. B*, *Colloids and Surfaces B*, *Langmuir*, and *J. Drug Deliv. Sci. Tech.*, many of which appear in the top quartile of their respective scientific fields and have had a significant impact on citation impact. Her recent research activities are centred on the design, synthesis, and evaluation of nanostructured carriers such as calixarene based systems, metallomicelles, liposomes, carbon nanotubes, and metal–organic frameworks, for the delivery of genetic material, antineoplastic drugs, antiviral agents, and antimicrobial compounds. These investigations integrate kinetic and thermodynamic methodologies, electrochemical and spectroscopic techniques, and computational approaches, yielding fundamental insights into DNA compaction, ligand/receptor interactions, and supramolecular self assembly. She has served as Principal Investigator in multiple competitive national and regional research projects addressing innovative nanotechnological strategies for HIV eradication, biocompatible nanoformulations, and functional materials for biomedical and biotechnological applications.

Her supervision of several doctoral theses, as well as of numerous undergraduate and master's theses, and her active collaboration with interdisciplinary and international research groups underscore her commitment to scientific development and academic excellence.

*pharmaceutics*

MDPI

*Article*

# Antifungal Potential of Synthetic Peptides against *Cryptococcus neoformans*: Mechanism of Action Studies Reveal Synthetic Peptides Induce Membrane–Pore Formation, DNA Degradation, and Apoptosis

**Tawanny K. B. Aguiar [1,†], Nilton A. S. Neto [1,†], Cleverson D. T. Freitas [1], Ayrles F. B. Silva [1], Leandro P. Bezerra [2], Ellen A. Malveira [1], Levi A. C. Branco [1], Felipe P. Mesquita [3], Gustavo H. Goldman [4], Luciana M. R. Alencar [5], Jose T. A. Oliveira [1], Ralph Santos-Oliveira [6,7] and Pedro F. N. Souza [1,3,*]**

1 Department of Biochemistry and Molecular Biology, Federal University of Ceará, Fortaleza 60451-970, CE, Brazil
2 Department of Fisheries Engineering, Federal University of Ceará, Fortaleza 60455-970, CE, Brazil
3 Drug Research and Development Center, Department of Physiology and Pharmacology, Federal University of Ceará, Fortaleza 60430-275, CE, Brazil
4 Faculty of Pharmaceutical Sciences of Ribeirão Preto, University of São Paulo, São Paulo 14040-903, SP, Brazil
5 Department of Physics, Laboratory of Biophysics and Nanosystems, Federal University of Maranhão, São Luís 65080-805, MA, Brazil
6 Laboratory of Nanoradiopharmaceuticals and Radiopharmacy, Zona Oeste State University, Rio de Janeiro 23070-200, RJ, Brazil
7 Brazilian Nuclear Energy Commission, Nuclear Engineering Institute, Rio de Janeiro 21941-906, RJ, Brazil
* Correspondence: pedrofilhobio@gmail.com
† These authors contributed equally to this work.

**Abstract:** *Cryptococcus neoformans* is a human-pathogenic yeast responsible for pneumonia and meningitis, mainly in patients immunocompromised. Infections caused by *C. neoformans* are a global health concern. Synthetic antimicrobial peptides (SAMPs) have emerged as alternative molecules to cope with fungal infections, including *C. neoformans*. Here, eight SAMPs were tested regarding their antifungal potential against *C. neoformans* and had their mechanisms of action elucidated by fluorescence and scanning electron microscopies. Five SAMPs showed an inhibitory effect ($MIC_{50}$) on *C. neoformans* growth at low concentrations. Fluorescence microscope (FM) revealed that SAMPs induced 6-kDa pores in the *C. neoformans* membrane. Inhibitory assays in the presence of ergosterol revealed that some peptides lost their activity, suggesting interaction with it. Furthermore, FM analysis revealed that SAMPs induced caspase 3/7-mediated apoptosis and DNA degradation in *C. neoformans* cells. Scanning Electron Microscopy (SEM) analysis revealed that peptides induced many morphological alterations such as cell membrane, wall damage, and loss of internal content on *C. neoformans* cells. Our results strongly suggest synthetic peptides are potential alternative molecules to control *C. neoformans* growth and treat the cryptococcal infection.

**Keywords:** synthetic antifungal peptides; *Cryptococcus neoformans*; cryptococcal meningitis; inhibition; apoptosis induction

## 1. Introduction

Fungi cause various diseases, from mild superficial mycoses on the skin to severe invasive lung infections. Fungal infections can cause more than 50% mortality, especially those caused by fungi from genus *Cryptococcus*, *Candida*, *Aspergillus*, and *Pneumocystis*, among the most lethal human pathogens [1–3]. The ability to treat those infections was revolutionary to medicine. However, in the past 80 years, fungi have become resistant to most or even all available antifungal agents. Thus, this creates an urgent need for new molecules to overcome the resistance and develop novel treatments for fungal infectious diseases [2,4].

Among those human-pathogenic fungi, *C. neoformans* is a yeast responsible for pneumonia and meningitis. *C. neoformans* is mostly common in immunocompromised patients, organ transplanted patients, those submitted to cancer chemotherapy, and HIV+ patients [5]. *Cryptococcus* strains have evolved virulence traits that make it a unique and highly resistant fungal pathogen, such as a capsule, which protects against phagocytosis [6]. In addition, the inappropriate use of antifungal agents accelerated the development of antifungal resistance. The resistance of *C. neoformans* to echinocandins, the newest fungicidal drug class, is a huge problem, leading public health systems worldwide without an option to treat *C. neoformans* infections [7]. This has driven the need for new molecules to cope with *C. neoformans* infection and develop new therapies [8–10]. Therefore, seeking and developing new molecules effective against *C. neoformans* is imperative to produce a new drug to treat cryptococcal infections. Several research groups worldwide have been seeking new alternatives to overcome the threat imposed by *C. neoformans* [9,10].

Thus, searching for new compounds with different mechanisms than conventional drugs to inhibit fungal growth is urgently required. Recently, two sequential studies showed the potential of Ellagic acid (EA), a polyphenolic compound present in plants, which has presented high activity against *C. neoformans* [9,10]. In the first study, the authors showed that mice treated with EA presented a survival rate of 70% toward *C. neoformans* infection. In contrast, mice treated with fluconazole had only 20% survival [9]. In the second study [10], it was shown in silico and in vitro that EA interacts and inhibits the laccase from *C. neoformans*, thus indicating that laccase is an excellent target to focus on the treatment of *C. neoformans* infection. Antimicrobial peptides are also potential alternative molecules. For instance, Mahindra et al. [11] reported many natural peptides that present activity against *C. neoformans*. However, some natural peptides presented in the study were toxic to kidney cells, making them inappropriate for further studies. The natural antimicrobial peptides presented several problems to clinical application. Usually, the natural peptides are toxic to human cells, are fairly susceptible to proteolysis, and have a high production cost [12].

In this scenario, synthetic antimicrobial peptides (SAMPs) are a potential alternative to overcoming infections caused by *C. neoformans*. Compared to natural peptides, SAMPs are rationally designed to enhance their antimicrobial activity and remove limitations of natural peptides (e.g., toxicity) [12]. This makes SAMPs good candidates for new antifungal drugs. For example, our research group has designed eight synthetic peptides that present no toxicity to human erythrocytes, fibroblast, keratinocytes, and even zebrafish embryos, in addition, to being resistant to proteolysis [12,13].

Therefore, it was hypothesized that synthetic antimicrobial peptides, which had no toxicity as discussed before, have antifungal activity against *C. neoformans* by damaging cell membranes, making the development of resistance hard. Based on that, here, these eight are bioinspired from three antimicrobial plant proteins, *Mo*-CBP3 (SAMPs named *Mo*-CBP$_3$-PepI, *Mo*-CBP$_3$-PepII, and *Mo*-CBP$_3$-PepIII) from *Moringa oleifera* seeds [14]. *Rc*-2S-Alb (SAMPs named *Rc*Alb-PepI, *Rc*Alb-PepII, and *Rc*Alb-PepIII) [12] from *Ricinus communis*. Chitinase (SAMPs named PepGAT and PepKAA) [15] from *Arabidopsis thaliana* with proven antifungal, antibacterial, antibiofilm, and antiviral activity against different human pathogens [12,13] had their antifungal potential tested against *C. neoformans*. Of the eight, five SAMPs presented great inhibitory activity against *C. neoformans*, and investigation of the mechanism of action revealed those peptides targeted cell membrane and induced *C. neoformans* apoptosis. The great importance of this work is that synthetic peptides, which are not toxic, present activity against *C. neoformans* and can potentially be used in developing new drugs to overcome *C. neoformans* resistance to drugs.

## 2. Materials and Methods

### 2.1. Fungal Strains, Chemicals, and Synthetic Peptides

*Cryptococcus neoformans* (ATCC 32045) was gently provided by the Department of Pathology of the Federal University of Ceará (UFC), Fortaleza, Brazil. All the chemicals used in the experiments were obtained from Sigma Aldrich (São Paulo, SP, Brazil).

*2.2. Peptide Synthesis*

The synthetic peptides Mo-CBP3-PepI, Mo-CBP3-PepII, Mo-CBP3-PepIII, RcAlb-PepI, RcAlb-PepII, RcAlb-PepIII, PepGAT, and PepKAA were chemically synthesized by the company Chempeptide (Shanghai, China). The quality and purity (≥95%) were analyzed by reverse-phase high-performance liquid chromatography (RP-HPLC, Jasco, Easton, MD, USA) and mass spectrometry (Waltham, MA, USA).

*2.3. The Minimum Inhibitory Concentration Assay*

The minimum inhibitory concentration (MIC) assay was performed using a broth microdilution test using 96-well plates [12]. The cells were grown on YPD agar for approximately 15 days, and subsequently, cryptococcal cells were resuspended in YPD medium and standardized at $10^6$ cells $mL^{-1}$. In 96-well plates, 25 μL of YPD with cryptococcal cells and 25 μL of each synthetic peptide at different concentrations (50 to 0.004 μg $mL^{-1}$) were added. The microplates were incubated for 24 h. Then, the absorbance was measured at 600 nm using an automated microplate reader (Epoch, Biotek, Santa Clara, CA, USA). The negative control for inhibition of *C. neoformans* was 5% DMSO. The positive control for inhibition was made by two antifungal drugs, Nystatin (NYS, 1000 μg $mL^{-1}$) and Itraconazole (ITR, 1000 μg $mL^{-1}$).

*2.4. Mechanisms of Action Employed by Peptides*

2.4.1. Ergosterol Interaction Assay

The interaction of peptides with ergosterol was evaluated following [16]. Cryptococcal cells ($10^6$ cells $mL^{-1}$) and ergosterol (0.02, 0.04, and 0.08 mg $mL^{-1}$), *Mo*-CBP$_3$-PepII, *Rc*Alb-PepII, *Rc*Alb-PepIII, PepGAT and PepKAA (MIC50) and YPD medium (1:1:1:1 $v/v$) were incubated in 96-well plates at 30 °C for 24 h. Next, fungal growth was measured at 620 nm using an automated microplate reader. DMSO-NaCl and Nystatin were used as controls.

2.4.2. Cell Membrane Integrity Assay

To evaluate the pore formation induced by peptides on the *C. neoformans* membrane, the methodology described by Dias et al. [12] was used. After the antifungal assay (under the same conditions described above), the samples were washed with 0.15 M NaCl, centrifuged (5000× *g* 5 min at 4 °C), and incubated with PI at 1 μM for 30 min at room temperature in the dark. After that, the cells were analyzed under a fluorescence microscope (Olympus System BX60, Olympus, Tokyo, Japan) with an excitation wavelength of 488 nm and an emission wavelength of 525 nm. Fluorescent *C. neoformans* cells were counted using ImageJ software using the Cell Counter plugin [17]. The same picture has the cells counted in the bright and fluorescent field. The number of cells in the bright field was considered 100%. In the fluorescent field, cells that released fluorescent were called positive cells, and those without fluorescence were called negative cells. The following equation reached the % of positive cells: Number of positive cells × 100/number of cells in bright field. The number of negative cells was calculated following the equation: number of cells in the bright field—number of positive cells. Three different images were used to count cells.

Additionally, the methodology described by Dias et al. [12] was used to evaluate the size of pores formed. The cells of *C. neoformans* were treated as above and incubated with 10 μM of conjugated fluorescein isothiocyanate (FITC)-Dextran with 6 kDa (Sigma Aldrich, São Paulo, SP, Brazil). After incubation for 30 min at 25 °C in the dark, the cells were washed as above and observed under a fluorescence microscope (Olympus System BX60) with an excitation wavelength of 490 nm and emission wavelength of 520 nm. Fluorescent *C. neoformans* cells were counted using ImageJ software using the Cell Counter plugin [17]. The same picture has the cells counted in the bright and fluorescent fields, and the number of cells in the bright field was considered 100%. In the fluorescent field, cells that released fluorescent were called positive cells, and those without fluorescence were called negative cells. The following equation reached the % of positive cells: Number of positive cells × 100/number of cells in bright field. The number of negative cells was calculated following the equation: number of cells in the bright field—number of positive cells. Three different images were used to count cells.

2.4.3. DNA Degradation on *C. neoformans* Induced by Peptides

The kit DeadEnd™ Fluorometric TUNEL System (Promega, São Paulo, SP, Brazil) followed the manufacturer's instructions to evaluate the DNA degradation induced by peptides. Fluorescent *C. neoformans* cells were counted using ImageJ software using the Cell Counter plugin [17] described above in the cell membrane assay.

2.4.4. Caspase 3/7 Assay

The caspase activity was measured after cell incubation for 24 h, in the presence and absence of synthetic peptides, according to the methodology described by Qorri and Harless [18], with some modifications. The cells were treated as above and then incubated using a 3 µL CellEvent® reagent (ThermoFisher, São Paulo, SP, Brazil) for 30 min in the dark. Afterwards, cells were washed and centrifuged as mentioned above. Finally, the cells were observed under a fluorescence microscope (Olympus System BX60) with an excitation wavelength of 342 nm and an emission wavelength of 441 nm. Fluorescent C. neoformans cells were counted using ImageJ software using the Cell Counter plugin [17]. The same picture has the cells counted in the bright and fluorescent field. The number of cells in the bright field was considered 100%. In the fluorescent field, cells that released fluorescent were called positive cells, and those without fluorescence were called negative cells. The following equation reached the % of positive cells: Number of positive cells × 100/number of cells in bright field. The number of negative cells was calculated following the equation: number of cells in the bright field—number of positive cells. Three different images were used to count cells.

2.4.5. Scanning Electron Microscopy (SEM)

The cells of *C. neoformans* untreated and treated with peptides were prepared and analyzed by SEM following Staniszewska et al. [19], with some adaptions. After the antifungal assay described previously in Section 2.3, cells were fixed with 1% (*v*/*v*) glutaraldehyde in 0.15 M sodium phosphate buffer at pH 7.2 for 16 h. Next, the cells were washed with sodium phosphate buffer at pH 7.2 and centrifuged (5000× *g* for 5 min at 4 °C) each time. Then, samples were dehydrated with increased ethanol concentrations (30%, 50%, 70%, 100%, and 100% [*v*/*v*]) for 10 min each at 25 °C and centrifuged as above each time. The final dehydration was performed with 50% (*v*/*v*) hexamethyldisilane (HDMS, Sigma, St. Louis, MI, USA) diluted in ethanol for 10 min, centrifuged as above, and then dehydrated with 100% HDMS. The dried cells were placed into a cover glass and covered with gold using a coating machine (Emitech-Q150TES, Quorum Technologies, Lewes, England) coupled with positron-emission tomography (PET). SEM analysis ran in a scanning electron microscope (Quanta 450 FEG, FEI, Waltham, MA, USA) with a magnification of 20,000×.

### *2.5. Statistical Analysis*

All experiments were performed three times independently, and the values are expressed as the mean ± standard error. GraphPad Prism 5.01 (GraphPad Software company, Santa Clara, CA, USA) for Microsoft Windows was used to run the statistical analyses. All data obtained in the assays were submitted to ANOVA, followed by the Tukey test ($p < 0.05$).

## 3. Results

### *3.1. Antifungal Activity*

Five of eight peptides were tested in 12 serial dilutions to reach the Minimum Inhibitory Concentration of peptides required to inhibit 50% of yeast growth ($MIC_{50}$) (Table 1), *Mo*-CBP$_3$-PepII, *Rc*Alb-PepII, *Rc*Alb-PepIII, PepGAT, and PepKAA presented an $MIC_{50}$, respectively, of 25, 0.04, 0.04, 0.04, and 0.04 µg mL$^{-1}$ (Table 1). Although Mo-CBP3-PepI, Mo-CBP3-PepIII, and RcAlb-PepI inhibited *C. neoformans* growth, none of them reached

50% of inhibition in all concentrations tested (Table 1). The peptides that reached the $MIC_{50}$ were chosen to investigate the mechanism of action.

**Table 1.** Minimum inhibitory concentration (MIC) of synthetic against *C. neoformans*.

| Peptides | $MIC_{50}$ ($\mu g\ mL^{-1}$) against *C. neoformans* |
|---|---|
| *Mo*-CBP$_3$-PepI | [a] ND |
| *Mo*-CBP$_3$-PepII | 25 |
| *Mo*-CBP$_3$-PepIII | ND |
| *Rc*Alb-PepI | ND |
| *Rc*Alb-PepII | 0.04 |
| *Rc*Alb-PepIII | 0.04 |
| PepGAT | 0.04 |
| PepKAA | 0.04 |
| Nystatin | 250 |
| Itraconazole | 500 |

[a] ND means that $MIC_{50}$ was not reached.

### 3.2. Ergosterol Interactions

We further investigated if peptides could interact with ergosterol in the membrane of C. neoformans. To evaluate that, peptides at $MIC_{50}$ concentration were assayed against *C. neoformans* in the presence of ergosterol at concentrations of 20, 40, and 80 $\mu g\ mL^{-1}$. To some extent, all peptides had antifungal activity against *C. neoformans* affected by the presence of ergosterol (Figure 1). For instance, *Mo*-CBP$_3$-PepII and *Rc*Alb-PepIII completely lost their activity against *C. neoformans* in the presence of ergosterol at 40 $\mu g\ mL^{-1}$ (Figure 1A,C). In contrast, *Rc*Alb-PepII lost activity in the presence of 80 $\mu g\ mL^{-1}$ of ergosterol (Figure 1B). PepGAT and PepKAA were the most affected by the presence of ergosterol, losing the inhibitory activity in all tested concentrations (Figure 1D,E).

### 3.3. Membrane Pore Formation

The presence of pores on *C. neoformans* membranes was confirmed by propidium iodide (PI) uptake assay. PI interacts with DNA releasing red fluorescence but cannot pass through a healthy membrane. As expected, the healthy membrane of control *C. neoformans* did not allow the passage of PI and had no red fluorescence (Figure 2). In contrast, the PI uptake and red fluorescence showed that all peptides could induce pore formation on the *C. neoformans* membrane (Figure 2).

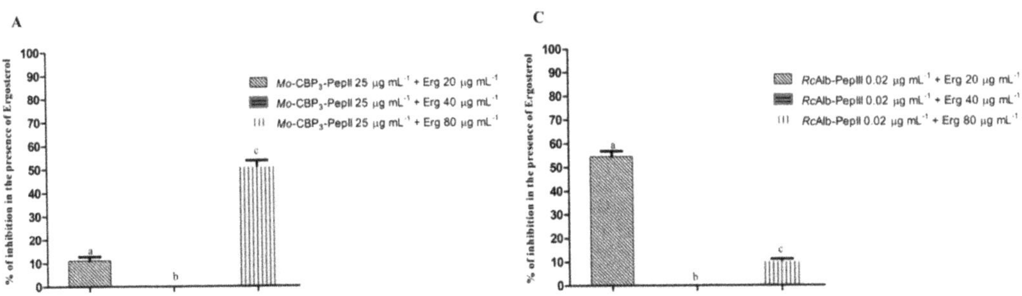


**Figure 1.** *Cont.*

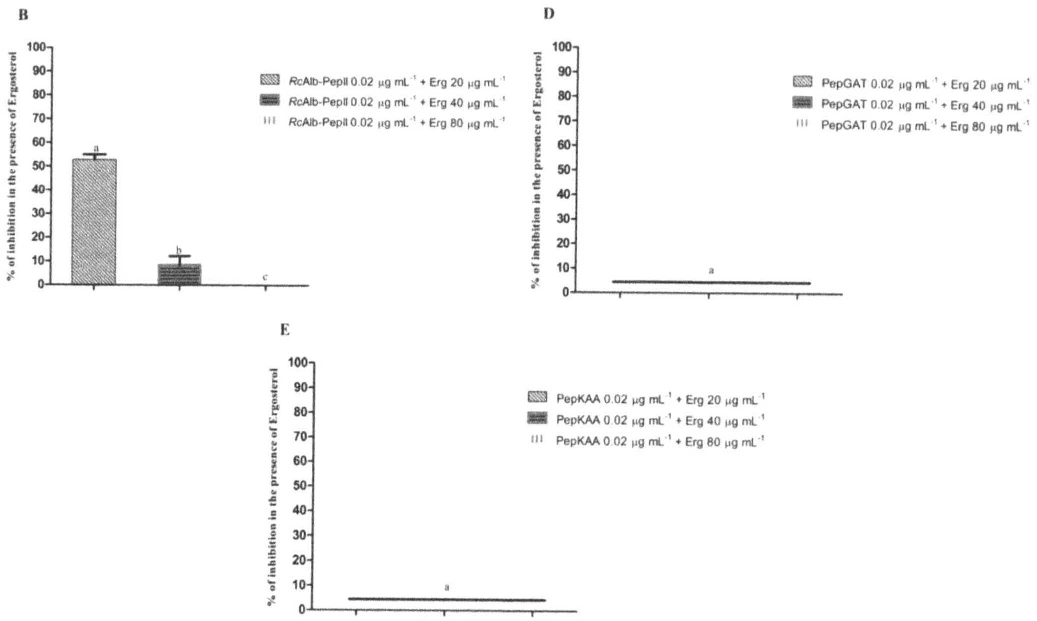


**Figure 1.** The interaction of ergosterol and its role in the antifungal activity of synthetic peptides. (**A**) *Mo*-CBP$_3$-PepII, (**B**) *Rc*Alb-PepII, (**C**) *Rc*Alb-PepIII, (**D**) PepGAT, and (**E**) PepKAA DMSO-NaCl was used as a negative control. Data are presented as mean ± standard deviation (SD). Using the Tukey test, different letters represent the statistical difference ($p < 0.05$). The experiment was repeated three times.

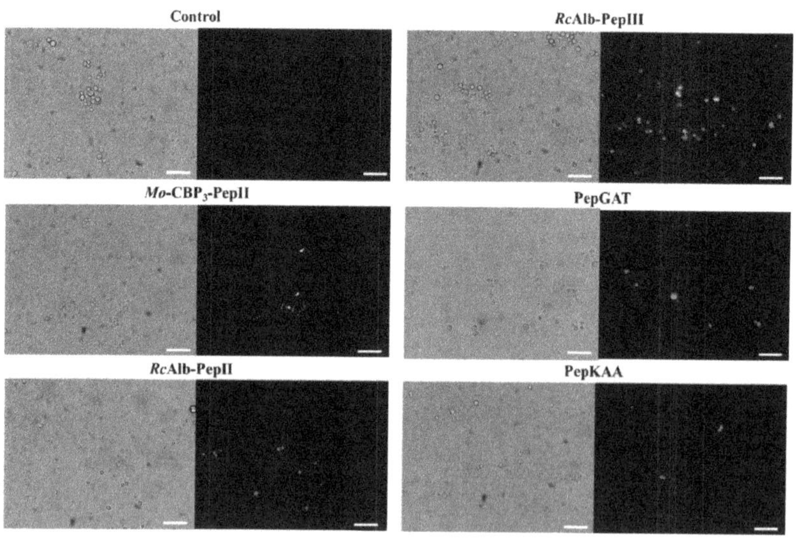


**Figure 2.** Fluorescence images showing membrane pore formation induced by *Mo*-CBP$_3$-PepII, *Rc*Alb-PepII, *Rc*Alb-PepIII, PepGAT, and PepKAA, respectively, at 25, 0.04, 0.04, 0.04, and 0.04 μg mL$^{-1}$. Detection of red fluorescence in the peptide-treated cells indicates that PI was internalized. In control (DMSO-NaCl), the absence of PI fluorescence indicates the integrity of the cell membrane. Bars: 100 μm.

PI assay only provides information about the pores on the membrane without any clue about their size. An additional experiment using dextran with a size of 6 kDa conjugated with FITC (Fluorescein isothiocyanate—green fluorescence, Figure 3) revealed all peptides induced pore with a size of at least 6 kDa, which allows the movement of dextran by the membrane of *C. neoformans*.

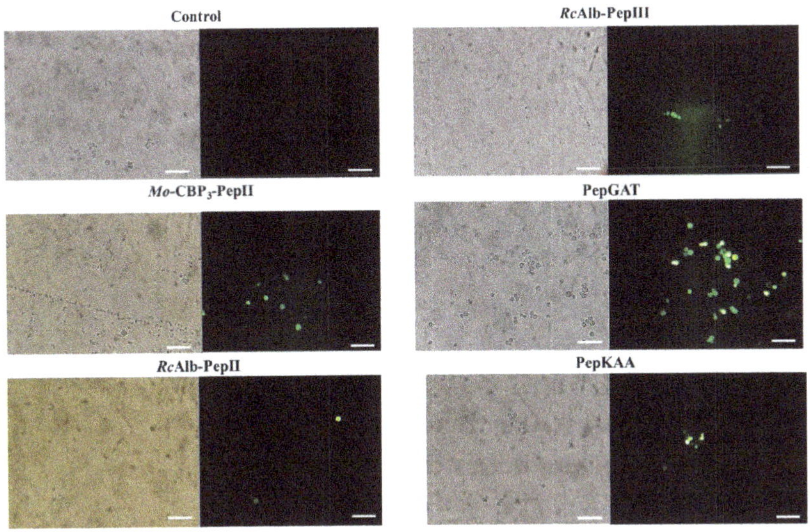


**Figure 3.** Fluorescence images showing membrane pore formation using fluorescein isothiocyanate (FITC)-dextran (6 kDa) induced by *Mo*-CBP$_3$-PepII, *Rc*Alb-PepII, *Rc*Alb-PepIII, PepGAT, and PepKAA, respectively, at 25, 0.04, 0.04, 0.04, and 0.04 µg mL$^{-1}$. *C. neoformans* cells were incubated with peptides and DMSO-NaCl. Detection of green fluorescence indicates that cells internalized FITC-dextran. Bars: 100 µm.

### *3.4. DNA Degradation and Apoptosis in C. neoformans Cells Induced by Peptides*

The *C. neoformans* cells treated with synthetics peptides at MIC$_{50}$ concentration showed yellow fluorescence, indicating DNA degradation and fragmentation induced by peptides. The same was not observed in the control (Figure 4).

As peptides induced DNA degradation in *C. neoformans*, we reasoned that the peptides could also induce apoptosis in *C. neoformans* cells. A Caspase-3/7 Green Detection kit evaluated the activity of caspases. The activity of caspase-3/7, which suggests that the cell is in apoptosis, was observed in all the cells treated with synthetics peptides (MIC$_{50}$) (Figure 5). The control, as expected, was not observed in fluorescence.

### *3.5. Counting Cells*

The counting of PI-fluorescent cells (positive cells) using the ImageJ program [17] revealed that 98% of cells treated with *Rc*Alb-PepIII presented a PI-fluorescence (Figure 6A). The evaluation of dextran-FITC-fluorescent cells using the ImageJ program revealed that after treatment with PepGAT and PepKAA, 86 and 85% of cells presented dextran-FITC-fluorescent (Figure 6B). The quantitative evaluation of TUNNEL-fluorescent cells revealed no difference in TUNNEL-fluorescent cells. All peptides induced fluorescence in around 97% of cells presented TUNNEL-fluorescence, indicating DNA damage after treatment (Figure 6C). The analysis on ImageJ program revealed *Mo*-CBP$_3$-PepII was the most potent, with 90% of treated cells releasing fluorescence, indicating apoptosis establishment. All other peptides induced apoptosis to a different extent (Figure 6D).

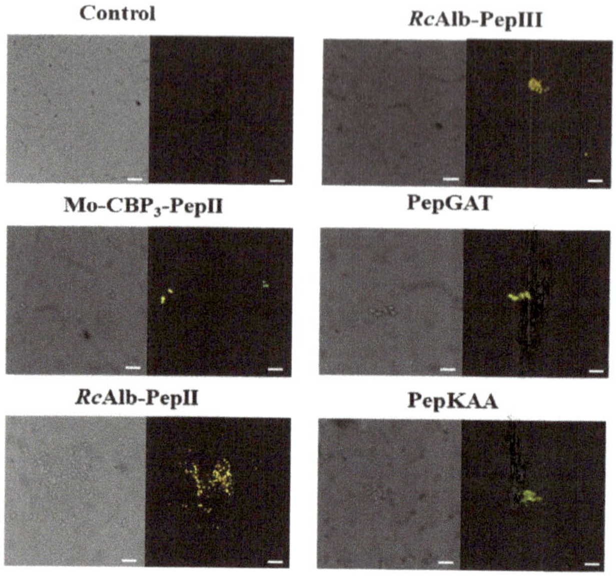


**Figure 4.** DNA fragmentation in *C. neoformans* cells induced by *Mo*-CBP$_3$-PepII, *Rc*AlbPepII, *Rc*Alb-PepIII, PepGAT, and PepKAA, respectively, at 25, 0.04, 0.04, 0.04, and 0.04 μg mL$^{-1}$. The cells were treated with peptides, and the control negative was DMSONaCl. Bars: 100 μm.

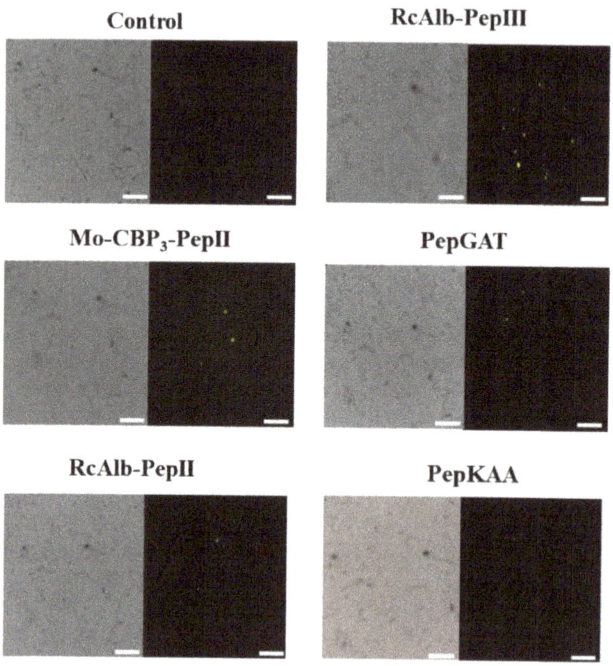


**Figure 5.** Apoptosis induction in *C. neoformans* cells by *Mo*-CBP$_3$-PepII, *Rc*Alb-PepII, *Rc*Alb-PepIII, PepGAT, and PepKAA, respectively, at 25, 0.04, 0.04, 0.04, and 0.04 μg mL$^{-1}$. Green fluorescence images show that treatment with the peptides (MIC$_{50}$) activates caspases involved in programmed cell death. Control: DMSO-NaCl. Bars: 100 μm.

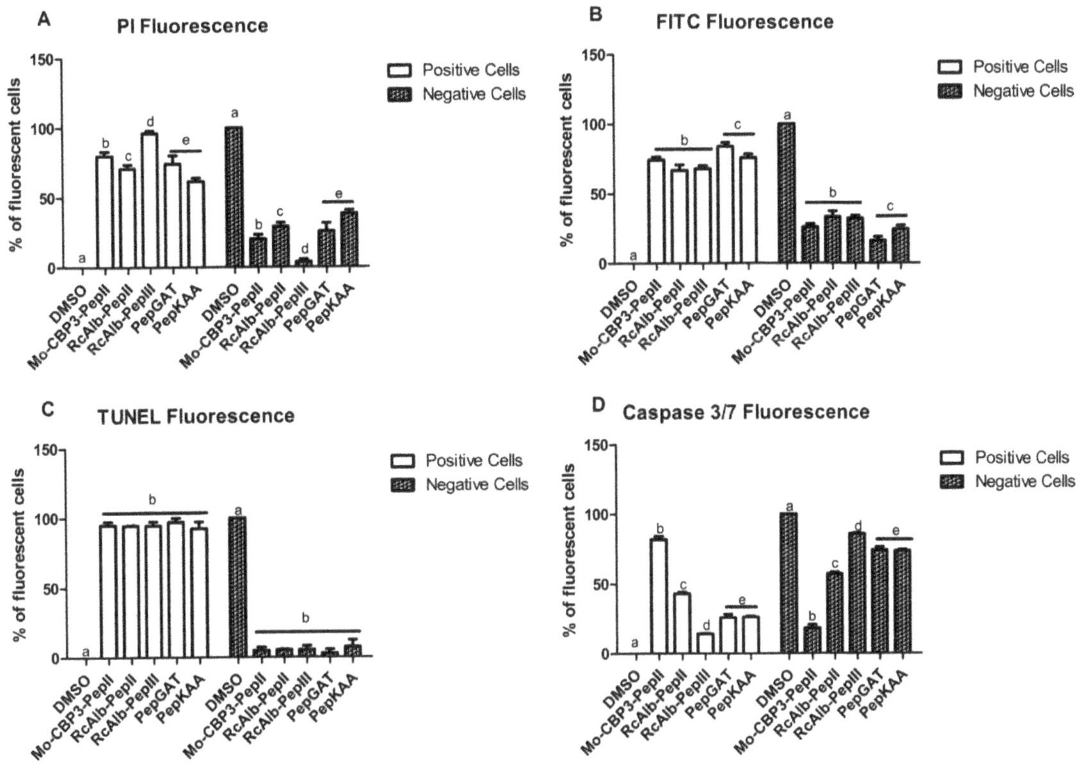


**Figure 6.** The number of fluorescent *C. neoformans* cells PI (**A**), Dextran-FITC (**B**), DNA fragmentation (**C**), and apoptosis (**D**). The letters represent the mean ± standard deviation of three replicates. Different lowercase letters indicate statically significant difference compared to DMSO-NaCl by analysis of variance ($p < 0.05$). The concentration of peptides was 25, 0.04, 0.04, 0.04, and 0.04 μg $mL^{-1}$, respectively, for *Mo*-$CBP_3$-PepII, *Rc*Alb-PepII, *Rc*Alb-PepIII, PepGAT, and PepKAA.

### 3.6. SEM Analysis of *C. neoformans* Cells Morphology

SEM analysis was performed to evaluate the possible damage to *C. neoformans* morphology caused by synthetic peptides. SEM images revealed that control cells of *C. neoformans* are healthy with a standard spherical shape with the absence of any damage on a surface such as cracks and scars (Figure 7). In contrast, all peptides damaged *C. neoformans* cells (Figure 7). The peptides-treated cells presented deformation in cell morphology (Figure 7—white arrows), scars, cracks, broken cell wall, depression, distortion (Figure 7—white arrowhead), and loss of internal content (Figure 7 red arrowhead). The loss of internal content presented in SEM images confirmed the fluorescence assays (Figures 2 and 3), showing damage to the membrane of *C. neoformans*.

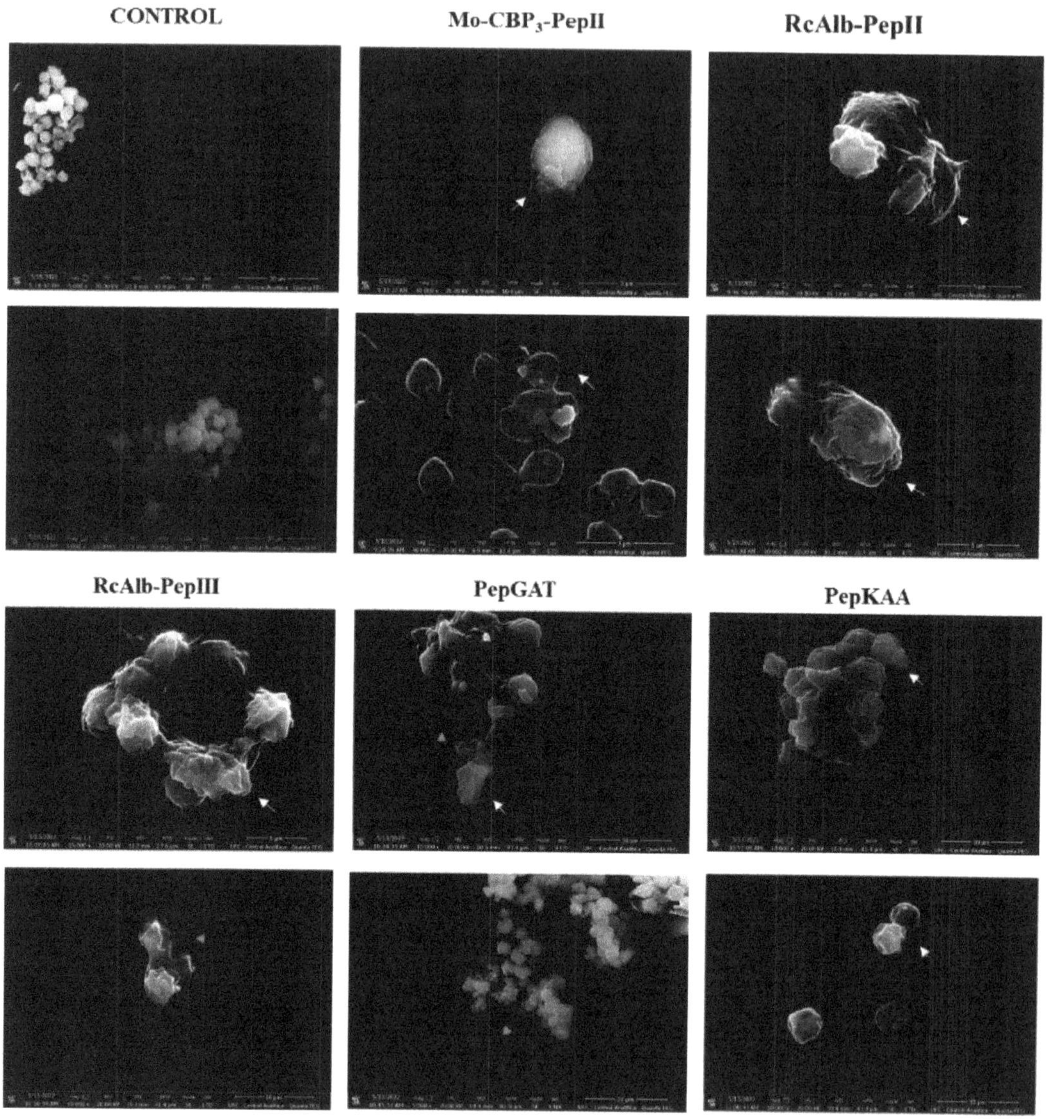


**Figure 7.** SEM images showing *C. neoformans* cells after treatment with *Mo*-CBP$_3$-PepII, *Rc*Alb-PepII, *Rc*Alb-PepIII, PepGAT, and PepKAA, respectively, at 25, 0.04, 0.04, 0.04, and 0.04 μg mL$^{-1}$ Control: DMSO-NaCl solution. White arrows show damage to cellular structure, and red arrows indicate cytoplasmic leakage.

## 4. Discussion

*C. neoformans* is a highly problematic echinocandin-resistant yeast, affecting immunocompromised patients such as transplanted patients, those under cancer chemotherapy, and HIV+. *C. neoformans* is responsible for a high number of fungal meningitis in immunocompromised patients and ∼15% of deaths in HIV+ patients each year [20,21]. In this sense, rationally designed synthetic peptides present high activity without the associated toxicity or susceptibility to proteolysis. In addition, the advances in chemical synthesis have made synthetic peptides application affordable [22]. Recently, a synthetic peptide AW9-Ma showed an $MIC_{50}$ against *C. neoformans* at a concentration of 64 µg $mL^{-1}$ [23], which is higher than all concentrations presented by the synthetic peptides (Table 1). However, the same peptide presented toxicity to human cells. Our previous works showed the peptides used here were not toxic to human erythrocytes (types A, B, and O), fibroblasts, and keratinocytes. Experiments also showed that peptides were not toxic to embryos of zebrafish. Additionally, our peptides prove to be resistant to proteolysis. Besides activity against *C. neoformans*, peptides must be considered as potential molecules against *C. neoformans* [12–14].

The peptides *Mo*-$CBP_3$-PepII, *Rc*Alb-PepII, *Rc*Alb-PepIII, PepGAT, and PepKAA, presented here, reached an $MIC_{50}$ against *C. neoformans* at low concentrations in addition to acting by multiple mechanisms of actions to damage *C. neoformans* cells. The minimum inhibitory concentration of peptides that inhibited 50% of *C. neoformans* growth was determined (Table 1). These concentrations defined for five peptides were used to study the mechanism of action employed by peptides against *C. neoformans*. For example, we provide an experiment showing that our peptides have their anti-cryptococcal activity affected when the cultures were supplied with different concentrations of exogenous ergosterol (Figure 1). The activity reduction strongly indicates that these peptides have a higher affinity for free-ergosterol than the ergosterol in the membrane of fungi. This result indicates that in normal conditions, in the absence of free ergosterol, peptides can target the ergosterol in the membrane of fungal cells.

The cell membrane is a complex system composed of many lipids, complete embedded or anchored proteins, and sterol types that act as stabilizers. In fungal membranes, ergosterol is the primary compound of sterols, making it the target of many antifungal drugs. For example, itraconazole targets the enzyme lanosterol 14-α-demethylase involved in ergosterol biosynthesis, blocking its production and leading to cell death [24].

We have shown that some of our peptides have an affinity for ergosterol. One of the consequences of the interaction of the peptides with ergosterol is the destabilization of the plasma membrane, often leading to pore formation. In literature, a work shows that an anticandida protein, *Mo*-$CBP_2$, exerts its activity by interacting with ergosterol [16]. Nevertheless, to the best of our knowledge, no study discussed the anti-cryptococcal activity of synthetic peptides interacting with ergosterol. *Mo*-$CBP_3$-PepII [14], *Rc*Alb-PepII and *Rc*Alb-PepIII [12], PepGAT, and PepKAA [15] proved experimentally that they can induce pore formation in other human pathogenic yeasts. This study was not different, as revealed by the PI influx assay (Figure 2).

Plasma membrane remodeling upon external insults is metabolically expensive [15]. To target and induce pore formation in membranes is not new for synthetic peptides. For instance, MSI-1, a synthetic cationic peptide, demonstrated membrane disruption by pore formation, resulting from its interaction with the membrane [25]. The ability to form pores in the membrane is not prevalent in all synthetic peptides. Still, it is an important mechanism, as they compromise the development of fungal resistance since changes in membrane composition can be dangerous for cellular life [15].

The PI uptake assay is a standard assay to show the membrane pore formation. However, it only indicates the presence of a tiny pore on the membrane, which sometimes does not necessarily result in cell death. To move forward on the damage to the membrane, we provide an experiment that revealed all peptides induced pore formation of size, at least 6 kDa (Figure 3). Different from the pore size that allows the movement of PI, a pore 6 kDa-sized on the membrane is a huge problem that cells have to deal with. A big pore allows the movement of small molecules and other peptides and proteins. The question arises: how do small synthetic peptides induce a pore of at least 6 kDa on *C. neoformans* membranes? We have a hypothesis that could explain that.

We suggest the big pore formed by peptides on the membrane is due to self-association ability once inserted into the membrane. Self-association is a vital characteristic of antimicrobial peptides and is responsible for the ability to induce pore formation [26]. With a big pore, we reasoned that those peptides could be internalized by an energy-independent mechanism and find a target in the cytoplasm. After reaching the cytoplasm, peptides could interfere in dozens of cellular pathways that drive cell death. For instance, Maurya et al. [27] described two synthetic peptides, VS2 and VS3, which can induce pore formation on *C. albicans* membranes and move through them, reaching the target on the cytoplasm.

In addition to membrane destabilization, the peptides were able to induce DNA fragmentation (Figure 4), followed by caspase-mediated programmed cell death (cmPCD) (Figure 5). These results are consonant because caspase-3 is responsible for initiating apoptosis by inducing DNA fragmentation [28]. Caspase-3 starts apoptotic DNA fragmentation by inactivating a protein called DNA fragmentation factor-45 (DFF45) and an inhibitor of caspase-activated DNase (ICAD). This releases a caspase-3-activated DNase, which starts DNA fragmentation.

We have four possible explanations for these sequential events involving DNA fragmentation and cmPCD. First, peptides interact with an unknown target outside the cell and trigger signaling inside the cell leading to DNA fragmentation and cmPCD. Second, these events were triggered by the damage caused by peptides on the cell membrane leading to cytoplasmic stress, and thus DNA fragmentation and cmPCD. Third, peptides move through the huge pore formed, and once inside the cell-induced, those events lead to cell death. Fourth, considering all this is a dynamic process, it is possible to suggest that all three explained above could happen simultaneously, giving no chance to *C. neoformans* cells to survive.

The SEM analysis corroborates all those damages caused by peptides to *C. neoformans* cells (Figure 6). Peptides-treated cells showed severe morphological alterations such as the loss of intracellular content, broken cell wall, and depression-like cavities in the cell, probably due to the pores caused by the interaction of the peptides in the membrane. Here, it was shown that synthetic peptides have different targets in potential as candidates in the treatment of fungal infections are fascinating, since the fungus would need to develop different strategies to resist.

## 5. Conclusions

Our results revealed that five synthetic antimicrobial peptides are active against *C. neoformans* at very low concentrations. Studies of mechanisms of action revealed those peptides damage the membrane and cell wall of *C. neoformans* cells and induce DNA fragmentation leading to apoptosis. These results revealed the peptides as alternative molecules to treat cryptococcal infection, with multiple mechanisms of action supporting anti-cryptococcal activity, making the development of resistance difficult. Based on the mechanisms employed by the peptides, it is feasible to suggest that peptides also have the potential to synergize drugs that are not effective anymore against *C. neoformans*.

**Author Contributions:** All authors made substantial contributions. The conception and design of the study and acquisition of data, analysis, and interpretation were performed by T.K.B.A., C.D.T.F., A.F.B.S., N.A.S.N., E.A.M., L.P.B., L.A.C.B., J.T.A.O., F.P.M. and P.F.N.S. Microscopic analyses were carried out by L.M.R.A., R.S.-O., E.A.M., F.P.M. and A.F.B.S. Writing or revising the article was done by T.K.B.A., C.D.T.F., G.H.G., L.M.R.A., R.S.-O. and P.F.N.S. Final approval and submission P.F.N.S. All authors have read and agreed to the published version of the manuscript.

**Funding:** This study was funded by Carlos Chagas Filho Foundation for Research Support of Rio de Janeiro State (FAPERJ) (Cientista do Nosso Estado: E-26/200.815/2021; Rede NanoSaude: E-26/010.000981/2019, Pesquisa na UEZO: E-26/010.002362/2019; Temáticos: E-26/211.269/2021, Infraestrutura e Pesquisa na UEZO e UERJ: E-26//211.207/2021, Bolsa de Pós Doutorado Senior (PDS): E-26/202.320/2021) CNPq (Bolsa de Produtividade 1B: 301069/2018-2) to Ralph Santos-Oliveira.

**Informed Consent Statement:** Not applicable.

**Data Availability Statement:** The data supporting this study's findings are available on request from the corresponding author.

**Acknowledgments:** Special thanks to CAPES for providing the postdoctoral grant to Pedro F. N. Souza (grant number 88887.318820/2019-00). We are also grateful to the staff of the central analytical facilities of UFC, Brazil.

**Conflicts of Interest:** The authors report no conflict of interest. The authors alone are responsible for the content and the writing of the paper.

## References


1. Bastos, R.W.; Rossato, L.; Goldman, G.H.; Santos, D.A. Fungicide Effects on Human Fungal Pathogens: Cross-Resistance to Medical Drugs and Beyond. *PLOS Pathog.* **2021**, *17*, e1010073. [CrossRef] [PubMed]
2. Fisher, M.C.; Alastruey-Izquierdo, A.; Berman, J.; Bicanic, T.; Bignell, E.M.; Bowyer, P.; Bromley, M.; Brüggemann, R.; Garber, G.; Cornely, O.A.; et al. Tackling the Emerging Threat of Antifungal Resistance to Human Health. *Nat. Rev. Microbiol.* **2022**, *20*, 557–571. [CrossRef]
3. Van Daele, R.; Spriet, I.; Wauters, J.; Maertens, J.; Mercier, T.; Van Hecke, S.; Brüggemann, R. Antifungal Drugs: What Brings the Future? *Med. Mycol.* **2019**, *57*, S328–S343. [CrossRef]
4. Robbins, N.; Caplan, T.; Cowen, L.E. Molecular Evolution of Antifungal Drug Resistance. *Annu. Rev. Microbiol.* **2017**, *71*, 753–775. [CrossRef] [PubMed]
5. Zafar, H.; Altamirano, S.; Ballou, E.R.; Nielsen, K. A Titanic Drug Resistance Threat in Cryptococcus Neoformans. *Curr. Opin. Microbiol.* **2019**, *52*, 158–164. [CrossRef] [PubMed]
6. Lin, X. Cryptococcus Neoformans: Morphogenesis, Infection, and Evolution. *Infect. Genet. Evol.* **2009**, *9*, 401–416. [CrossRef]
7. Huang, Y.S.; Liu, C.E.; Lin, S.P.; Lee, C.H.; Yang, C.J.; Lin, C.Y.; Tang, H.J.; Lee, Y.C.; Lin, Y.C.; Lee, Y.T.; et al. Echinocandins as Alternative Treatment for HIV-Infected Patients with Pneumocystis Pneumonia. *AIDS* **2019**, *33*, 1345–1351. [CrossRef]
8. Gutierrez-Gongora, D.; Geddes-McAlister, J. Peptidases: Promising Antifungal Targets of the Human Fungal Pathogen, *Cryptococcus Neoformans*. *FACETS* **2022**, *7*, 319–342. [CrossRef]
9. Khan, M.A.; Khan, A.; Azam, M.; Allemailem, K.S.; Alrumaihi, F.; Almatroudi, A.; Alhumaydhi, F.A.; Azam, F.; Khan, S.H.; Zofair, S.F.F.; et al. Liposomal Ellagic Acid Alleviates Cyclophosphamide-Induced Toxicity and Eliminates the Systemic Cryptococcus Neoformans Infection in Leukopenic Mice. *Pharmaceutics* **2021**, *13*, 882. [CrossRef] [PubMed]
10. Azam, F.; Khan, M.A.; Khan, A.; Ahmad, S.; Zofair, S.F.F.; Younus, H. In Silico and in Vitro Studies on the Inhibition of Laccase Activity by Ellagic Acid: Implications in Drug Designing for the Treatment of Cryptococcal Infections. *Int. J. Biol. Macromol.* **2022**, *209*, 642–654. [CrossRef]
11. Mahindra, A.; Bagra, N.; Wangoo, N.; Khan, S.I.; Jacob, M.R.; Jain, R. Discovery of Short Peptides Exhibiting High Potencyagainst Cryptococcus Neoformans. *ACS Med. Chem. Lett.* **2014**, *5*, 315. [CrossRef]
12. Dias, L.P.; Souza, P.F.N.; Oliveira, J.T.A.; Vasconcelos, I.M.; Araújo, N.M.S.; Tilburg, M.F.V.; Guedes, M.I.F.; Carneiro, R.F.; Lopes, J.L.S.; Sousa, D.O.B. RcAlb-PepII, a Synthetic Small Peptide Bioinspired in the 2S Albumin from the Seed Cake of Ricinus Communis, Is a Potent Antimicrobial Agent against Klebsiella Pneumoniae and Candida Parapsilosis. *Biochim. Biophys. Acta-Biomembr.* **2020**, *1862*, 183092. [CrossRef] [PubMed]
13. Souza, P.F.N.; vanTilburg, M.F.; Mesquita, F.P.; Amaral, J.L.; Lima, L.B.; Montenegro, R.C.; Lopes, F.E.S.; Martins, R.X.; Vieira, L.; Farias, D.F.; et al. Neutralizing Effect of Synthetic Peptides toward SARS-CoV-2. *ACS Omega* **2022**, *7*, 16222–16234. [CrossRef] [PubMed]
14. Oliveira, J.T.A.; Souza, P.F.N.; Vasconcelos, I.M.; Dias, L.P.; Martins, T.F.; Van Tilburg, M.F.; Guedes, M.I.F.; Sousa, D.O.B. Mo-CBP3-PepI, Mo-CBP3-PepII, and Mo-CBP3-PepIII Are Synthetic Antimicrobial Peptides Active against Human Pathogens by Stimulating ROS Generation and Increasing Plasma Membrane Permeability. *Biochimie* **2019**, *157*, 10–21. [CrossRef]
15. Souza, P.F.N.; Marques, L.S.M.; Oliveira, J.T.A.; Lima, P.G.; Dias, L.P.; Neto, N.A.S.; Lopes, F.E.S.; Sousa, J.S.; Silva, A.F.B.; Caneiro, R.F.; et al. Synthetic Antimicrobial Peptides: From Choice of the Best Sequences to Action Mechanisms. *Biochimie* **2020**, *175*, 132–145. [CrossRef]
16. da Silva Neto, J.X.; da Costa, H.P.S.; Vasconcelos, I.M.; Pereira, M.L.; Oliveira, J.T.A.; Lopes, T.D.P.; Dias, L.P.; Araújo, N.M.S.; Moura, L.F.W.G.; Van Tilburg, M.F.; et al. Role of Membrane Sterol and Redox System in the Anti-Candida Activity Reported for Mo-CBP2, a Protein from Moringa Oleifera Seeds. *Int. J. Biol. Macromol.* **2020**, *143*, 814–824. [CrossRef] [PubMed]
17. Schneider, C.A.; Rasband, W.S.; Eliceiri, K.W. NIH Image to ImageJ: 25 Years of Image Analysis. *Nat. Methods* **2012**, *9*, 671–675. [CrossRef] [PubMed]
18. Qorri, B.; Harless, W.; Szewczuk, M.R. Novel Molecular Mechanism of Aspirin and Celecoxib Targeting Mammalian Neuraminidase-1 Impedes Epidermal Growth Factor Receptor Signaling Axis and Induces Apoptosis in Pancreatic Cancer Cells. *Drug Des. Dev. Ther.* **2020**, *14*, 4149–4167. [CrossRef] [PubMed]
19. Staniszewska, M.; Bondaryk, M.; Swoboda-Kopec, E.; Siennicka, K.; Sygitowicz, G.; Kurzatkowski, W. Candida Albicans Morphologies Revealed by Scanning Electron Microscopy Analysis. *Braz. J. Microbiol.* **2013**, *44*, 813–821. [CrossRef]
20. Rajasingham, R.; Smith, R.M.; Park, B.J.; Jarvis, J.N.; Govender, N.P.; Chiller, T.M.; Denning, D.W.; Loyse, A.; Boulware, D.R. Global Burden of Disease of HIV-Associated Cryptococcal Meningitis: An Updated Analysis. *Lancet Infect. Dis.* **2017**, *17*, 873–881. [CrossRef]
21. Marty, F.; Mylonakis, E. Antifungal Use in HIV Infection. *Expert Opin. Pharmacother.* **2002**, *3*, 91–102. [CrossRef]
22. Zhang, T.; Chen, Z.; Tian, Y.; Han, B.; Zhang, N.; Song, W.; Liu, Z.; Zhao, J.; Liu, J. Kilogram-Scale Synthesis of Osteogenic Growth Peptide (10–14) Using a Fragment Coupling Approach. *Org. Process Res. Dev.* **2015**, *19*, 1257–1262. [CrossRef]

23. Tancer, R.J.; Wang, Y.; Pawar, S.; Xue, C.; Wiedman, G.R. Development of Antifungal Peptides against Cryptococcus Neoformans; Leveraging Knowledge about the Cdc50Δ Mutant Susceptibility for Lead Compound Development. *Microbiol. Spectr.* **2022**, *10*, e00439-22. [CrossRef]
24. Ermakova, E.; Zuev, Y. Effect of Ergosterol on the Fungal Membrane Properties. All-Atom and Coarse-Grained Molecular Dynamics Study. *Chem. Phys. Lipids* **2017**, *209*, 45–53. [CrossRef]
25. Ma, L.; Wei, S.; Ye, X.; Xu, P.; Chen, H.; Liu, Z.; Zhou, C. Antifungal Activity of Peptide MSI-1 against Cryptococcus Neoformans Infection in Vitro and in Murine Cryptococcal Meningoencephalitis. *Peptides* **2020**, *130*, 170334. [CrossRef]
26. Huang, Y.; Huang, J.; Chen, Y. Alpha-Helical Cationic Antimicrobial Peptides: Relationships of Structure and Function. *Protein Cell* **2010**, *1*, 143–152. [CrossRef]
27. Maurya, I.K.; Pathak, S.; Sharma, M.; Sanwal, H.; Chaudhary, P.; Tupe, S.; Deshpande, M.; Chauhan, V.S.; Prasad, R. Antifungal Activity of Novel Synthetic Peptides by Accumulation of Reactive Oxygen Species (ROS) and Disruption of Cell Wall against Candida Albicans. *Peptides* **2011**, *32*, 1732–1740. [CrossRef]
28. Janssens, S.; Tinel, A. The PIDDosome, DNA-Damage-Induced Apoptosis and Beyond. *Cell Death Differ.* **2011**, *19*, 13–20. [CrossRef]

pharmaceutics

MDPI

Review

# An Overview of the Supramolecular Systems for Gene and Drug Delivery in Tissue Regeneration


**Saketh Reddy Ranamalla [1,2], Alina Silvia Porfire [1,*], Ioan Tomuță [1,†] and Manuela Banciu [3,†]**

1 Department of Pharmaceutical Technology and Bio Pharmacy, Faculty of Pharmacy, "Iuliu Hațieganu" University of Medicine and Pharmacy, 400010 Cluj-Napoca, Romania
2 Doctoral School in Integrative Biology, Faculty of Biology and Geology, "Babeș-Bolyai" University, 400015 Cluj-Napoca, Romania
3 Department of Molecular Biology and Biotechnology, Center of Systems Biology, Biodiversity and Bioresources, Faculty of Biology and Geology, "Babeș-Bolyai" University, 400015 Cluj-Napoca, Romania
* Correspondence: aporfire@umfcluj.ro
† These authors contributed equally to this work.


**Abstract:** Tissue regeneration is a prominent area of research, developing biomaterials aimed to be tunable, mechanistic scaffolds that mimic the physiological environment of the tissue. These biomaterials are projected to effectively possess similar chemical and biological properties, while at the same time are required to be safely and quickly degradable in the body once the desired restoration is achieved. Supramolecular systems composed of reversible, non-covalently connected, self-assembly units that respond to biological stimuli and signal cells have efficiently been developed as preferred biomaterials. Their biocompatibility and the ability to engineer the functionality have led to promising results in regenerative therapy. This review was intended to illuminate those who wish to envisage the niche translational research in regenerative therapy by summarizing the various explored types, chemistry, mechanisms, stimuli receptivity, and other advancements of supramolecular systems.

**Keywords:** supramolecular; self-assembling; non-covalent interactions; hydrogels; nanofibers; drug delivery; gene delivery; tissue regeneration

## 1. Introduction

Tissue regeneration has been an area of prominent research in the twenty-first century that emphasizes the regeneration of human cells, tissues, or whole organs for reestablishing structural and physiological functions [1]. The targeted physiological areas of this interdisciplinary research field are widespread, including dermal, cardiovascular, musculoskeletal, gastrointestinal, and nervous systems, and most of the medications being developed are cell and gene therapy-based medications [2]. In most scenarios such as injuries where regenerative strategies are followed, the extracellular matrix is either partly or completely lost [3]. The extracellular matrix (ECM), which is a three-dimensionally arranged interwoven network of fibers derived from the proteins, proteoglycans and glycosaminoglycans act as structural supports and as media for the transfer of oxygen and nutrients [4]. This ECM is highly dynamic and undergoes remodeling and serves the purpose of being a tissue-specific substrate that allows cell attachment, migration, and proliferation. In the cases of injuries or pathological conditions, the ECM acts as a base for the signaling molecules such as growth factors and morphogens, thereby creating a microenvironment for the cells to differentiate and function [5].

In conditions where ECM is lost, the design and manufacturing of a similar mechanistic scaffold that can simulate the biological environment of the damaged tissues is a major challenge. The biomimetic scaffolds should be able to either reproduce the ECM or be able to substitute it by providing the required physical support that is usually provided by the various proteins for the cells and the signaling molecules to regenerate or repair the part of the tissue. The scaffolds should also be capable of supporting the normal functioning of the targeted tissue and improve the quality of life for the patients.

Biomolecules such as proteins, receptors, enzymes, and many small molecules have often been observed to self-assemble themselves, and to form supramolecular complexes that allow them to regulate a variety of biological functions [6]. This phenomenon of self-assembly backed up by non-covalent intermolecular forces is attributed to Supramolecular chemistry coined by Jean-Marie Lehn, who received the Nobel prize in 1987 with Donald J. Cram and Charles J. Pedersenn for their contribution to the field. He defined it as the "chemistry beyond the molecule", where molecules are held together by non-covalent interactions such as hydrogen bonds, van der Waals forces, and ion or dipole interactions [7].

Attributed to this non-covalent chemistry, many supramolecular bio-functional materials have been developed in the past three decades for regenerative medicine. These materials, while acting as a mechanistic scaffold, are aimed to deliver therapeutic molecules/genes and at the same time try to mimic the functional properties of the tissue. These bio-functional materials have proven advantages of safety, response to external stimuli, reversibility, biomimicry, and many other benefits in in vitro and in vivo conditions [8]. Researchers have reviewed both the scaffold and scaffold-free approaches that mimic the biological processes for regenerative medicine taking in account of the spatiotemporal data that occur in in vitro organogenesis and in vivo conditions [9,10]. With this due diligence, the researchers have instituted confidence in this platform and are working towards making technological advances and bringing these systems closer to the patients [11]. This article uniquely reviewed the supramolecular systems that have been applied for tissue regeneration with their types based on origin, fundamentals of mechanism, technical aspects of synthesis and characterization, and innovations to improve clinical applicability.

## 2. Types of Supramolecular Systems Used for Tissue Regeneration

There has been a plethora of work carried out on supramolecular systems owing to their tunability and adaptability for regenerative medicine. For the sake of simplicity, we classified the systems into two groups based on their origin: bio-macromolecule-based and synthetic-based systems, as shown in Figure 1. In addition to these systems, there are also supramolecular systems derived from the natural biomaterials.

### *2.1. Bio-Macromolecule-Based Systems*

This category of supramolecular systems uses the advantage of natural biomimicry offered by the materials as they are also inherently synthesized and circulated amongst the cells and tissues. Based on the type of macromolecules used, it can be further classified into lipids, peptides, and nucleic acid-based systems, as illustrated in Figure 2.

#### 2.1.1. Lipid-Based Systems

Glycerides and fatty acids are the structural units of the lipids and usually do not form self-assembling structures until the former ones are in an aqueous environment, but the lipids, due to their significant hydrophobicity, tend to form supramolecular systems much more easily. The lipids can be modified to form supramolecular delivery systems such as nanoparticles [12], micelles [13], liposomes [14], hydrogels [15], and dendrimers [16]. Lipids, in combination with other bio-macromolecules such as nucleic acids [17] and proteins [12], tend to act as a scaffold in the place of the lost tissue in the regenerative medicine domain. These supramolecular-based systems are used majorly for the delivery of drugs and genetic material to the targeted tissues.

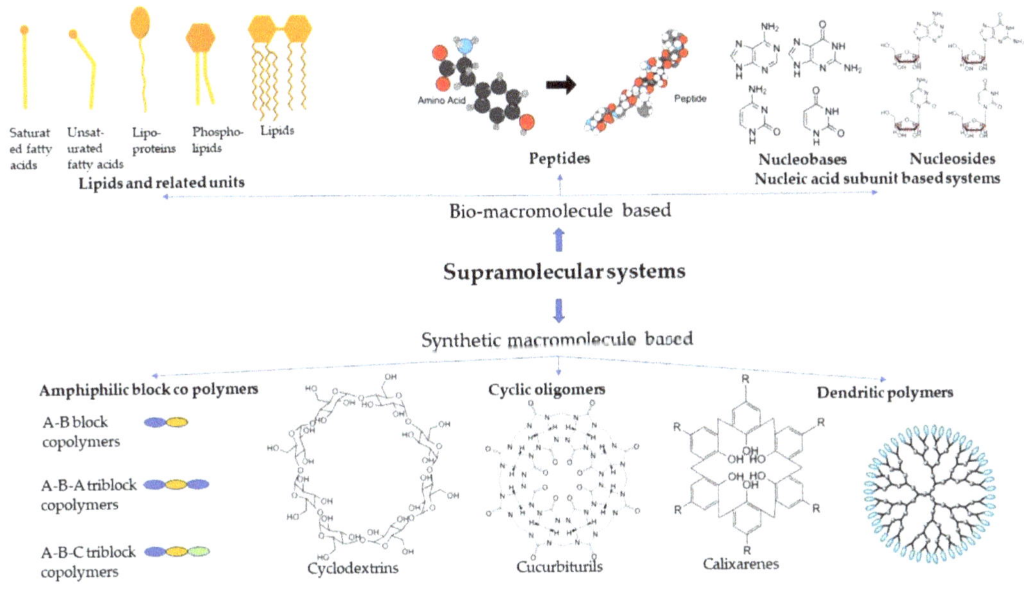


**Figure 1.** Types of supramolecular systems used for tissue regeneration (created with Biorender.com [accessed on 30 June 2022]).

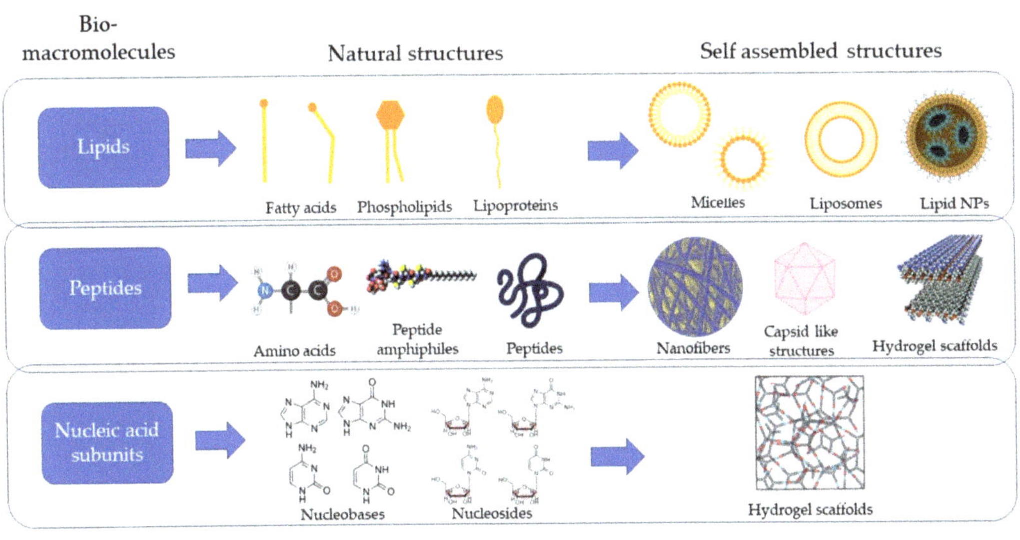


**Figure 2.** Biomacromolecule based self-assembly structures (created with Biorender.com [accessed on 30 June 2022]).

Henrich et al. reported the synthesis of soft-core nanoparticles with a diameter of about 10 nm that are similar in size, shape, composition, protein structure and surface chemistry to human High-Density Lipoproteins (HDL). These self-assembled phospholipid particles can carry out most of the HDL functions such as those of the cholesterol efflux from macrophages, cholesterol delivery to hepatocytes, lecithin: cholesterol acyltransferase activity support, and inflammation suppression. These synthetic HDLs have immense potential to function as therapeutic agents [12]. Additionally, utilization of biologically active monoglycerides such as glycerol monolaurate (GML) or its ether derivative 1-O-dodecyl- rac -glycerol (DDG) to form supramolecular assemblies producing nano micelles was reported by Yoon et al. These micelles can modulate the membrane interactions with cell-membrane-mimicking giant unilamellar vesicles that can assist in nanomedicine [13].

Liposomes are self-assembled phospholipid membranes that can deliver therapeutically active compounds which could be drug molecules, cells, growth factors, genetic material, and others. Tremendous research involving liposomes has been documented in the last three decades and a lot of modifications have been made to the structure of the liposomes to regulate the release of the therapeutic materials. Hu et al. in their research work on the poly(lactic-co-glycolic acid)-liposomes delivered both microRNA 145 and the platelet-derived growth factor, which helped in the cell differentiation of the mesenchymal stromal cells into vascular smooth muscle cells. Though the mesenchymal stromal cells have differentiation ability, the efficiency of differentiation is low. However, the research team could translate these results in the in vivo skin wound healing models using male Sprague–Dawley rats, providing new insights into utilizing the liposomes as a multi-delivery system [18].

Liposomes also have been integrated onto biomaterial scaffolds to release drug or genetic material load to be dually efficient as a mechanical support and to achieve the desired therapeutic effect. Lee et al. demonstrated the use of liposomes loaded with smoothened agonists for the Hedgehog signaling pathway responsible for endochondral bone healing. These liposomes are then adhered to using biocompatible polydopamine adhesive onto the trabecular bone mimetic apatite-coated scaffolds. The in vitro experiments in the mouse bone marrow stem cells and the in vivo experiments using the parietal bone defect model have suggested successful cell adhesion and cell proliferation [19]. Another similar example is from the research by Mohammadi et al., where the team achieved a sustained release of the BMP-2 peptide over 21 days from the liposomes attached to the poly L-lactic acid nanofibers coated with hydroxyapatite nanoparticles. The in vitro studies have confirmed the cell proliferation and cell differentiation of the mesenchymal stem cells. The in vivo osteoinduction efficiency was evaluated by the subcutaneous implantation of the scaffolds in the in vitro rat models, which revealed primary ossification with the liposomes [20].

### 2.1.2. Peptide-Based Systems

Peptides are unique biomolecules placed between the small molecules (<500 Da) which could be easily developed, and the large molecules (>5000 Da) can be specific and potent at the same time [21]. Tissue regeneration, in a sense, necessitates the use of two complementary vital elements. The first element is a physiologically compatible scaffold that could be easily absorbed by the body without causing injury, and the second is appropriate cells, such as stem cells and primary cells, which can successfully replace damaged tissues without causing harm. It would be beneficial for tissue healing if suitable biological scaffolding could be used to drive cell differentiation. Many scaffold-forming self-assembling peptides have been examined for this purpose, with peptide amphiphiles being one of the most well-studied groups [22].

Self-assembling peptide amphiphiles consist of these hydrophilic and hydrophobic moieties that tend to form secondary structural motifs such as β-sheets and α-helices [23]. These secondary structures are backed by hydrogen bonding and van der Waals forces and the electrostatic associations assemble to form 1 D nanostructures. When the amphiphilic structures are placed in water, the hydrophobicity of aliphatic chains triggers the formation of lower surface area and high-aspect-ratio 3 D structures such as nanofibers. Peptide nanofibers have been researched and been employed for the regeneration of every tissue in the body, owing to their promising results in mimicking the complex organization of tissues [24]. One such application was studied by Mansukhani et al., who investigated the use of peptide amphiphile nanofibers containing the apolipoprotein A1 (Apo A1)-derived targeting peptide 4F as nanocarriers for Liver X receptor (LXR) delivery (ApoA1-LXR PA) in vivo and showed that supramolecular nanostructures can be used as safe and effective drug nanocarriers in the treatment of atherosclerosis [25].

The supramolecular behavior of the peptides has also been advantageous in designing the nanocarrier systems in the form of dendritic structures which can engulf the drug or genetic material and deliver it to selective tissue. Li et al. used the self-assembly of poly(L-lysine) dendrimers to form pH-responsive capsid-like nanocarriers which could enhance the penetration and accumulation of doxorubicin in multicellular tumor spheroids mimicking solid tumor tissues [26].

Any biomaterial that is being developed for tissue regeneration should be physically and chemically equivalent to that of the extracellular matrix of the tissue [27]. Peptides, peptide conjugates, and peptide aggregates, due to their supramolecular capability, better biocompatibility, and biodegradability than the synthetic supramolecular systems, are the preferred scaffolds by researchers [28]. They are preferred over polymeric scaffolds due to the ability of angiogenic sprouting and vascularization. This was extensively studied by Siddiqui et al. in their research article, where microporous polymeric scaffolds and viscoelastic nano porous peptide hydrogels were used to create two-component scaffolds. The implant vascularization and cellular infiltration were measured by the bioactive moieties in the primary sequences of the peptide monomers, hence showing the utility of soft supramolecular peptide hydrogels for designing multi-component regenerative scaffolds [29].

Amino acids such as tyrosine and phenylalanine form hydrogels readily through π–π interactions and are being majorly used for external stimuli-triggered delivery systems. Just like the naturally occurring amino acids, there are synthetic amino acids that form small molecular hydrogels such as diphenylalanine which undergo the π–π stacking of amino acids to form the hydrogels. The utilization of self-assembling peptides to form such hydrogels through non-covalent interactions helps in delivering biologics such as antibodies, growth factors, genes etc. [30]. Abraham et al. showed, in their research article, the improved versions of the Phenylalanine-derived gelators that are protected by Fluorenyl methoxycarbonyl (Fmoc) form some of the most stable hydrogels from the low molecular weight gelators [31]. Synthetic amino acids such as diphenylalanine also have been used in combination with some cyclic macromolecules such as β-cyclodextrin to form supramolecular nanospheres that can be reversibly assembled and disassembled into nanofibers. Zhang et al. used ferrocene-modified diphenylalanine that can reversibly assemble and dissemble by the chemical redox reactions of ferrocene groups, therefore demonstrating a redox-sensitive peptide supramolecular system [32].

#### 2.1.3. Nucleic Acid Subunit-Based Systems

The building blocks of the nucleic acids such as nucleosides and nucleotides have recently been widely explored as diagnostics, tissue scaffolding, and targeted drug release systems due to their capability of self-assembly. All the nucleosides and nucleotides contain the nucleobases and ribose or a deoxy ribose sugar molecule. Nucleosides are differentiated from the nucleotides by consisting of phosphate groups in addition to the nucleobases and the ribose sugar molecule. The nucleobases are nitrogen-containing heterocyclic compounds which can be purines (Adenine {A} and Guanine {G}) and pyrimidines (Uracil {U}, Thymine {T}, and Cytosine {C}). Due to their aromatic nature, these nucleobases naturally exhibit π–π stacking and, additionally, there are hydrogen bond acceptors and donors in both types of nucleobases favoring hydrogen bonding. These non-covalent interactions, called Watson–Crick base pairing and Hoogsteen base pairing, help to form the supramolecular systems. These nucleobases are attached to a ribose sugar molecule via glycosidic linkages which are further connected to a phosphoryl group constituting the nucleic acids DNA and RNA. The phosphoryl group bears an anionic charge which further strengthens the supramolecular system by electrostatic interactions [33].

The nucleic acid subunit-based systems tend to form gels when supramolecular assembly is induced. The induction process typically takes place in the presence of lipophilic groups which increase the hydrophobicity appending the self-association. Among these types, guanosine and its derivative-based organogels have been much focused on lately. Zhao et al. have carried out immense research on the supramolecular nucleoside-based hydrogels and reported on the applications in drug delivery, regenerative medicine, and theranostic devices. Zhao et al. used Isoguanosine and its derivatives such as the 2′-deoxyribonucleoside and the 2′-deoxy-2′-fluoro ribonucleoside to form hydrogels in alkali metal salt solutions, which had excellent long-term stability with good loading efficiencies for small molecules [34]. Their recent article mentioned the dual functional supramolecular hydrogel made from Isoguanosine-borate-guanosine prepared by a one-pot procedure that can be used for small molecule delivery [35]. Other derivatives of adenine and cytosine have also been employed, but little literature is available on the application for regenerative medicine [36]. Cheng et al. invented self-assembling physically cross-linked supramolecular polymers composed of cytosine, poly(ethylene glycol) (PEG), and hydrophobic poly(epichlorohydrin). They observed that the cytosine functionalized substrates improved wound healing by promoting quick cell migration into the injured cellular surface [37].

### 2.2. Synthetic Supramolecular Systems

These groups of synthetically produced macromolecules that are being used for tissue regeneration mostly include block copolymers, dendritic polymers, or cyclic oligomers. The subtypes are diagrammatically represented in Figure 3. Block copolymers that are usually used for regenerative medicine comprise diblock, triblock, and other multiblock copolymers, whereas cyclic oligomers comprise cyclodextrins, calixarenes, and cucurbit(8)urils. Then there are dendritic polymers, which are mostly classified by the type of subunits that comprise them. The synthetic supramolecular systems have flexibility over biomacromolecule-based systems for being able to be manufactured as required by the tissue to be mimicked.

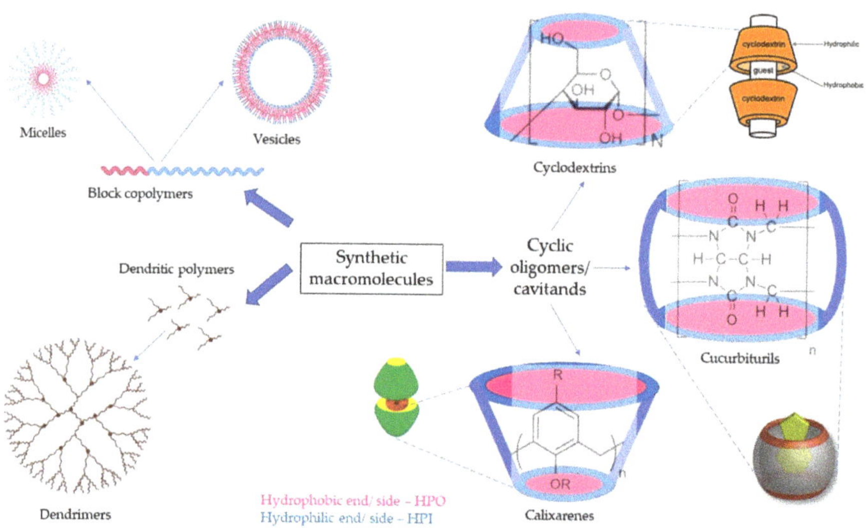


**Figure 3.** Sub-types of synthetic macromolecule-based supramolecular systems and their self-assembly structures (created with Biorender.com [accessed on 30 June 2022]).

#### 2.2.1. Block Copolymers

Block copolymers, as the name suggests, consist of a linear arrangement of blocks of two or more polymers connected end-to-end. Based on their sequential arrangement of blocks, they can vary from the di-block (A-B) consisting of two blocks, to tri-block (A-B-C or A-B-A) consisting of three blocks, to multi-block $(A\text{-}B)_n$ consisting of multiple blocks. The synthesis of these block copolymers is performed by polymerization techniques utilizing ions, free radicals, and metal catalysts. The polymers are then electro spun into nanofibers or are employed in techniques such as bio-printing to form tissue scaffolds. The block copolymers majorly act as substitutes for the natural scaffold, possessing most of the necessary characteristics such as porosity for cell attachment, angiogenesis, nutrients transfer, biodegradability, and biocompatibility [38].

Rico et al. listed the utility of poly(ethylene oxide)-poly(propylene oxide)-poly(ethylene oxide) tri-block copolymers for gene delivery in human regenerative medicine. They reviewed the formation of micellae and hydrogels, their applications, and their limitations [39]. Other ABA tri-block copolymers such as poly(propylene fumarate)-polyethylene glycol-poly(propylene fumarate) have been used for three-dimensional (3D) printing of amphiphilic hydrogels with demonstrated mechanical stability and tolerance for degradation [40].

These amphiphilic block copolymers can also be made stimuli-responsive to physiological conditions, making them more functional for tissue regeneration. Lee et al. synthesized poly(ε-caprolactone) block copolymers and proposed them as a model for drug and gene delivery with demonstrated thermo-responsive phase transition and in vitro biodegradability [41]. Biodegradable amphiphilic poly (ethylene glycol) (PEG)-based ether-anhydride terpolymer was synthesized to form different-shaped self-assembling micelles and they were assessed for cellular internalization rate. Through this research, Yang et al. found that comb-shaped micelles had a high blood circulation rate, thereby acting as a suitable drug carrier system for regenerative medicine [42].

2.2.2. Dendritic Polymers

Dendrimers are a class of synthetic polymers that have evolved over the past two decades. The term is derived from Greek, which means Dendra—tree and meros—part of which suggests the architecture of these polymeric macromolecules that resemble a tree. As in a tree, several branching units originate from a multi-functional core unit and end with a capping unit. These repetitive branching monomer units of the synthetic macromolecules from the core are organized into layers called generations. These systems can be surface modified for many applications including reducing the cytotoxicity, clearance, and increasing biodistribution. Among the wide variety of dendrimers being researched, glycodendrimers and peptide dendrimers are found to be more predominant. The glycodendrimers are derived from the repetitive carbohydrate units and the peptide dendrimers have a peptidyl core with functional branching units. In contrast with the polymers acting as a natural scaffold, they act as efficient delivery systems for small molecules, proteins, and genetic material [43]. To form the scaffold, they use non-covalent interactions such as hydrogen bonds, van der Waals forces, and electrostatic interactions in addition to covalent bonds [44].

Bai et al. reported a self-reinforcing hydrogel for bone repair by utilizing non-covalent interactions between β-cyclodextrin-graft-poly(N-isopropyl acrylamide) as host and adamantane decorated generation 2.5 poly(amidoamine)s dendrimer as guest polymer. Furfuryl amine grafted chondroitin sulfate (ChS-F) and maleimido-terminated poly(ethylene glycol) (PEG2K–AMI) were then chemically cross-linked to the hydrogel to obtain a scaffold with high water content and mechanical strength [45]. Dendrimer nanoparticles made up of carboxymethyl chitosan/poly(amidoamine) were used to observe the cell internalization in neurons, astrocytes, oligodendrocytes, and microglial cells using fluorescent probes. These systems can be further used for the delivery of drugs to the damaged parts of the central nervous system [46].

The delivery of genetic material by dendritic systems has also been a widely researched topic. Bi et al. proposed hydrogels made up of poly(amidoamine) (PAMAM), hyaluronic acid (HA) and arginyl glycyl aspartic acid (RGD) peptide with reliable results in cell viability, proliferation, and attachment demonstrated in vitro in the bone marrow stem cells [47]. Zhu et al. used dendrimers for the delivery of a single plasmid construct carrying Yamanaka factors that can generate pluripotent stem cells from mouse embryonic fibroblasts [48]. Other plasmid DNA was shown to be delivered efficiently with functionalized generation 5 (G5) dendrimers of PAMAM with hydrophobic chains that have reduced cell cytotoxicity in mesenchymal stem cells (MSC) [49].

Researchers have also come up with new strategies such as the layer-by-layer (LbL) technique for the supramolecular dendrimers that can be used for the inclusion and modulation of the release of pharmaceutical compounds or various bioactive substances [50].

#### 2.2.3. Cyclic Oligomers

Cyclic oligomers are the class of synthetic self-assembly systems that consist of cyclic polymers that use non-covalent interactions to form container-shaped structures. These structures are also called cavitands and allow them to act as hosts for many guest molecules including small and macromolecules. The most widely used supramolecular cyclic oligomers for regenerative medicine are cyclodextrins, calixarenes, and cucurbiturils [51].

Cyclodextrins (CD) are a group of oligosaccharides arranged cyclically to have a hydrophobic cavity and a hydrophilic external face. They are formed by the enzymatic conversion of starch and are named α, β, and γ cyclodextrins constituting 6,7 and 8 glucose subunits linked by α-1,4-linkages respectively [52]. Cyclodextrin use in regenerative medicine has been an extensively researched topic with a wide range of applications ranging from serving as scaffolds for cartilage, bone, and other tissues to vehicle/vectors for genes and drugs. For regeneration of cartilaginous tissues and wound healing, a combination of CD (especially β-CD) with hyaluronic acid (HA) has been widely investigated. For example, Zhao et al. studied the photo-responsive reversible supramolecular interactions between the azobenzene and these complexes cyclodextrin-bearing hyaluronic acid host polymer (HA-CD) for wound healing [53]. Zhang et al. prepared the biocompatible supramolecular polymeric nanofibers that comprise a network of the HA-CD and magnetic field facilitated self-assembly of magnetic nanoparticles made up of adamantane and actin-binding peptide. These nanofibers are capable of cellular internalization and polarizing mammalian cells in the presence of external magnetic field [54]. CD can also play the role of stabilizers in the supramolecular systems as demonstrated by Milcovich et al., who used β-CD as a stabilizer for unilamellar catanionic vesicles, which could deliver bioactive molecules [55].

Some researchers have used the host–guest chemistry of these macromolecules copolymerized with derivatives of adamantane and acrylamide and molded into functional 3D constructs to deliver therapeutic cells (MSC), growth factors (TGF-β1), and other molecules that can help in the regeneration of damaged tissues [56,57]. By incorporation of cationic groups such as ethanolamine functionalized poly(glycidyl methacrylate) to the cyclodextrin host modules, they can also be used as gene vectors as reported by Zhang et al. with good transfection results [58]. Cyclodextrins have also been proven as a delivery system for small molecules such as dexamethasone for regeneration of cartilaginous tissues [59], resveratrol for preventing osteoporosis in postmenopausal women [60], simvastatin to improve water solubility, and osteo differentiation efficiency in bone regenerative therapy [61].

Cucurbit(n)urils (CB[n]) are also a group of "n" number of repetitive macrocyclic glycoluril molecules linked by methylene groups, which possess a hydrophobic cavity such as that of cyclodextrins formed by the carbonyl groups. The number of molecules determines the dimensions of the cavities of these host molecules, where a single guest molecule would require CB(5–7) whereas CB(>8) would be required to host more than 2 guest molecules [62]. As cyclodextrins, cucurbiturils are mostly employed as delivery systems for small and large molecules to the damaged tissues.

Calix(n)arenes are another type of cavitand molecule that form hydrophobic cavities and are named due to their cyclical structural arrangement similar to the form of a Greek Calix-krater vessel [63]. These supramolecular hosts are very flexible with easily modifiable and controllable conformations. Due to this reason, they can be tuned into scaffolds and used as delivery and diagnostic agents.

## 2.3. Natural Biomaterials

### 2.3.1. Collagen

Collagen is one of the most used biomaterials due to its biocompatibility and being one of the most abundant proteins in the extracellular matrix. Collagen is present in large quantities in bones, skin, tendon, blood vessels, intestine, and cornea. Therefore, it can be used to fabricate diverse types of tissues. The collagen can be either used as the decellularized extracellular matrix or can be used in several types of regenerated collagen biomaterials in the form of hydrogels, scaffolds, or microspheres [64]. Due to its abundance in the bone matrix, collagen is mostly used for cartilaginous tissue and bone regeneration [65,66].

### 2.3.2. Alginate

Alginate, being a water-soluble polysaccharide, readily forms hydrogels that are biocompatible and biodegradable in the physiological medium. The hydrogels could be formed from the alginate in the presence of bivalent and trivalent cations forming a 3D structure that can carry substantial amounts of water. These hydrogels can carry small molecules, cells, and other delivery systems such as nanoparticles [67]. Martine et al. reviewed the combinations and strategies to make the alginate composites that could promote corneal regeneration [68]. Zhai et al. reported the co-assembled supramolecular structures made up of cell adhesive peptide and the alginate that could promote accelerated wound healing and has haemostatic control [69]. Piras et al. demonstrated a stem cell-compatible dual-network hybrid calcium alginate gel loaded with silver nanoparticles [70].

### 2.3.3. Gelatin

Gelatin itself is a product of the partial hydrolysis of collagen, which is a major component in the extracellular matrix. Being partially hydrolyzed, it contains a mixture of polypeptide chains. Gelatin also shares the same advantages as collagen by being biocompatible, nonimmunogenic, and being soluble at physiological temperature. Gelatin is also mostly sought out biomaterial used for regenerative medicine, but researchers have been using with synthetic macromolecules to form host–guest interactions that assist in cell filtration. Feng et al. used aromatic residues of gelatin with β-cyclodextrin to form hydrogels that help in cell adhesion and enhance the delivery of hydrophobic drugs. In another study, Zeinab et al. made self-healable biomimetic hydrogel using gelatin, molybdenum disulphide and β-cyclodextrin, which could be used for regeneration of extracellular matrix [71]. Madl et al. prepared the gelatin hydrogels with Cucurbit(8)uril and encapsulated human fibroblast cells, demonstrating its potential application in bioprinting [72].

### 2.3.4. Hyaluronic Acid

Hyaluronic acid, also a naturally occurring polysaccharide, is also a primary component of the extracellular matrix of the human connective tissue. Hyaluronic acid in physiological conditions undergoes enzymatic degradation in the presence of hyaluronidase and hydrolysis. Hence, hyaluronic acid is made to react with crosslinking agents to form covalent bonds to improve the stability in the physiological conditions. So, HA is used in combination with nucleobases such as cytosine, guanosine to form hydrogen bonding, or combined with Poly(N-isopropylacrylamide) to form hydrophobic bonds making the supramolecular hydrogels. They can form metal co-ordination supramolecular complexes with metal ions such as $Mg^{2+}$, $Zn^{2+}$, $Ca^{2+}$, and $Ag^{2+}$ or also inclusion complexes with Cucurbit(8)urils, adamantane, or β-cyclodextrin [73]. Jung et al. made supramolecular hydrogels that can encapsulate human MSCs and demonstrated chondrogenic differentiation, indicating its use in the cartilage regeneration and other tissue engineering applications [74].

Fernandes et al. prepared supramolecular hydrogels containing HA and cyclodextrin or adamantane for corneal wound healing [75].

## 3. Self-Assembly Mechanism and the Driving Forces

The kinetics of the drug or gene release from the architecture of the supramolecular systems is dependent on the kinetics of the self-assembly mechanism of the systems. Hence, emphasis has been put on the self-assembly mechanism of the various non-covalent bonds that help in the process.

*Lipids:* The kinetics of lipoplex formation has been critically examined by researchers, and the nucleation and growth processes such as that of the adsorption of the polyelectrolytes on oppositely charged colloidal particles were discovered. Lipid aggregates are amphiphilic and form vesicles or phases/lamellae due to the van der Waals forces between the hydrophobic molecules and the hydrogen bonding between the hydrophilic molecules. When cationic lipids are mixed with negatively charged nucleic acids, rearrangement takes place due to the electrostatic interactions, thus forming multilamellar lipoplexes, as shown in Figure 4a [17].

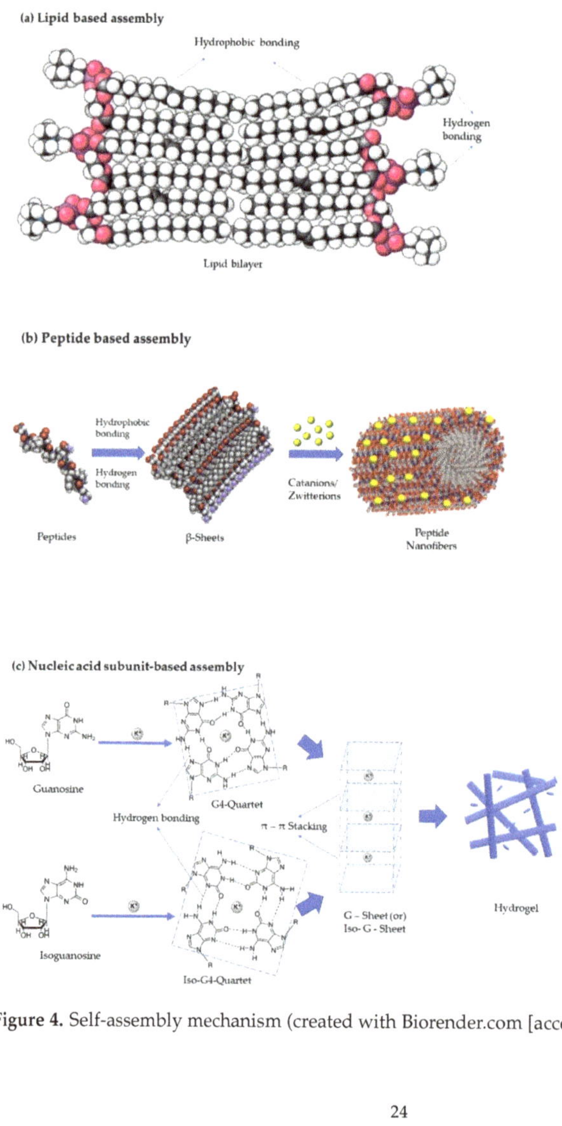


Figure 4. Self-assembly mechanism (created with Biorender.com [accessed on 30 June 2022]).

*Peptides*: Peptide assembly is influenced by noncovalent interactions such as hydrophobic effects, electrostatic interactions, and π–π stacking. Mostly, the amphiphilic peptides that have been used for the self-assembly processes have a surfactant-like structure composed of a hydrophobic tail with many hydrophobic amino acids such as Gly, Ala, Val, Leu, and Ile, and a hydrophilic core represented by one or two hydrophilic amino acids, either negatively charged (Asp or Glu) or positively charged (Lys, His or Arg), resulting in anionic or cationic surfactant-like peptides, respectively. The hydrophobic interaction and hydrogen bonding are the most important driving forces for amphiphilic peptide self-assembly, which lead to the formation of β-sheets that in turn helps in the formation of vesicles or nanofibers. It has also been demonstrated that the addition of an extra ionic bond has a substantial effect on the self-assembling structures. Catanionic and zwitterionic surfactants are the other two forms of surfactants, in addition to typical anionic and cationic surfactants. The former is a mixed system of anionic and cationic surfactants, whilst the latter is made up of surfactants with both positive and negative charges combined in a single hydrophilic head. These materials form lamellar structures, nanotubes, nanovesicles, and micelles, as shown in Figure 4b [22].

Self-assembly peptides that form hydrogels are also widely researched. Hydrogen bonding can occur spontaneously in systems that generate supramolecular fibrils capable of noncovalent cross-linking. Water-soluble fibrils can be made up of either covalently linked polymers or noncovalently linked supramolecular assemblies, with cross-linking occurring via both covalent bonds and noncovalent interactions such as hydrogen bonding, stacking, and van der Waals forces. Braun et al. discovered that the hydrogel-forming peptide SgI37-49 self-assembly is governed by the secondary nucleation of monomers on the surface of pre-existing fibrils. The rate of nucleation in this catalytic nucleation process exhibits enzyme-like saturation effects, with the rate of nucleation being highly concentration-dependent below 50 M and effectively concentration-independent at higher concentrations [76].

*Nucleic acid subunit based self-assemblies*: All the nucleic acid sub-components, namely nucleobases, nucleosides, and nucleotides, serve as supramolecular motifs in the construction of complex architectures via non-covalent interactions such as hydrogen bonding, electrostatic effects, π–π stacking, hydrophobic interactions, and metal coordination. Different structural properties endow them with varying binding abilities. Because of the non-covalent interactions between the components, the resulting assemblies have controllable morphology, physico-chemical properties, and stimuli responsiveness. Commonly used nucleosides for hydrogels are guanosine, Isoguanosine, and ureidopyrimidine, which form quartets by intermolecular hydrogen bonding [77,78]. The molecules in the quartet with the double bonds undergo π–π stacking to form G-Sheets or quadruplexes, as presented in Figure 4c. Such quadruplexes are further grouped to form hydrogels which can be used in regenerative medicine as a delivery vehicle and as a scaffold [79].

*Block co-polymers:* One of the most fundamental driving mechanisms in the supramolecular assembly of tissue engineering complexes is based on hydrophobic interactions. These interactions can cause the association and subsequent self-assembly of supramolecular polymer fibers, or they can produce physical cross-links between polymer chains, which are critical in the self-assembly of biological materials such as fibrillar proteins. There is an increase in the entropy that occurs due to the repulsion of hydrophobic faces away from the hydrophilic environment of the swelling hydrogel and the surface-bound water molecules. This substantial gain in net entropy with a minor amount of enthalpy drives the hydrophobic interactions, which can self-assemble or support the physical structure in the polymer chains. This mechanism is frequently used in conjunction with chemical cross-linking to improve the mechanical properties of the resulting gels, and unlike other supramolecular motifs, it may be used to make robust self-healing hydrogels. Amphiphilic block copolymers that use these hydrophobic bonds to form supramolecular structures are often used for drug delivery, cell encapsulation, and cartilage regeneration. These hydrogel matrices self-assemble in aqueous conditions and dissolve hydrophobic compounds, allowing therapeutic doses of tiny molecules to be delivered locally. In the end, these scaffolds increased cell infiltration, reduced inflammation, and promoted wound healing in vivo, making them one of the few systems whose therapeutic applicability has been proven [80–84].

*Dendrimers:* Amphiphilic supramolecular dendrimers were researched as an alternative for covalently bound dendrimers for biomedical applications. The most widely used dendritic polymers contain small amphiphilic dendrimers containing a hydrophobic alkyl chain and hydrophilic PAMAM dendron. These dendrons can be easily synthesized in large quantities, with high purity, utilizing divergent or convergent methods or a mix of the two. The dendron with both the hydrophilic and the hydrophobic part can self-assemble into stable and resilient noncovalent supramolecular dendrimers. Due to their amphipathic nature, they can have hydrophobic interactions in their core regions, and hydrogen bonds inside their dendron shells. The simplicity to change the length and nature of the hydrophobic chain, as well as the creation of the hydrophilic PAMAM dendron and the varied terminal functions, provides unique structural flexibility and diversity for a diverse range of biological applications [85].

*Host–guest chemistry in cyclic oligomers:* Host–guest interactions in the macrocyclic molecules are one of the most studied non-covalent techniques for forming supramolecular hydrogels. As previously described, most of the cyclic oligomers that are being used for tissue regeneration are cavitands meaning that they have a cavity constructed by the repeating monomer units. In the cyclodextrins, calixarenes, and cucurbiturils, the cavity is hydrophobic due to the aromatic rings and the surface is hydrophilic due to the hydroxyl groups or other hydrophilic moieties protruding at the ends of the cavities. The hydrophobic groups of the monomer units are responsible for the hydrophobic interactions, which are critical in the formation of the host cavity. Guest molecules or the hydrophobically modified polymers are then physically entrapped, forming supramolecular hydrogels. The stimuli-responsive cyclic oligomers contain stimuli-responsive moieties/polymers that initiate the formation of the inclusion complexes without affecting the bulk properties of the oligomers. At the induction of stimuli, these moieties help in the formation of the host–guest interactions. These phenomena were explained well by Saunders et al. by relevant examples [86].

*Natural Biomaterials*

*Collagen:* Collagen-based biomaterials, which are majorly fabricated in the form of de-cellularized ECM, have the advantage of less risk of immunological rejection. The collagen is either obtained by decellularization of the organ and recellularized before implantation or is decellularized and stored desperately in distinct biomaterial forms such as gels, for ease of use for in vitro and in vivo applications. This decellularization process preserves the original structure of the collagen, but the major hurdles are to understand the molecular mechanism and to achieve the consistency of the biomaterials during the recellularization process. So, the regenerated collagen biomaterials are often used for the regenerative medicine. One of the most widely used forms of this biomaterial is the hydrogel, prepared by self-assembly process triggered especially by temperature rise to physiological temperatures. To form hydrogels, the collagen solution is mixed with the therapeutic agent and the temperature is adjusted for the physical transition into gels. Another type of collagen-based delivery system is represented by microspheres, prepared by direct aliquoting, or emulsifying the polymer solution, followed by temperature adjustment to form the microspheres and subsequent encapsulation of cells or therapeutic material into the microspheres. Collagen is also used in the form of a scaffold, built three-dimensionally by lyophilization, electrospinning, or 3D printing, to which other cells, genes, or drugs are attached [64].

*Alginate:* Alginate is a biopolymer that readily dissolves in water and forms gels through electrostatic interactions influenced by the electrolytes used. Apart from the gels, alginate has also been used in the preparation of nanofibers, nanocoatings, and nanoparticles, which could be used for therapeutic material delivery. Alginate macromolecules are amphiphilic and generally undergo intra- or intermolecular hydrophobic interactions and hydrogen bonding to form self-assembled nanostructures such as nanoparticles and nanofibers that can carry either drugs or genetic material. Alginate is also used with other supramolecular systems listed earlier in this section such as the cyclic oligomers, peptides, and other natural biomaterials to form these self-assembled systems. Characteristics of alginate, such as the resemblances to the native ECM and ability for permeation of gases and small molecules through it when prepared in the form of tissue-engineered scaffolds are the major reasons that it has been extensively researched for potential in tissue regeneration and wound healing [87].

*Gelatin:* Generally, gelatin does not form supramolecular systems on its own and therefore it is used in combination with other supramolecular systems. Cross-linking is generally carried out in the presence of chemical reagents that form covalent bonds or by the dehydrothermal method that uses vacuum heating for the formation of gelatin microparticles. These systems have been used for various regenerative medicine applications reviewed by Nii et al. [88]. There are studies that use these biomaterials with cyclic oligomers or other reagents employing host–guest chemistry to form inclusion complexes and other supramolecular structures [71,72,89–91].

*Hyaluronic acid:* Hyaluronic acid, which is hydrophilic and can be easily chemically modified, generally forms supramolecular hydrogels which are used as scaffolds for tissue engineering and regenerative medicine. Hyaluronic acid readily forms hydrogen bonding to form these reversible hydrogels, but the interactions in water or aqueous solution weaken the bong. Hence, HA is often combined with materials such as poly(N-isopropylacrylamide) (PNIPAM) to form hydrophobic interactions and to obtain stronger hydrogels. Possessing negatively charged carboxyl groups at physiological pH, HA can interact electrostatically with positively charged groups such as carboxymethyl hexanyl chitosan or chondroitin sulfate. It is also reported that HA forms coordination bonds with bivalent and trivalent metal ions such as the Mg2+, Cu2+, Fe2+, Ba2+, and Ca2+. Recently, the most extensively researched hydrogels have been those based on HA with cyclic oligomers such as β-CD or Cucurbiturils, which use the host–guest chemistry to form the inclusion complexes [73].

## 4. Preparation Techniques and Formulation Considerations

### *4.1. Lipid-Based Systems*

When lipids are immersed in an aqueous environment, their amphiphilic nature allows them to form structured assemblies such as vesicles or membranes. Lipid bi-layer sheets and liposomes are being researched majorly as a delivery vehicle for the small and large molecules rather than a biomimetic scaffold. In regenerative medicine, they have been applied to deliver the stem cells with growth/differentiation factors, DNA, or interference RNA (RNAi) and in combination with scaffolds. Preparation of liposomes can be performed by a conventional method of thin-film hydration, and then loading is performed actively or passively with small drug molecules or biologically active macromolecules. The passive loading mechanisms such as the mechanical dispersion method, solvent dispersion method, and detergent removal method are commonly followed. There are many types of mechanical dispersion such as French press extrusion, freeze-thaw, micro-emulsification, membrane extrusion, and others [92]. Many new techniques have been employed lately, which were reviewed by Has et al., for both hydration and loading techniques. Modified methods include electro formation, microfluidics-assisted methods, curvature tuning method, packed bed-assisted hydration, osmotic shock method, dual asymmetric centrifugation, spray-drying, and lyophilization [93]. The schematic representation of the preparation of liposomes is given in Figure 5.

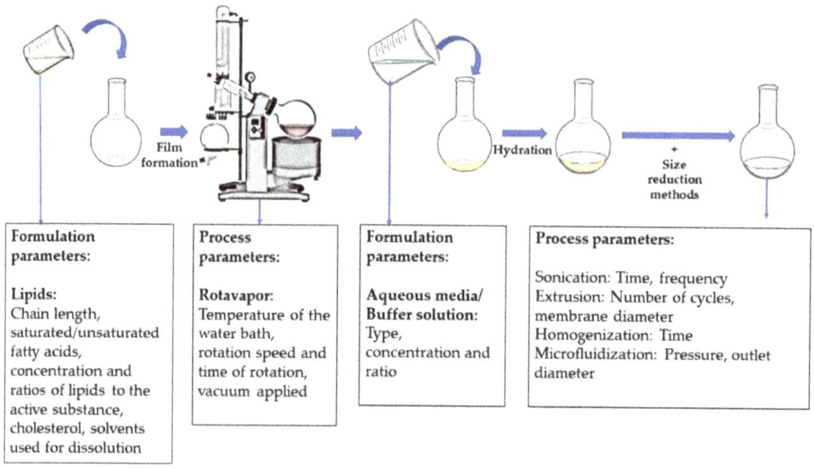


**Figure 5.** Schematic representation of the preparation of liposomes, highlighting the formulation and process parameters involved (created with Biorender.com [accessed on 30 June 2022]).

In the conventional hydration techniques, usually, the essential materials are lipids, active substances, and the buffer solution. The critical quality attributes of the liposomes are majorly affected by the physiochemical properties of these components. Porfire et al. discussed the critical material and process attributes that influence the liposome properties. They discussed that saturated fatty acids have a higher transition temperature and do not undergo oxidative or hydrolytic degradation such as unsaturated fatty acids. The chain length of the lipids will influence the thickness of the lipid bilayer which is inversely proportional to the internal vesicular volume for encapsulation of the therapeutic molecules. The lipids also impact the fluidity and permeability of the bilayer and the charge. Cholesterol used usually for mechanically supporting the lipid bilayer also impacts the encapsulation efficiency. The solvents used, the concentrations and ratios of lipids, solvents, and active substances have a profound effect on the target profile of the liposomes [94].

In addition, many material attributes vary according to the type of preparation process selected. For the thin-film hydration technique, the temperature of the water bath, the speed and time of rotation of the flask, and the vacuum applied might influence the liposome size, but it is the type of the size reduction methods employed that has a greater impact on the final properties of the liposomes. For example, if the liposomes are extruded for size reduction, the diameter of the extrusion membrane and the number of cycles influence the particle size of the liposomes.

### *4.2. Peptide-Based Systems*

Peptide nanofibers and hydrogels have been used in regenerative medicine due to their ability to exhibit bioactive signals, which can be performed by integrating the bioactive component within the peptide sequence or co-assembling the peptide with the bioactive signal. Hence, these two types of delivery systems are much more focused on by the scientists to improve their applicability as not only an extracellular matrix scaffold but also as a delivery vehicle for small and large molecules in the biomedical domain. Peptides and peptide amphiphiles, as discussed earlier, form multiple conformational structures such as micelles, β-sheets, and nanofibers when influenced by the external environment subjected to changes in pH, temperature, and electrolyte ions. Nanofibers have been the most applicable form in tissue engineering. There are various methods of manufacturing nanofibers such as template synthesis, phase separation, melt-blown technology, force spinning, and freeze-drying, but electrospinning is mostly preferred for peptide nanofibers [95].

Electrospinning is a low-cost and easily accessible method for producing nanofibers using electrical forces and polymer solutions, in a short amount of time with surface control of nanofibers [96]. A spinneret, a high voltage power supply, and a grounded collecting plate are the three fundamental components of an electrospinning apparatus (usually a metal screen, plate, or rotating mandrel). The principle of this technology is to apply high voltage to a polymer solution to generate electrical field jets, and then evaporate the solvent while the formed jets flow to a grounded collector to obtain nanofibers. The process is diagrammatically represented in Figure 6.

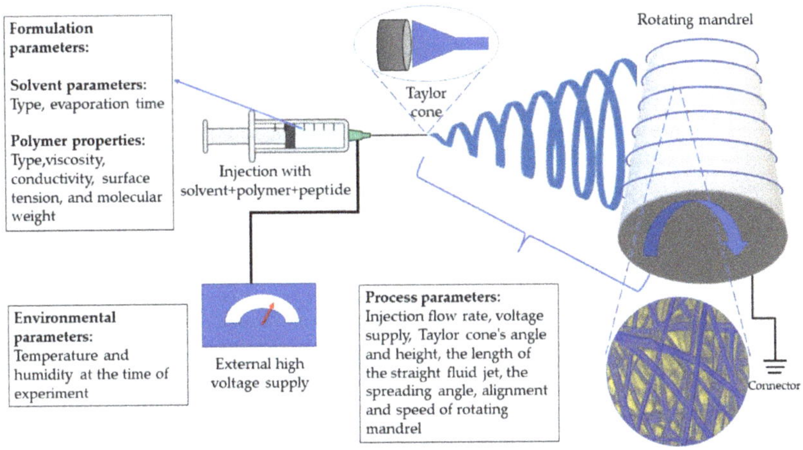


**Figure 6.** Pictorial representation of electrospinning process.

Parameters related to the polymer solution, process parameters, and environmental conditions affect the electrospinning process. The viscosity, conductivity, surface tension, and molecular weight of the polymer are all formulation factors that have a substantial impact on the morphology and size of the fibers. The process parameters are the applied electrical force, tip to distance collector, and feed/flow rate. The electrospinning process is also influenced by environmental circumstances, which include the temperature and humidity at which the operation is carried out, to avoid degradation of the peptides. In addition to these parameters, the formulation additives such as the type of organic solvent used to dissolve the peptides and to enhance the spinnability. To improve mechanical qualities, peptide/proteins can be combined with natural and synthetic polymers such as Eudragit®, poly-L-lactic acid (PLLA), polycaprolactone (PCL), chitosan, polylactic acid (PLA), and PEO. Morphology, fiber stability, decreased degradation in the physiological environment, increased biological function, and increased spinnability are examples of these features. Glutaraldehyde, formaldehyde, genipin, proanthocyanin, and chlorination are examples of cross-linkers that can be utilized for this purpose [95].

*4.3. Nucleic Acid Subunit-Based Systems*

Nucleosides such as guanosine and Isoguanosine assemble in quartet structures to form hydrogels which can be used for regenerative medicine. The nucleobases associate through Hoogsteen hydrogen bonding to form vertical stacks of square-shaped quartet aromatic structures and grow into wires or fibrous structures which drive the gelation process. These self-assembled hydrogels are either stabilized by cations or anions. Many different preparation methods have been reported by researchers. The common main components are the gelator molecules, which are the nucleosides such as guanosine or Isoguanosine in their stable forms such as hydrazides or aldehydes which, in the presence of monovalent or bi-valent cations and anions, yield self-assembling structures [77].

### 4.4. Block Copolymers (BCP)

Amphiphilic block copolymers majorly form three types of assembled structures, for example micelles, polymerosomes, and nanoparticles. Micelles are self-assembled nanostructures formed when the concentration of the BCP in dilute solutions is above the critical micellar concentration (CMC). These micelles serve as excellent carrier systems for drugs and biomolecules. Polymerosomes are also self-assembled structures and differ from the micelles by being double-layered vesicular structures [97–99].

### 4.5. Dendrimers

The dendrimers are either prepared by convergent or divergent methods consisting of a multifunctional central core with branching dendritic polymers involving the formation of covalent bonds. Due to this covalent synthesis, the higher generation of dendrimers, which have many branches, often has structural defects due to incomplete reactions. In the case of amphiphilic dendritic polymers, dendrons are also manufactured either by convergent or divergent methods. However, then the hydrophilic dendrons have hydrophobic alkyl chains that form the core by electrostatic and hydrophobic interactions. This problem could be overcome by the non-covalent synthesis using the amphiphilic dendritic polymers with hydrophobic alkyl chains and the hydrophilic dendrons consisting of PAMAM. The hydrophilic dendrons are directed towards the outer surface, while the hydrophobic alkyl chain is directed towards the center, as shown in Figure 7. The hydrophobic alkyl chains from various dendrons form the core by electrostatic and hydrophobic interactions [44].

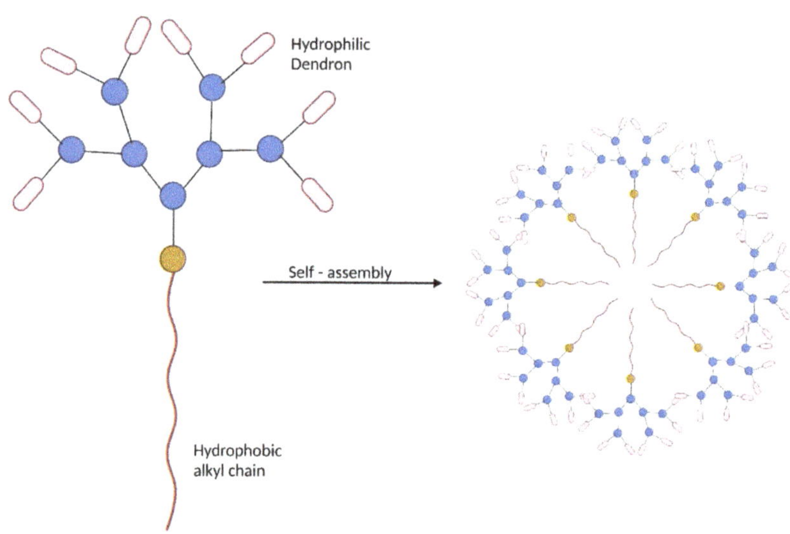


**Figure 7.** Amphiphilic dendritic copolymers (created with Biorender.com [accessed on 30 June 2022]).

Chen et al. synthesized cationic dendrimers with hydrophilic PAMAM dendrons with seven tertiary amines in the inner structure and eight of them on the terminals using click chemistry with triethanolamine as the core. They observed that the longer alkyl chains improve the hydrophobic interaction and the stability of the complex. Additionally, the dendrimers with fewer generations or shorter alkyl chains led to insufficient genetic material loading. This might be due to the lesser hydrophobic groups when compared with the longer alkyl chains, which impacts the electrostatic interaction with the genetic material [100].

### 4.6. Cyclic Oligomers

Cyclic oligomers being used in regenerative medicine are synthesized mostly chemically, and then the inclusion complexes are formed through various preparation methods to host the guest molecules of drugs and other biomacromolecules. Cyclodextrins are prepared by the enzymatic degradation of starch by using glucosyltransferase.

The preparation of inclusion complexes of cyclic oligomers is critical in the performance, morphology, and stability of the delivery systems. The inclusion complexes are prepared by many methods, namely co-precipitation methods, kneading, grinding, spray drying, irradiating by microwaves, and by the utilization of super critical fluids [101]. Co-precipitation is one of the most simplistic and efficient methods where the guest molecule to be hosted is dissolved in organic solvents to which solution containing the cyclic oligomer is added and agitated. The solution is then cooled until crystallization occurs. The crystals are then washed with organic solvents and dried [102–104]. A simple method called the kneading method consists of making a paste of cyclodextrins with a small amount of water and adding the guest molecules with thorough mixing. Then the resultant paste is washed off with solvents to obtain the solid form of the inclusion complex [105]. An alternative method to the above two techniques is the utilization of super critical fluids. Most commonly, super critical carbon dioxide is used, which is maintained at super critical conditions of temperature and pressure in an autoclave, with the cyclodextrins and the guest molecules. A rapid pressure drop occurs due to which carbon dioxide is then vaporized, and the inclusion complex is formed. A more simplistic method is the grinding method, which involves mechanical energy that gives sufficient intensity to the guest molecules to become trapped in the host molecules. Some methods employ microwaves to blend guest molecules and the host molecules in a minimum amount of solvent such as ethanol [106,107]. For water-soluble or water-dispersible guest and host molecules, spray drying could be utilized to form the inclusion complexes. In this technique, the liquid containing the molecules is atomized into fine droplets which are then dried by a heated air stream and separated from the air.

## 5. Characterization

Supramolecular-based systems usually involve self-assembling units (both biomacromolecule based as well as synthetic) whose equilibrium constant varies with the varying chain lengths. For such dynamic systems, a single characterization technique might often not be sufficient, and a combination of techniques would be required to evaluate them qualitatively and quantitatively [108]. Additionally, these systems are mostly produced in the form of gels that mimics the extracellular matrix of the target tissue or act as delivery systems to carry therapeutic material to the targeted site. So, the characterization mostly involves similar testing methods as that of viscous gels. The general characterization of other delivery systems would also be taken into consideration, but majorly the supramolecular mechanism was studied and represented in Table 1.

### 5.1. Rheology

Rheology in practical terms can be defined as the study of the flow and deformation of materials under the applied external forces [109]. It is primarily focused on relating the force with the deformation in materials such as liquids and semisolids, which in turn can provide valuable information about dynamics and structural assemblies. The researchers test the elastic storage modulus ($G'$), the measure of energy stored during a strain cycle, and elastic loss modulus ($G''$), the measure of energy lost during a strain cycle, to assess the nature of the supramolecular structure and assemblies. Dawn et al. detailed frequency sweep experiments, and time-dependent experiments, about the determination of yield stress and linear viscoelastic region. According to the $G'$ and $G''$ the supramolecular gels were categorized into healable and non-healable. Further healable systems were sub-categorized into fibrous, non-fibrous, self-healing, and stereochemistry-based systems based on the type of framework [110].

**Table 1.** Characterization techniques and information obtained.

| Characterization Technique | Evaluated Parameters | Information Obtained |
|---|---|---|
| **Rheology** | Elastic storage modulus (G′), elastic loss modulus (G″), | Stability of the supramolecular gel at induced strain and temporal variation. Structural assembly of the monomers [109,110] |
| **Chromatography** | Retention or exclusion time | The average molecular weight of the monomers [108] |
| **Spectroscopy:** | | |
| Infrared | Vibrations of atoms and shifts in the characteristic peaks | Non-covalent interactions that appear during sol–gel transition/supramolecular assembly [111] |
| UV/Visible | Absorption wavelengths | Quantitative determination of non-covalent interactions that appear during sol–gel transition/supramolecular assembly [53,112,113] |
| Fluorescence | Loss of vibrational energy in the form of fluorescence | Quantitative determination of non-covalent interactions [114–116] |
| Nuclear magnetic resonance | Chemical shift, coupling constant, line widths, peak integral, relaxation time, and the nuclear Over Hauser effect (NOE) | Chemical structure and formation of non-covalent interactions in cavitands [56,117–123] |
| Mass spectrometry | Mass-to-charge ratio ($m/z$) of one or more molecules | Chemical structure and end groups identification [111,124–126] |
| Circular dichroism | The difference in absorbance of right- and left-circularly polarized light | The intra- and intermolecular interactions in chiral supramolecules with changes in temperature and time [115,126] |
| **Dynamic light scattering** | Intensity fluctuations during Brownian motion | Particle size [127–131] |
| **X-ray light scattering** | Intensities of X-rays scattered | Shape, conformation, and assembly of supramolecular complexes [77,125,132] |
| **Thermal analysis:** Isothermal titration calorimetry (ITC) | Various thermodynamic parameters—enthalpy (ΔH), entropy (ΔS), free energy (ΔG) | Binding affinity between the molecules and stoichiometry |
| Differential scanning calorimetry | Heat flow | Sol–gel transition enthalpy [130,133] |
| **Microscopy** | Topography of materials | Shape and size of the supramolecular delivery systems [77,111,118,134–137] |

### *5.2. Chromatography Techniques*

Chromatographic techniques such as size exclusion chromatography have often been used for polymer characterization and to provide information about the molecular mass distribution of the polymers. Gel permeation chromatography was reviewed by Liu et al., where they considered research on supramolecular systems such as dendrimers with multiple hydrogen-bonding arrays [108]. These techniques, when combined with light scattering and x-ray scattering techniques, will provide the average molecular weight of the polymer.

### *5.3. Spectroscopy Techniques*

Based on the information sought regarding self-assembled polymer structures, a variety of spectroscopic techniques are available for characterization. All the spectroscopic techniques used for supramolecular systems are reviewed in this section.

Infrared spectroscopy could be used to characterize the non-covalent interactions behind the gelling process of supramolecular systems. IR spectroscopy can be used to explain the formation of intermolecular hydrogen bonding during aggregation, and the formation of new bands in the CH stretching areas because of the packing of aliphatic chain molecules [111].

Ultraviolet and visible light is often absorbed by molecules to excite the electrons from the π bonds or the nonbonding electrons to higher antibonding molecular orbitals. In supramolecular systems, non-covalent interactions can also cause physical changes, for example, in the case of gelation, the interactions increase the hydrophobicity of the surroundings [112,113]. In the case of stimuli-responsive supramolecular systems, where physical changes are influenced by external stimuli, UV/Visible spectroscopy can be used to quantitatively determine the non-covalent interactions [53].

Fluorescence spectroscopy is another type of electromagnetic spectroscopy that is used for the quantitative determination of supramolecular systems. The principle differs from the UV/Vis by analyzing the fluorescence of the electrons that are previously excited and lose their vibrational energy to come to the ground state [114,115]. It can also provide details regarding the inclusion of complexation by cyclic oligomers [116].

$^1$H NMR probes hydrogen nuclei within the molecules of a substance to determine the structure and the interactions of its molecules. In the supramolecular systems, the chemical shift changes that are driven by noncovalent interactions can be monitored [117]. Diffusion-ordered NMR spectroscopy (DOSY) has become significant in the characterization of self-assembly systems for being able to measure translational diffusion coefficient that accounts for the net result of thermal motion induced in solution by particles or molecules [118,119]. This coefficient can provide accurate hydrodynamic dimensions of the systems by using the Stokes–Einstein equation as well as the thermodynamic parameters. Nuclear Over Hauser effect spectroscopy (NOESY) [56,120] and rotating frame nuclear Over Hauser effect spectroscopy (ROESY) [121–123] have also been used to obtain information about the relative positions of the building components in host–guest interactions of cyclic oligomers by employing two-dimensional NMR.

Mass spectrometry has been employed in some situations where chemical composition and end group identification for supramolecular polymers had to be determined [111,124–126].

Circular dichroism spectroscopy is a technique that involves the study of the stereo structures and the intra- and intermolecular interactions of various classes of chiral supramolecules. This technique always is used to monitor the thermal responsive changes in nanoscale chiral aggregates assemblies [115,126].

### 5.4. Dynamic Light Scattering and X-ray Scattering Techniques

The dynamic light scattering technique (DLS) is used to determine the size distribution profile, structural formation, and interactions of small particles in suspension or small polymers in the solution. When a particle is irradiated and subjected to Brownian motion, two frequencies of equal intensity, including a positive and negative Doppler shift proportionate to the particle velocity, are generated in addition to the frequency that would usually be scattered. Brownian motion causes interference between the non-shifted wave (proton re-emission) and the two waves, resulting in microscopic intensity changes. The scattered intensity is measured as a function of time and self-correlated after that. The relaxation time due to Brownian motion is obtained, and the particle size is determined using hydrodynamic models of the diffusion coefficients. The diffusion coefficient can also be calculated using DLS, which simply monitors changes in the scattered light intensity of diffusing particles. The study of light scattering by structures with diameters in the sub-micrometer range allows key features such as shape and internal structure to be determined. Because the size (or diffusion coefficient) increases drastically when 3D networks grow, DLS is an effective tool for the characterization of supramolecular gels [127–129,131].

X-ray techniques have been transformed significantly over the past two decades to cater for the characterization of structural motifs of the supramolecular assemblies and to understand the weak intermolecular interactions and the local packing of the molecules. To determine the arrangement of atoms, a beam of X-rays impacts the material and causes the beam of light to spread out in many different directions. A crystallographer can create a three-dimensional picture of the density of electrons within the system by measuring the angles and intensities of these diffracted beams. The mean locations of the atoms in the system, as well as their chemical bonds, disorder, and other information, may be deduced using this electron density [77]. This X-ray diffraction method was employed by Hwang et al. in the characterization of cucurbiturils to determine the layer structure and the alignment of the fibrils during self-assembly [132]. Angelerou et al. used this technique in the characterization of nucleoside-based supramolecular gel to check the local packing of the molecules in N4-octanoyl-2′-deoxycytidine xerogels [125].

### 5.5. Thermal Analysis

In supramolecular chemistry, noncovalent interactions involve energy and momentum transfers between molecules. Isothermal titration calorimetry can be used to determine these thermodynamic parameters such as binding affinity, enthalpy changes, and the stoichiometry of the interaction between the molecules. Differential scanning calorimetry (DSC) is a thermoanalytical technique that measures the difference in the amount of heat required to raise the temperature of a sample and a reference as a function of temperature. These techniques can not only determine the sol–gel transition enthalpy but also the thermal stability of the supramolecular gel. Xia et al. obtained enthalpy changes and the thermal stability of the oligopeptide hybrid films using DSC [133]. Park et al., used this technique to explain the reversible phase transition of their β-cyclodextrin-based noncovalent, double-network hydrogel [130].

### 5.6. Microscopic Techniques

Microscopy techniques are mostly used together with other characterization techniques and often a combination of microscopic techniques is used to understand the morphology of the sample. Scanning electron microscopy (SEM) is a type of electron microscopy that uses a focused beam of electrons to scan across the material to create images. These electrons interact with the electrons in the sample, resulting in a variety of signals that may be detected and carry information on the surface topography and composition of the sample [111,134,135]. In most cases, the electron beam is scanned in a raster scan pattern, and the position of the beam is coupled with the detected signal to create a picture. Another microscopy technique is transmission electron microscopy (TEM), in which a beam of electrons interacts with the object as it goes through. The interaction of the electrons with the specimen can result in the formation of an image. An imaging device, such as a fluorescent screen, a layer of photographic film, or a sensor, is used to magnify and focus the image (CCD camera). In theory, TEM has enough resolution to detect molecules at the sub-nanometer scale [111,136,137]. One of the most important tools for photographing, measuring, and manipulating materials at the nanoscale is the atomic force microscope (AFM). The data are collected by "feeling" the surface with an extremely sensitive "spring-board-like" cantilever. Attractive or repulsive interactions that influence the tip at the end of the cantilever as it is moved over a sample cause the cantilever to bend, thereby providing a mechanical means to probe local nanoscale effects [77,118,136]. These techniques have been used widely to study the structural and morphological details of the materials. In the supramolecular systems, the individual fibers that self-assemble to form the hydrogels could be visualized with higher levels of a resolution, allowing the user to determine the structural changes with and without the therapeutic molecules. This electron microscopy when coupled with a focus ion beam allows 3D imaging of the supramolecular systems. Cryo-electron microscopy techniques step up in providing the observations of the hydrogels at different gelator concentrations and observing the nano-structural changes during their synthesis.

## 6. In Vitro and In Vivo Biocompatibility Studies

One of the most important characteristics of any delivery system is its biocompatibility and, since it is being employed in regenerative medicine, the supramolecular systems need to be more bio-compliant than other delivery systems. Most of the prototypes successful in the in vitro studies usually become phased out due to their inability to prove their efficacy in in vivo models. Hence, a major emphasis has been given to the successful prototypes and research activities held previously, proving the biocompatibility of both the biomacromolecule-based and synthetic macromolecule-based supramolecular systems.

Some of the most recent development and studies regarding the biocompatibility of the supramolecular systems with the various tissues are tabulated in Table 2 and Figure 8.

**Table 2.** Research on stability and biocompatibility.

| Type of Tissue | Type of Supramolecular System | Application |
|---|---|---|
| Nervous tissue | Peptide-based hydrogels | Wang et al. proposed self-assembling peptides RADA16 with osteopontin-derived angiogenic motif SVVYGLR that helped in the angiogenesis and promoted the reconstruction of the neural tissue and recovery of the reflexive responses to the motion in a zebrafish model [138] |
| | | Ma et al. proposed a self-assembling peptide hydrogel named Slanc with chemically synthesized oligopeptide sequence K(SL)3RG(SL)3K–G–KLTWQELYQLKYKGI with vascular endothelial growth factor. These hydrogels were first checked for the cytocompatibility using in vitro methods and then checked in fluid percussion injury models in vivo in Sprague–Dawley rats. The in vivo results have shown angiogenesis, neuroprotection and axonal outgrowth around the hydrogels indicating regeneration of the brain injury [139]. |
| | Nucleic acid-based hydrogels | Yuan et al. made a highly permeable supramolecular DNA hydrogel matrix with homologous neural stem cells to regenerate severe spinal cord injury. The hydrogels were tested using in vivo rat models and have been evaluated for the migration, proliferation, and differentiation of the stem cells. It was found that the hydrogel-treated groups showed regeneration in the form of newborn oligodendrocytes and the myelin structure regeneration [140]. |
| | Cyclic oligomer-based hydrogels | An injectable composite hydrogel made from gelatin acrylated β-cyclodextrin polyethylene glycol was prepared to carry motor neurons from embryonic stem cells by Wang et al. In their research, they demonstrated neuroinflammation response to the transplanted composite gels and a functional recovery in the behavior of the spinal cord injured rat models [141]. |
| Cardiovascular tissue | Supramolecular peptide nanofibers | A zymogen activator peptide Nap-FFEG-IVGGYPWWMDV which can activate the hepatocyte growth factor precursor (pro-HGF) is made into self-assembled nanofibers to perform anti-apoptosis and pro-angiogenesis. This has helped to demonstrate regeneration of the infarct area of the heart affected due to acute myocardial infarction in the adult male C57 BL/6 mice [142] |
| | | In another similar example, a self-assembling peptide Nap-pD-E7, that enables a sheet of mesenchymal stem cells, was isolated from the bone marrow to form cell spheroids. The peptide loaded with MSC spheroids is then checked in vivo in myocardial infarction-induced mice models. It was seen that the phosphopeptide promoted the paracrine effect and lead to neovascularization [143]. |
| | Nucleic acid subunit-based systems | Growth factors are incorporated into supramolecular ureidopyrimidinone (Upy) hydrogel exhibiting sol–gel behavior that forms a gel at neutral pH. Intramyocardial delivery in a porcine model of myocardial infarction showed improved blood flow and the formation of new cardiomyocytes [144]. A similar study using chain extended ureidopyrimidinone polymers was functionalized with heparin and Interleukin 4 for in-situ arterial tissue regeneration in rat models [145]. |
| Renal system | Supramolecular self-assembly β-sheet peptide hydrogel | A functional peptide-based scaffold containing Naphthalene (Nap) covalently conjugated to a short D-form peptide (Nap-DFDFG) and C domain of insulin-like growth factor-1 (IGF-1C) has been prepared to deliver the human placenta-derived mesenchymal stem cells. These hydrogels showed endogenous regeneration and improved blood flow when tested in a murine acute kidney model [146] |
| | Peptide nanofibers | Nanofibers derived from Arg-Gly-Asp peptides adhere readily to the integrins derived from the extracellular vesicles from the mesenchymal stem cells (MSCs). This system, when intrarenally injected into the acute kidney-injured rat models, was observed to determine an increase in proliferation, autophagy, and renal function [147]. The same research group also tested a hydrogel made by the combination of Tyr-Ile-Gly-Ser-Arg and Arg-Gly-Asp peptides and combined it with a biocompatible biotin-D-amino acid for carrying MSCs. The group reported the enhanced paracrine function of the MSCs in the acute kidney injured rat models [148]. |
| | Cyclic oligomers | Cheng et al. proposed hypoxia-sensitive Azocalix(5)arenes co-assembled with mesenchymal stem cell-derived extracellular vesicles for targeted therapy in kidney injury. They reported the inhibition of HIF-1α expression in hypoxic renal tubular epithelial cells (TECs). This delivery system could be used further for delivering therapeutic and diagnostic agents [149]. |
| Digestive system | Cyclic oligomers | In the cases of treatment of type 1 diabetes, the transplanted pancreatic islets suffer from oxidative stress and inflammation. Delivery of bilirubin with the help of poly lysine conjugated cyclodextrin was attempted in a diabetic mice model. This system helped in the reduction of the oxidative stress and inflammation, promoted angiogenesis, and strengthened the function of the transplanted islets [150]. |
| | Amphiphilic block copolymers | For tissue repair in gastric environments, Wang et al. developed an anti-biofouling and biocompatible hydrogel based on ABA triblock copolymers. This hydrogel was checked in the in vivo gastric perforation repair model, and the results suggested a constrained inflammation and an increase in the vascular density. The reduced inflammation was explained due to the anti-biofouling capacity, which is the ability to prevent the accumulation of the microbes during the wound healing process, which makes it an ideal material for postoperative wound dressing for tissue regeneration [151]. |

**Table 2.** *Cont.*

| Type of Tissue | Type of Supramolecular System | Application |
| --- | --- | --- |
| Muscle/ Connective | Peptide nanofibers | In the case of muscle regeneration, the basal lamina plays a significant role. The laminin mimetic peptide nanofibers lauryl-VVAGKKIKVAV-Am mimics the muscle basal lamina environment. It significantly promoted satellite cell activation in skeletal muscle and myogenic differentiation and accelerated myofibrillar regeneration in the in vivo acute muscle injury model in Sprague–Dawley rats [152]. |
| | | In conditions such as sarcopenia, which is described by a rapid loss of muscle mass and function, delivery of growth factor-like Insulin-like growth factor -1 (IGF-1) has proven beneficial. Shang et al. attempted muscle repair by using IGF-1mimicking peptide sequence Nap-FFGSSSR which forms a supramolecular hydrogel, which could promote myoblast proliferation and promoted muscle regeneration in glucocorticoid-induced sarcopenia rat models. Further RNA sequencing was performed to elucidate the similarity in the activation of the Akt signaling pathway by IGF-1 to that of the peptide hydrogel [153]. |
| | Nucleic acid subunit-based systems | Mori et al. described a supramolecular material with polycarbonate and ureidopyrimidinone functionalized with UPy-modified cyclic arginine-glycine-aspartic acid (cRGD) peptide additives. This material promoted myogenesis and neovascularization in the rat hernia model accelerating the tissue growth and regeneration of the abdominal wall [154]. |
| Bone/ Cartilaginous | Peptide amphiphiles | Histidine-containing peptides incorporated with a dicarboxylic acid-like succinic acid have been used for three-dimensional cell culture using a mouse fibroblast cell line. In vitro studies revealed the growth and nourishment of cells in the presence of the peptide gel [155,156] |
| | Cyclic oligomer-based systems | β-cyclodextrin—gellan gum complex hydrogel was developed to enhance the affinity of the anti-inflammatory drug dexamethasone known for improving the chondrogenesis and decreasing the inflammatory response in the cartilage defected rabbit model [59]. Another such example was described in the research by Jeong et al., where mesenchymal stem cells were encapsulated in β-cyclodextrin modified hyaluronic acid and adamantane modified Hyaluronic acid. |
| | Nucleic acid-based systems | Yan et al. proposed a DNA-based hydrogel with isolated mesenchymal stem cells (MSC) and tested it in vitro to check for cell proliferation and chondrogenic differentiation. Upon confirmation of the differentiation, the hydrogels were injected into severe osteoarthritis rabbit models which supported the MSC in a high-friction environment and showed signs of cartilage regeneration [156]. |
| | Lipid-based systems | Molecules such as Rhein and other therapeutic agents which possess chondroprotective action are very poorly bioavailable when taken through the oral route. Ebada et al., in their research, made cationic solid lipid nanoparticles entrapped with rhein and which could be injected directly into the articular joints. The lipid-based systems proved efficient in inhibition of inflammation, and cartilage deterioration in the Monoiodoacetate induced arthritic rat models [157]. |
| Dental | Peptide-based hydrogels | Siddiqui et al. made a self-assembling peptide SLan angiogenic target peptide with K(SL)6K–G–KLTWQELYQLKYKGI sequence for dental pulp revascularization. They checked for biocompatibility with subcutaneous administration of the peptides to the female wistar rats and then in adult beagle dogs as pulp revascularization models. The growth factor mimetic peptide was found to be the material of choice for tissue regeneration, promoting angiogenesis in cases of pulpectomy [158]. |
| | | Biocompatible hydrogelator Nap-Phe-Phe-Tyr-OH (NapFFY) was co-assembled with stromal cell-derived factor-1 (SDF-1) and bone morphogenetic proteins (BMPs) and studied for periodontal bone regeneration by Tan et al. The team observed that the hydrogel has increased the cell proliferation of the endogenous bone marrow mesenchymal stem cells due to the SDF-1, and in vivo models of the critical-sized periodontal bone defect models of maxillae in rats suggested the accelerated osteogenesis [159]. |
| | Nucleic acid subunit-based systems | Wang et al. used a monomeric nucleoside molecular gelator 2-amino-2′-fluoro-2′-deoxyadenosine, which is self-healable, shear-thinning, and injectable to the tooth sockets directly. After checking for the biocompatibility, the team checked the anti-bacterial activity against the streptococcus mutans and the porphyromonas gingivalis and observed reduced inflammation at the sites of application in the in vivo rat models, thereby helping in the regeneration of the tooth socket [160]. |
| Skin | Nucleic acid subunit-based systems | For accelerated wound healing and skin regeneration, guanosine quartet hydrogels loaded with recombinant human-sourced collagen (G4-RHC) are used as medical patches. The RHC that is integrated into the gel engages macrophages and fibroblasts at the injury site and supports the formation of new connective tissue for skin regeneration [161]. |
| | Peptide amphiphile nanofibers | To heal wounds made by burns, bioactive Arg-Gly-Asp-Ser (RGDS) modified peptide amphiphilic gels seeded with thermally damaged fibroblasts and human umbilical vein endothelial cells were used in a rat burn model. Pathological and histological examinations have been done in the injured area, which showed significant re-epithelialization and capillary formation supporting the burn wound closure [162]. |
| | Peptide hydrogels | Jian et al. designed a platelet-derived growth factor (PDGF) mimicking peptide by connecting a self-assembling motif derived from β-amyloid peptide and the PDGF epitope VRKIEIVRKK. Upon checking for cell proliferation of fibroblasts and keratinocytes and cell migration, the formulation was tested in a full-thickness skin wound model. The collagen disposition and the angiogenesis in the in vivo model support the finding of this material as a suitable biomaterial for chronic wound healing [163]. |

**Table 2.** *Cont.*

| Type of Tissue | Type of Supramolecular System | Application |
|---|---|---|
| | Cyclic oligomer-based hydrogels | To enhance wound healing, epidermal growth factor (EGF) was delivered using supramolecular polysaccharide hydrogels consisting of cyclic oligomer β-cyclodextrin and azobenzene groups conjugated to hyaluronic acid chains. The formulation was tested on a full-thickness skin defect model and showed an increase in growth factor levels, granulation tissue formation, and angiogenesis [53]. |
| | | For wound healing, supramolecular hydrogels were made with cyclodextrin-modified gelatin and adamantane-modified hyaluronate, with encapsulated fibroblasts and conjugated with human growth factor. After checking for cytocompatibility and cell proliferation, the mice were injected with fibroblasts mixed with these hydrogels and checked for skin regeneration for 21 days. The research group found that fibroblast proliferation from the hydrogels has helped in angiogenesis and skin regeneration [164]. |

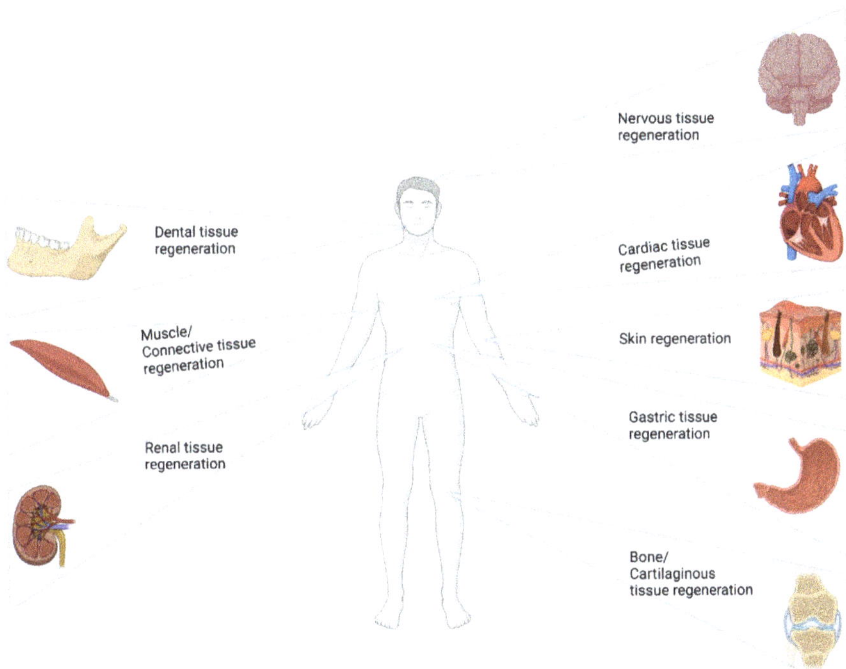


**Figure 8.** Targeted tissues for regeneration using supramolecular systems (created with Biorender.com [accessed on 30 June 2022]).

## 7. Innovations and Future Approaches to Improving Clinical Applicability

### *7.1. Stimuli Responsivity—Control Using Various Factors Such as pH, Temperature, Light, Enzymes and Others*

Despite enormous research in drug research and development, more than half of potential treatments fail in clinical trials due to a lack of therapeutic efficacy and unacceptable safety. The therapeutic effectiveness and safety of a pharmacological agent are heavily influenced by drug formulation and delivery techniques. The use of stimuli-responsive triggers to modulate drug biodistribution such that a drug acts both when it is needed and at the place where it is needed is one commonly researched way toward more efficient delivery systems. Supramolecular systems can be designed to accompany stimuli-responsive moieties that can define their mechanism of action and the kinetics in the human body. When external stimuli such as changes in pH, temperature, light, electrical activity, or enzymes are detected, these stimuli-responsive systems change their shape or volume which causes them to grow or decrease in volume and consequently release the therapeutically active substance [165].

Alternatively, the process might be made more restricted by incorporating the ability to respond to pathophysiologic markers, such as changes in blood pressure, pH, an increase in redox activity, or a rise in enzyme concentrations. Injectable hydrogels that are responsive to pH, temperature, and enzymes have been studied for site-specific controlled drug delivery since any illness in the body induces conditions of low pH, increased temperature, and varying glucose concentrations. For targeted delivery systems, light and enzyme-responsive hydrogels are preferred, whereas pH-, temperature-, electric-, and light-responsive hydrogels can be employed for controlled release delivery systems [166].

#### 7.1.1. Temperature Responsive Systems

Temperature-responsive supramolecular hydrogels are the most researched stimuli responsive systems in the supramolecular systems due to their applicability. They undergo sol–gel or gel–sol transitions in response to minor changes in their surrounding temperature. The temperature-dependent phase changes of supramolecular hydrogels are predominantly driven by hydrophilic and hydrophobic interactions, like thermoreversible hydrogels. Biomaterials that display a sol–gel transition at physiological temperatures (37 °C) are ideal for use as scaffolds and for delivering biomolecules in tissue engineering [167]. Hao et al. designed a flexible self-assembling system formed from the complexation of a long-chain amino amide and a trifunctional carboxylic acid. This supramolecular system forms a reversible thermo-responsive gel with the sol–gel transition ranging between 23 and 76 °C [168]. In another example, self-assembling biomimetic β-sheet rich peptides when complexed with polysaccharides such as guar gum resulted in a thermoresponsive hydrogel that undergoes the sol–gel transition at variable temperatures [169]. A self-healing gel made from the ABA triblock copolymer was prepared by Wang et al. for postoperative tissue regeneration for gastric perforation [151].

#### 7.1.2. Light Responsive Systems

The employment of hydrogelators encoded with light-sensitive groups (e.g., photo-cleavable groups, photo-isomerizable groups, photo-dimerizable groups) to cause phase transitions is another strategy to design the stimuli-responsive systems [170,171]. Light-induced cis-trans isomerization is also termed photo isomerization and involves groups such as azobenzene and spiropyran. Zhao et al. used photo-responsive supramolecular hydrogels made up of azobenzene and α-cyclodextrin groups attached to hyaluronic acid chains, forming host–guest interactions. The azobenzene undergoes cis-trans isomerization upon application of the UV light and the epidermal growth factor (EGF) is released at the wound site for accelerated wound healing [53]. Photocleavable hydrogels employ o-nitrobenzyl, coumarin, or other groups which could be easily dissociated with exposure to UV light. Upon cleavage, the active biomacromolecules or drugs can be released from the hydrogels [172]. There are also photodimerizable groups, which have been used to make these photo-responsive systems, which could be either crosslinked or de-crosslinked, and readily transition to gel or sol upon light irradiation. Coumarin, cinnamic acid, and anthracene are some of the groups that exhibit photodimerization [173].

#### 7.1.3. Electric and Magnetic Responsive Systems

Hydrogelators containing magnetically active cores, such as paramagnetic or diamagnetic species (e.g., metal ions, aromatic moieties) that form aligned fibrillar structures in the presence of an external magnetic field, are used to create magnetic field-responsive supramolecular hydrogels. In most cases, magnetic nanoparticles are incorporated into the hydrogel matrix to produce these magnetic hydrogels. Zhang et al. developed a system based on biocompatible supramolecular polymeric nanofibers. They developed magnetic nanoparticles modified with actin-binding peptide, adamantane (MS-ABPAda), and cyclodextrin-bearing hyaluronic acid host polymer (HACD) that could remodel the stem cell polarization and could be applicable for tissue regeneration [54]. Another example is the inclusion of magnetic nanoparticles in peptide hydrogels made up of Fmoc-diphenylalanine and Fmoc−arginine−glycine−aspartic acid (Fmoc-RGD) short peptides which were tested in vivo in mice and were biocompatible and biodegradable [174]. Another category of stimuli-responsive hydrogels which are closely linked to magnetic responsive hydrogels are the electro-sensitive supramolecular hydrogels based on compounds such as (poly(3,4-ethylene dioxythiophene) polystyrene sulfonate), 3,4-dihydroxyphenylalanine (DOPA), diketopyrrolopyrrole which are incorporated into peptide-based hydrogels. These systems are applied in biomedical fields such as biosensing, drug delivery, and tissue engineering domains [175].

#### 7.1.4. Chemical/pH-Responsive Systems

The use of pH as a stimulus is one of the most effective ways to start supramolecular hydrogelation since a small amount of acid or base can cause a substantial pH shift by fast diffusion of protons or hydroxide ions. Because biological tissues have varying pH levels (gastric pH of 1–3 vs. intestinal pH of 6.1–7), pH-responsive supramolecular hydrogels can be employed as smart drug delivery vehicles. In addition, several diseased diseases, such as cancer, have been shown to have a different extracellular pH than the healthy state. The transport of active substances has often been aided by the difference in pH within the damaged tissues. Ghosh et al. prepared supramolecular hydrogel based on PEP-1, which is an octapeptide containing pH-responsive Aspartic acid and Leucine residues, which could host water-soluble guest molecules. These residues were responsible for the disassembly of the structure of the peptides in the acidic pH, thereby releasing the guest molecule into the vicinity [176]. Similar, hydrogels were made from peptides whose structural assembly can be modified with the change in the pH capable of forming an extracellular matrix with selective cell proliferation and cell adhesion ideal for tissue regeneration [177,178].

Another way to make supramolecular hydrogels is to use certain chemical compounds as a trigger for self-assembly. The use of specific small molecules as a trigger to drive/disrupt self-assembly is difficult because it requires strong molecular recognition to ensure efficacy and avoids nontarget effects. For example, reactive oxygen species (ROS), which are a major cause of oxidative stress and are associated with a range of diseases such as cancer and intervertebral disc degeneration, can be used as a trigger to release the drugs. Functional groups such as ferrocenyl groups when attached to the supramolecular systems can respond to the redox changes in the system [179]. Milcovich et al. fabricated ECM-inspired hybrid microspheres that are made up of collagen 1 and polypropylene sulfide (PPS), which exhibited high responsiveness to ROS, and that could be used as a platform to deliver drugs and other biomolecules [180]. The release of doxorubicin has been demonstrated by Zuo et al. from the star-shaped amphiphilic co-polymers with β-cyclodextrin and ferrocene pair which are dissociated due to the oxidation caused by ROS [181].

#### 7.1.5. Biological/Enzyme Responsive Systems

Biological responses and enzymatic reactions play a crucial part in the creation of hierarchical structures in nature. The supramolecular systems that are influenced by these biological stimuli and enzymes have gained a lot of interest in recent years due to their inherent flexibility to easily undergo structural or phase transition changes in-situ, thereby releasing the genes or drugs at the target organ [182,183].

There are many research publications citing this enzyme responsivity, one of the first one being from Vemula et al.'s group, who prepared supramolecular hydrogels with curcumin encapsulated in them. Using enzymes such as hydrolase, they demonstrated the release of curcumin from the hydrogels [184]. Unlike the former group, Yang et al. made supramolecular hydrogels from pentapeptides hydrogelator, Nap−FFGEY attached with enzymes such as kinase or phosphatase, which can induce a sol–gel transition. In the presence of the adenosine triphosphates and kinase, the gel is transitioned into sol due to the conversion of tyrosine residue into a relatively hydrophilic tyrosine phosphate. The sol–gel transition is triggered when the phosphatase enzyme is added, which counteracts the former mechanism by making it more hydrophobic [184]. Yu et al. used polymeric cyclodextrin and acrylamide or N-vinyl pyrrolidinone to form a host–guest supramolecular hydrogel. The guest molecules with two adamantane moieties form crosslinking between the hydrophobic cavities of the cyclodextrin and the β-lactam core, which could be broken down in the presence of the β-lactamases enzymes. This phenomenon degrades the hydrogel, thereby releasing drugs or biomolecules [185].

#### 7.1.6. Multi-Stimuli Systems

Most biological systems can respond to a variety of stimuli. Supramolecular hydrogels with multi-stimuli responsiveness, including pH, temperature, light, enzymes, redox potential, electric or magnetic field, or tiny molecules, have received a lot of attention. These multi-stimuli-responsive hydrogels respond to two or more stimuli in a sequential or concerted manner and can be used to control phase transition behavior. By employing precursors that are responsive to multiple stimuli and harnessing host–guest interactions to generate supramolecular hydrogels, it is possible to create multi-stimuli-responsive systems. Supramolecular dendronized copolymers were prepared by Zou et al. that could be regulated by the pH and the temperature for applications in drug delivery and tissue engineering [186].

### 7.2. *Molecular Simulations*

The design of supramolecular systems was mostly carried out by trial and error, and now the researchers have been trying to find quantitative (molecular) structure–property relationships (QSPR) that would be useful in cases such as protein-drug binding. The spatial resolution of experimental techniques is insufficient to provide information on the exact conformation of the individual building blocks. In most cases, this means that the packing of molecules can only be explained by combining a variety of experimental techniques. The fact that the nanostructures frequently are dispersed in their solvent excludes the use of common structural determination techniques such as X-ray crystallography or solution-phase NMR. Hence, a variety of techniques such as light absorption (UV/Vis, infrared (IR) and circular dichroism) and scattering (dynamic and static light scattering (DLS/SLS)), wide or small-angle X-ray scattering (WAXS/SAXS), and small-angle neutron scattering (SANS) are needed to be applied to gather small molecular conformations information to determine the intermolecular interactions. As most of these techniques are time-consuming, measuring the averages and using empirical models developed to mimic the macromolecular systems, there are high chances that the potentially important information is missed, or false interpretations are made. Using classical molecular simulations is one way to overcome these barriers. This computational method follows the movement of individual atoms or molecules over time, eliminating the need for ensemble averaging and mechanistic limitations [187].

Molecular simulations help us to create new self-assembling biomolecular systems using in silico methods and directly validate spectroscopic or scattering results by directly linking molecular simulation output with experimental observations. The molecular dynamics technique (MD) can be employed to study the supramolecular self-assembly by non-covalent interactions. All atoms (AA) are treated as interaction centers in MD and related techniques, in which force fields such as AMBER, CHARMM, OPLS, and GROMOS are applied, which can specify the configuration of the supramolecular aggregate and can be calculated by quantum mechanics. Such techniques give us information about the packing motifs, self-assembly pathways, and starter molecules.

However, all-atom models are frequently insufficient for reproducing crystal packing and melting data, inefficient pH models, extensive sampling techniques, and the requirement of large computing resources. In such situations, coarse-grain (CG) force fields, which connect groups of atoms into effective interaction centers, are employed. These force field techniques can address the large-scale self-assembly and can execute high-throughput simulations. Often, both these force fields are compared and calibrated using the regular analytical techniques such as microscopy, scattering techniques, NMR, and Electron paramagnetic resonance (EPR) spectroscopies. They are also indirectly compared for certain quantitative measurements such as the peptide secondary structure through IR spectroscopy and electronic structure through UV/Vis spectroscopy [187].

### 7.3. 3-D Printing

3D printing is a rapidly evolving manufacturing technology that has the potential to create 3D objects by depositing multiple layers of material. It was previously thought to be primarily useful for prototyping, but recent advances in this field indicate that it is now emerging as a disruptive technology capable of large-scale production scenarios. In regenerative medicine, this technique can be instrumental in providing the solution for scaffolds that can be structurally designed with specificity to location and biocompatible by employing inks made up of safe biodegradable polymers. Owing to their tunable viscosities and reversible mechanical properties, supramolecular polymers are ideal candidates for use in hybrid jetting inks.

Moroni et al., in their review, described the biofabrication strategies that can be employed to construct in vitro 3D tissue models from the mixture of biomaterials and cells. They described that the supramolecular biomaterials are ideal bioinks for to their ability to undergo shear thinning during flow due to the physical non-covalent bonds. Materials such as β-cyclodextrin in modified hyaluronic acid polymers could be broken down during extrusion and rapidly stabilized when deposited. Genetic material such as DNA also can be used in combination with polypeptides, forming a supramolecular assembly that can be easily broken down by the proteases and the nucleases. Natural biomaterials such as alginate also can act as bases onto which the complimentary peptides can be grafted, which protects the cells from external pressure during the extrusion.

Such hydrogel-forming systems are utilized to form the in vitro 3D tissue models that could also be used to check the safety and efficacy of the therapeutic agents. These models are mostly prepared as the cellular spheroids or the cell-laden hydrogel constructs that mimic the native tissues structurally and functionally. For example, to prepare a skin model, a hydrogel containing layers of melanocytes and keratinocytes could be considered. This skin model could be used to study the safety of the chemical compounds. A bioink consisting of human induced pluripotent stem cells can be utilized for making a liver model and can be used for evaluating metabolic activities [188]. In addition to the tissue models, researchers have been making 3D culture systems which are inducted biologically with the ECM components such as chitosan, alginate, collagen, gelatin, or hyaluronic acid. These models are being used for drug screening in the cases of disorders and diseases such as cancers. The stromal cells such as fibroblasts, macrophages, mesenchymal stem cells, and endothelial cells are co-cultured with the cancer cells to create the 3D models, to create a more realistic tumor environment [189]. For example, to investigate tumor-targeting drugs for neuroblastoma, an in-vitro 3D model was created by Kock et al. by co-culturing neuroblastoma and fibroblast cell spheroids [190]. Similarly, a novel scaffold-free 3D model was developed by a combination of pancreatic cells (PANC-1), endothelial cells, and fibroblasts by Lazzari et al. They managed to combine the tumor and stromal components for creating tumor spheroids for preclinical screening of drugs for pancreatic cancer [191].

Hart et al. described the use of a biodegradable poly(caprolactone) diol [$M_n$ = 2000 Da] that was added to a series of hydrogen-bonding moieties, resulting in a supramolecular polymer with good solubility. A self-supporting twisted pyramid was also printed to show that the method could be used to deposit more detailed structures. The polymers' biocompatibility was also investigated, and cytotoxicity tests revealed that they were nontoxic following ISO 10993-5 and 10993-12. Cell attachment was also investigated, and confocal microscopy confirmed that the addition of hydrogen-bonding motifs to the biocompatible poly(caprolactone) did not affect cell attachment [192]. Several factors govern the printing process; an assessment has been carried out by Sather et al. to find what factors can contribute to the printability of the liquid crystalline supramolecular polymers. They discovered that pH and salt concentration govern intermolecular interactions among self-assembled structures, with lower charge densities on supramolecular polymers and higher charge screening from the electrolyte, resulting in higher viscosity inks using a combination of experimental techniques and molecular dynamics simulations [193]. Printing of the supramolecular networks may lead to phase separation due to shear-induced in the process. Rupp et al., in their research, found that the printability of the two poly(isobutylene) [$M_n$ = 8500–16,000 Da] can be enhanced by utilizing the nanocomposite form with silica nanoparticles with no phase separation [194].

The 3D-printed biomaterials for tissue regeneration need to undergo conformational changes according to the tissue structure with time. So, there has been a trend of 4D printing, utilizing the 3D-printed materials which could respond to the external stimuli or the internal tissue environment and transform over time. Many supramolecular systems could be used to print the cell-laden constructs and can be loaded with drugs or biomolecules and can be sensitized using various stimuli such as temperature, pH, electric fields, magnetic fields, and light to release them into the tissue environment [195].

## 8. Conclusions and Future Perspectives

Supramolecular systems which rely on non-covalent interactions are preferred for their unique properties such as thermodynamically reversible nature, self-healing properties, functionalization into bioactive materials, incorporation of stimuli responsivity, and others for tissue engineering. However, the challenge lies in the lack of robust materials that can be employed.

Bio-macromolecule-based supramolecular systems have resolved many issues that pertain to biocompatibility, but they are tough to produce at a larger scale with consistent properties. Synthetically derived supramolecular systems, on the other hand, have reduced batch-to-batch variations, and offer additional tailoring opportunities such as chemical signaling, delivery modulation, and others. The reproducibility and robustness of the preparation techniques affects the carrier capacity of these delivery systems and the interference with many material, formulation and process variables throughout the manufacturing and storage remains a bottleneck for these systems.

The preparation techniques are usually complicated and involve complex procedures that could be handled only by scientists who are well versed in polymer chemistry and medicine fields. The techniques are also required to be improved to increase the yield output and the rate of the reactions. Novel techniques need to be developed which can make scaffolds from a combination of the macromolecules which provide an easy translation into the healthcare industry. The use of technologies such as 3D printing, molecular simulations, and combinations thereof can further help the process of scalability and applicability in this regenerative medicine. The improvement in the accessibility of these systems will revolutionize the regenerative medicine field.

Even though there are many systems were successful in vitro and in vivo models, the clinical translation is still challenging. The clinical studies require the safety and efficacy to be evaluated and to take the long-term toxicity studies into consideration. Most of the polymers that have been synthesized are new and would require quite a large amount of significant clinical safety data in healthy volunteers before testing their efficacy on the patients, which also remains as a big hurdle for commercializing these novel therapeutic technologies.

Moving forward, these supramolecular systems may not only be limited to tissue regeneration but also would be applied to other ailments and for personalized medicine with the combination of medical devices and nanotheranostics. With the research on supramolecular systems increasing exponentially, many more advancements are anticipated in this emerging domain.

**Author Contributions:** Writing—original draft preparation, S.R.R.; writing—review and editing, S.R.R., A.S.P., M.B. and I.T.; supervision, I.T.; project administration, I.T.; funding acquisition, I.T. All authors have read and agreed to the published version of the manuscript.

**Funding:** This work was supported by CARTHAGO-ITN. This project has received funding from the European Union's Horizon 2020 research and innovation programme under the Marie Skłodowska-Curie (H2020-MSCA-ITN) grant agreement No 955335.

**Institutional Review Board Statement:** Not applicable.

**Informed Consent Statement:** Not applicable.

**Data Availability Statement:** Not applicable.

**Acknowledgments:** Parts of Figures 1 and 2 have been created with chem-space.com [accessed on 20 May 2022] (SIAChemspace, Riga, Latvia). Figures 1–5, 7 and 8 have been created with BioRender.com [accessed on 30 June 2022] (BioRender, Toronto, ON, Canada).

**Conflicts of Interest:** The authors declare no conflict of interest.

## Abbreviations

| | |
|---|---|
| ECM | Extracellular matrix |
| HDL | High density lipoproteins |
| GML | Glyceryl monolaurate |
| DDG | 1-O-dodecyl- rac -glycerol |
| BMP-2 | Bone morphogenetic protein 2 |
| Apo A1 | Apolipoprotein A1 |
| LXR | Liver X receptor |
| Fmoc | Fluorenyl methoxycarbonyl |
| A | Adenine |
| G | Guanine |
| U | Uracil |
| T | Thymine |
| C | Cytosine |
| PEG | Polyethylene glycol |
| ChS-F | Furfuryl amine grafted chondroitin sulfate |
| PAMAM | Polyamidoamine |
| HA | Hyaluronic acid |
| RGD | Arginyl glycyl aspartic acid |
| MSC | Mesenchymal stem cells |
| CD | Cyclodextrins |
| TGF-β1 | Transforming growth factor beta 1 |
| CB[n] | Cucurbit(n)urils |
| DNA | Deoxyribonucleic acid |
| RNA | Ribonucleic Acid |
| PLLA | poly-L-lactic acid |

| | |
|---|---|
| PCL | polycaprolactone |
| PLA | polylactic acid |
| PEO | polyethylene oxide |
| BCP | Block co-polymers |
| CMC | Critical micellar concentration |
| UV | Ultraviolet |
| NOE | Nuclear Over Hauser effect |
| DOSY | Diffusion-ordered NMR spectroscopy |
| NOESY | Nuclear Over Hauser effect spectroscopy |
| ROESY | Rotating frame nuclear Over Hauser effect spectroscopy |
| DLS | Dynamic light scattering |
| DSC | Differential scanning calorimetry |
| SEM | Scanning electron microscopy |
| TEM | Transmission electron microscopy |
| AFM | Atomic force microscope |
| HGF | hepatocyte growth factor |
| IGF-1 | Insulin-like growth factor -1 |
| TEC | tubular epithelial cells |
| PDGF | platelet-derived growth factor |
| EGF | epidermal growth factor |
| DOPA | 3,4-dihydroxyphenylalanine |
| ROS | Reactive oxygen species |
| MD | molecular dynamics |
| AMBER | Assisted Model Building with Energy Refinement |
| CHARMM | Chemistry at Harvard Macromolecular Mechanics |
| OPLS | optimized potentials for liquid simulations |
| GROMOS | Groningen Molecular Simulations |

## References


1. Mason, C.; Dunnill, P. A Brief Definition of Regenerative Medicine. *Regen. Med.* **2007**, *3*, 1–5. [CrossRef] [PubMed]
2. Qiu, T.; Hanna, E.; Dabbous, M.; Borislav, B.; Toumi, M. Regenerative Medicine Regulatory Policies: A Systematic Review and International Comparison. *Health Policy* **2020**, *124*, 701–713. [CrossRef] [PubMed]
3. Dimmeler, S.; Ding, S.; Rando, T.A.; Trounson, A. Translational Strategies and Challenges in Regenerative Medicine. *Nat. Publ. Group* **2014**, *20*, 814–821. [CrossRef]
4. Yue, B. Biology of the Extracellular Matrix: An Overview. *J. Glaucoma* **2014**, *23*, S20. [CrossRef] [PubMed]
5. Hussey, G.S.; Dziki, J.L.; Badylak, S.F. Extracellular Matrix-Based Materials for Regenerative Medicine. *Nat. Rev. Mater.* **2018**, *3*, 159–173. [CrossRef]
6. Feng, Z.; Zhang, T.; Wang, H.; Xu, B. Supramolecular Catalysis and Dynamic Assemblies for Medicine. *Chem. Soc. Rev.* **2017**, *46*, 6470–6479. [CrossRef] [PubMed]
7. Lehn, J. Supramolecular Chemistry: Where from? Where to? *Chem. Soc. Rev.* **2017**, *46*, 2378–2379. [CrossRef] [PubMed]
8. Zhou, J.; Li, J.; Du, X.; Xu, B. Supramolecular Biofunctional Materials. *Biomaterials* **2017**, *129*, 1–27. [CrossRef]
9. Thomas, D.; Gaspar, D.; Sorushanova, A.; Milcovich, G.; Spanoudes, K.; Mullen, A.M.; O'Brien, T.; Pandit, A.; Zeugolis, D.I. Scaffold and Scaffold-Free Self-Assembled Systems in Regenerative Medicine. *Biotechnol. Bioeng.* **2016**, *113*, 1155–1163. [CrossRef]
10. Milcovich, G.; Lettieri, S.; Antunes, F.E.; Medronho, B.; Fonseca, A.C.; Coelho, J.F.J.; Marizza, P.; Perrone, F.; Farra, R.; Dapas, B.; et al. Recent Advances in Smart Biotechnology: Hydrogels and Nanocarriers for Tailored Bioactive Molecules Depot. *Adv. Colloid Interface Sci.* **2017**, *249*, 163–180. [CrossRef]
11. Webber, M.J.; Appel, E.A.; Meijer, E.W.; Langer, R. Supramolecular Biomaterials. *Nat. Mater.* **2015**, *15*, 13–26. [CrossRef]
12. Henrich, S.E.; Hong, B.J.; Rink, J.S.; Nguyen, S.T.; Thaxton, C.S. Supramolecular Assembly of High-Density Lipoprotein Mimetic Nanoparticles Using Lipid-Conjugated Core Scaffolds. *J. Am. Chem. Soc.* **2019**, *141*, 9753–9757. [CrossRef]
13. Yoon, B.K.; Kim, M.C.; Jackman, J.A.; Cho, N.J. Dynamic Remodeling of Giant Unilamellar Vesicles Induced by Monoglyceride Nano-Micelles: Insights into Supramolecular Organization. *Appl. Mater. Today* **2021**, *24*, 101099. [CrossRef]
14. Monteiro, N.; Martins, A.; Reis, R.L.; Neves, N.M. Liposomes in Tissue Engineering and Regenerative Medicine. *J. R. Soc. Interface* **2014**, *11*, 20140459. [CrossRef]
15. Castelletto, V.; Kaur, A.; Kowalczyk, R.M.; Hamley, I.W.; Reza, M.; Ruokolainen, J. Supramolecular Hydrogel Formation in a Series of Self-Assembling Lipopeptides with Varying Lipid Chain Length. *Biomacromolecules* **2017**, *18*, 2013–2023. [CrossRef]
16. Yaddehige, M.L.; Chandrasiri, I.; Barker, A.; Kotha, A.K.; Williams, J.S.D.; Simms, B.; Kucheryavy, P.; Abebe, D.G.; Chougule, M.B.; Watkins, D.L. Structural and Surface Properties of Polyamidoamine (PAMAM)—Fatty Acid-Based Nanoaggregates Derived from Self-Assembling Janus Dendrimers. *Chem. Nano. Mat.* **2020**, *6*, 1833–1842. [CrossRef]

17. Dan, N.; Dan, N. Lipid-Nucleic Acid Supramolecular Complexes: Lipoplex Structure and the Kinetics of Formation. *AIMS Biophysics* **2015**, *2*, 163–183. [CrossRef]
18. Hu, K.; Xiang, L.; Chen, J.; Qu, H.; Wan, Y.; Xiang, D. PLGA-Liposome Electrospun Fiber Delivery of MiR-145 and PDGF-BB Synergistically Promoted Wound Healing. *Chem. Eng. J.* **2021**, *422*, 129951. [CrossRef]
19. Lee, C.S.; Hsu, G.C.Y.; Sono, T.; Lee, M.; James, A.W. Development of a Biomaterial Scaffold Integrated with Osteoinductive Oxysterol Liposomes to Enhance Hedgehog Signaling and Bone Repair. *Mol. Pharm.* **2021**, *18*, 1677–1689. [CrossRef]
20. Mohammadi, M.; Alibolandi, M.; Abnous, K.; Salmasi, Z.; Jaafari, M.R.; Ramezani, M. Fabrication of Hybrid Scaffold Based on Hydroxyapatite-Biodegradable Nanofibers Incorporated with Liposomal Formulation of BMP-2 Peptide for Bone Tissue Engineering. *Nanomed. Nanotechnol. Biol. Med.* **2018**, *14*, 1987–1997. [CrossRef]
21. Craik, D.J.; Fairlie, D.P.; Liras, S.; Price, D. The Future of Peptide-Based Drugs. *Chem. Biol. Drug Des.* **2013**, *81*, 136–147. [CrossRef] [PubMed]
22. Qiu, F.; Chen, Y.; Tang, C.; Zhao, X. Amphiphilic Peptides as Novel Nanomaterials: Design, Self-Assembly and Application. *Int. J. Nanomed.* **2018**, *13*, 5003–5022. [CrossRef]
23. Arslan, E.; Garip, I.C.; Gulseren, G.; Tekinay, A.B.; Guler, M.O. Bioactive Supramolecular Peptide Nanofibers for Regenerative Medicine. *Adv. Healthc. Mater.* **2014**, *3*, 1357–1376. [CrossRef] [PubMed]
24. Hendricks, M.P.; Sato, K.; Palmer, L.C.; Stupp, S.I. Supramolecular Assembly of Peptide Amphiphiles. *Acc. Chem. Res.* **2017**, *50*, 2440–2448. [CrossRef] [PubMed]
25. Mansukhani, N.A.; Peters, E.B.; So, M.M.; Albaghdadi, M.S.; Wang, Z.; Karver, M.R.; Clemons, T.D.; Laux, J.P.; Tsihlis, N.D.; Stupp, S.I.; et al. Peptide Amphiphile Supramolecular Nanostructures as a Targeted Therapy for Atherosclerosis. *Macromol. Biosci.* **2019**, *19*, 1900066. [CrossRef] [PubMed]
26. Li, Y.; Lai, Y.; Xu, X.; Zhang, X.; Wu, Y.; Hu, C.; Gu, Z. Capsid-like Supramolecular Dendritic Systems as PH-Responsive Nanocarriers for Drug Penetration and Site-Specific Delivery. *Nanomed. Nanotechnol. Biol. Med.* **2016**, *12*, 355–364. [CrossRef] [PubMed]
27. Rubert Pérez, C.M.; Stephanopoulos, N.; Sur, S.; Lee, S.S.; Newcomb, C.; Stupp, S.I. The Powerful Functions of Peptide-Based Bioactive Matrices for Regenerative Medicine. *Ann. Biomed. Eng.* **2014**, *43*, 501–514. [CrossRef]
28. Acar, H.; Srivastava, S.; Chung, E.J.; Schnorenberg, M.R.; Barrett, J.C.; LaBelle, J.L.; Tirrell, M. Self-Assembling Peptide-Based Building Blocks in Medical Applications. *Adv. Drug Deliv. Rev.* **2017**, *110–111*, 65–79. [CrossRef]
29. Siddiqui, Z.; Sarkar, B.; Kim, K.K.; Kumar, A.; Paul, R.; Mahajan, A.; Grasman, J.M.; Yang, J.; Kumar, V.A. Self-Assembling Peptide Hydrogels Facilitate Vascularization in Two-Component Scaffolds. *Chem. Eng. J.* **2021**, *422*, 130145. [CrossRef]
30. Zhang, Z.; Ai, S.; Yang, Z.; Li, X. Peptide-Based Supramolecular Hydrogels for Local Drug Delivery. *Adv. Drug Deliv. Rev.* **2021**, *174*, 482–503. [CrossRef]
31. Abraham, B.L.; Liyanage, W.; Nilsson, B.L. Strategy to Identify Improved N-Terminal Modifications for Supramolecular Phenylalanine-Derived Hydrogelators. *Langmuir* **2019**, *35*, 14939–14948. [CrossRef]
32. Zhang, L.; Zhang, Y.M.; Liu, G.; Liu, Y. Redox-Responsive Diphenylalanine Aggregate Mediated by Cyclodextrin. *Chin. Chem. Lett.* **2019**, *30*, 120–122. [CrossRef]
33. Peters, G.M.; Davis, J.T. Supramolecular Gels Made from Nucleobase, Nucleoside and Nucleotide Analogs. *Chem. Soc. Rev.* **2016**, *45*, 3188–3206. [CrossRef]
34. Zhao, H.; Schäfer, A.H.; Seela, F. Supramolecular Isoguanosine Assemblies Form Hydrogels with Excellent Long-Term Stability. *Chempluschem* **2017**, *82*, 826–833. [CrossRef]
35. Zhao, H.; Feng, H.; Liu, J.; Tang, F.; Du, Y.; Ji, N.; Xie, L.; Zhao, X.; Wang, Z.; Chen, Q. Dual-Functional Guanosine-Based Hydrogel Integrating Localized Delivery and Anticancer Activities for Cancer Therapy. *Biomaterials* **2020**, *230*, 119598. [CrossRef]
36. Chai, Y.; Zhou, X.; Li, C.; Ma, B.; Shen, Z.; Huang, R.; Chen, H.; Chen, B.; Li, W.; He, Y. Supermacrocyclic Assemblies by Hydrogen-Bond Codes of C7-Phenol Pyrazolo and Pyrrolo Derivatives of Adenine. *Chem. A Eur. J.* **2018**, *24*, 15495–15501. [CrossRef]
37. Cheng, C.-C.; Yang, X.-J.; Fan, W.-L.; Lee, A.-W.; Lai, J.-Y. Cytosine-Functionalized Supramolecular Polymer-Mediated Cellular Behavior and Wound Healing. *Biomacromolecules* **2020**, *21*, 3857–3866. [CrossRef]
38. Malik, S.; Sundarrajan, S.; Hussain, T.; Nazir, A.; Ramakrishna, S. Role of Block Copolymers in Tissue Engineering Applications. *Cells Tissues Organs* **2021**, *211*, 1–14. [CrossRef]
39. Rey-Rico, A.; Cucchiarini, M. PEO-PPO-PEO Tri-Block Copolymers for Gene Delivery Applications in Human Regenerative Medicine—An Overview. *Int. J. Mol. Sci.* **2018**, *19*, 775. [CrossRef]
40. Le Fer, G.; Dilla, R.A.; Wang, Z.; King, J.; Chuang, S.S.C.; Becker, M.L. Clustering and Hierarchical Organization of 3D Printed Poly(Propylene Fumarate)-Block-PEG-Block-Poly(Propylene Fumarate) ABA Triblock Copolymer Hydrogels. *Macromolecules* **2021**, *54*, 3458–3468. [CrossRef]
41. Lee, B.K.; Noh, J.H.; Park, J.H.; Park, S.H.; Kim, J.H.; Oh, S.H.; Kim, M.S. Thermoresponsive and Biodegradable Amphiphilic Block Copolymers with Pendant Functional Groups. *Tissue Eng. Regen. Med.* **2018**, *15*, 393–402. [CrossRef] [PubMed]
42. Yang, G.; Wang, J.; Li, D.; Zhou, S. Polyanhydride Micelles with Diverse Morphologies for Shape-Regulated Cellular Internalization and Blood Circulation. *Regen. Biomater.* **2017**, *4*, 149–157. [CrossRef] [PubMed]
43. Oliveira, J.M.; Salgado, A.J.; Sousa, N.; Mano, J.F.; Reis, R.L. Dendrimers and Derivatives as a Potential Therapeutic Tool in Regenerative Medicine Strategies—A Review. *Prog. Polym. Sci.* **2010**, *35*, 1163–1194. [CrossRef]

44. Lyu, Z.; Ding, L.; Tintaru, A.; Peng, L. Self-Assembling Supramolecular Dendrimers for Biomedical Applications: Lessons Learned from Poly(Amidoamine) Dendrimers. *Acc. Chem. Res.* **2020**, *53*, 2936–2949. [CrossRef]
45. Bai, X.; Lü, S.; Cao, Z.; Gao, C.; Duan, H.; Xu, X.; Sun, L.; Gao, N.; Feng, C.; Liu, M. Self-Reinforcing Injectable Hydrogel with Both High Water Content and Mechanical Strength for Bone Repair. *Chem. Eng. J.* **2016**, *288*, 546–556. [CrossRef]
46. Salgado, A.J.; Oliveira, J.M.; Pirraco, R.P.; Pereira, V.H.; Fraga, J.S.; Marques, A.P.; Neves, N.M.; Mano, J.F.; Reis, R.L.; Sousa, N. Carboxymethylchitosan/Poly(Amidoamine) Dendrimer Nanoparticles in Central Nervous Systems-Regenerative Medicine: Effects on Neuron/Glial Cell Viability and Internalization Efficiency. *Macromol. Biosci.* **2010**, *10*, 1130–1140. [CrossRef]
47. Bi, X.; Luckanagul, J.A.; Allen, A.; Ramaboli, M.; Campbell, E.; West, D.; Maturavongsadit, P.; Brummett, K.; Wang, Q. Synthesis of PAMAM Dendrimer-Based Fast Cross-Linking Hydrogel for Biofabrication. *J. Biomater. Sci. Polym. Ed.* **2015**, *26*, 669–682. [CrossRef]
48. Zhu, K.; Li, J.; Lai, H.; Yang, C.; Guo, C.; Wang, C. Reprogramming Fibroblasts to Pluripotency Using Arginine-Terminated Polyamidoamine Nanoparticles Based Non-Viral Gene Delivery System. *Int. J. Nanomed.* **2014**, *9*, 5837–5847. [CrossRef]
49. Santos, J.L.; Oliveira, H.; Pandita, D.; Rodrigues, J.; Pêgo, A.P.; Granja, P.L.; Tomás, H. Functionalization of Poly(Amidoamine) Dendrimers with Hydrophobic Chains for Improved Gene Delivery in Mesenchymal Stem Cells. *J. Control. Release* **2010**, *144*, 55–64. [CrossRef]
50. Sousa, C.F.v.; Fernandez-Megia, E.; Borges, J.; Mano, J.F. Supramolecular Dendrimer-Containing Layer-by-Layer Nanoassemblies for Bioapplications: Current Status and Future Prospects. *Polym. Chem.* **2021**, *12*, 5902–5930. [CrossRef]
51. Gangemi, C.M.A.; Puglisi, R.; Pappalardo, A.; Trusso Sfrazzetto, G. Supramolecular Complexes for Nanomedicine. *Bioorganic Med. Chem. Lett.* **2018**, *28*, 3290–3301. [CrossRef]
52. Alvarez-Lorenzo, C.; García-González, C.A.; Concheiro, A. Cyclodextrins as Versatile Building Blocks for Regenerative Medicine. *J. Control. Release* **2017**, *268*, 269–281. [CrossRef]
53. Zhao, W.; Li, Y.; Zhang, X.; Zhang, R.; Hu, Y.; Boyer, C.; Xu, F.J. Photo-Responsive Supramolecular Hyaluronic Acid Hydrogels for Accelerated Wound Healing. *J. Control. Release* **2020**, *323*, 24–35. [CrossRef]
54. Zhang, B.; Yu, Q.; Liu, Y. Polarization of Stem Cells Directed by Magnetic Field-Manipulated Supramolecular Polymeric Nanofibers. *ACS Appl. Mater. Interfaces* **2021**, *13*, 9580–9588. [CrossRef]
55. Milcovich, G.; Antunes, F.E.; Grassi, M.; Asaro, F. Stabilization of Unilamellar Catanionic Vesicles Induced by β-Cyclodextrins: A Strategy for a Tunable Drug Delivery Depot. *Int. J. Pharm.* **2018**, *548*, 474–479. [CrossRef]
56. Ren, P.; Wang, F.; Bernaerts, K.v.; Fu, Y.; Hu, W.; Zhou, N.; Dai, J.; Liang, M.; Zhang, T. Self-Assembled Supramolecular Hybrid Hydrogels Based on Host–Guest Interaction: Formation and Application in 3D Cell Culture. *ACS Appl. Bio Mater.* **2020**, *3*, 6768–6778. [CrossRef]
57. Wei, K.; Zhu, M.; Sun, Y.; Xu, J.; Feng, Q.; Lin, S.; Wu, T.; Xu, J.; Tian, F.; Xia, J.; et al. Robust Biopolymeric Supramolecular "Host−Guest Macromer" Hydrogels Reinforced by in Situ Formed Multivalent Nanoclusters for Cartilage Regeneration. *Macromolecules* **2016**, *49*, 866–875. [CrossRef]
58. Zhang, Y.; Jiang, Q.; Wojnilowicz, M.; Pan, S.; Ju, Y.; Zhang, W.; Liu, J.; Zhuo, R.; Jiang, X. Acid-Sensitive Poly(β-Cyclodextrin)-Based Multifunctional Supramolecular Gene Vector. *Polym. Chem.* **2018**, *9*, 450–462. [CrossRef]
59. Choi, J.H.; Park, A.; Lee, W.; Youn, J.; Rim, M.A.; Kim, W.; Kim, N.; Song, J.E.; Khang, G. Preparation and Characterization of an Injectable Dexamethasone-Cyclodextrin Complexes-Loaded Gellan Gum Hydrogel for Cartilage Tissue Engineering. *J. Control. Release* **2020**, *327*, 747–765. [CrossRef]
60. Shah, A.A.; Shah, A.; Lewis, S.; Ghate, V.; Saklani, R.; Narayana Kalkura, S.; Baby, C.; Singh, P.K.; Nayak, Y.; Chourasia, M.K. Cyclodextrin Based Bone Regenerative Inclusion Complex for Resveratrol in Postmenopausal Osteoporosis. *Eur. J. Pharm. Biopharm.* **2021**, *167*, 127–139. [CrossRef]
61. Terauchi, M.; Inada, T.; Tonegawa, A.; Tamura, A.; Yamaguchi, S.; Harada, K.; Yui, N. Supramolecular Inclusion Complexation of Simvastatin with Methylated β-Cyclodextrins for Promoting Osteogenic Differentiation. *Int. J. Biol. Macromol.* **2016**, *93*, 1492–1498. [CrossRef] [PubMed]
62. Das, D.; Assaf, K.I.; Nau, W.M. Applications of Cucurbiturils in Medicinal Chemistry and Chemical Biology. *Front. Chem.* **2019**, *7*, 619. [CrossRef]
63. Pan, Y.-C.; Hu, X.-Y.; Guo, D.-S. Biomedical Applications of Calixarenes: State of the Art and Perspectives. *Angew. Chem. Int. Ed.* **2021**, *60*, 2768–2794. [CrossRef]
64. Lin, K.; Zhang, D.; Macedo, M.H.; Cui, W.; Sarmento, B.; Shen, G. Advanced Collagen-Based Biomaterials for Regenerative Biomedicine. *Adv. Funct. Mater.* **2019**, *29*, 1804943. [CrossRef]
65. Pan, P.; Chen, X.; Metavarayuth, K.; Su, J.; Wang, Q. Self-Assembled Supramolecular Systems for Bone Engineering Applications. *Curr. Opin. Colloid Interface Sci.* **2018**, *35*, 104–111. [CrossRef]
66. Zheng, L.; Jiang, X.; Chen, X.; Fan, H.; Zhang, X. Evaluation of Novel in Situ Synthesized Nano-Hydroxyapatite/Collagen/Alginate Hydrogels for Osteochondral Tissue Engineering. *Biomed. Mater.* **2014**, *9*, 065004. [CrossRef]
67. Kaczmarek-Pawelska, A. Alginate-Based Hydrogels in Regenerative Medicine. In *Alginates Recent Uses of This Natural Polymer*; IntechOpen: London, UK, 2019.
68. Tarsitano, M.; Cristiano, M.C.; Fresta, M.; Paolino, D.; Rafaniello, C. Alginate-Based Composites for Corneal Regeneration: The Optimization of a Biomaterial to Overcome Its Limits. *Gels* **2022**, *8*, 431. [CrossRef]

69. Zhai, Z.; Xu, K.; Mei, L.; Wu, C.; Liu, J.; Liu, Z.; Wan, L.; Zhong, W. Co-Assembled Supramolecular Hydrogels of Cell Adhesive Peptide and Alginate for Rapid Hemostasis and Efficacious Wound Healing. *Soft Matter.* **2019**, *15*, 8603–8610. [CrossRef]
70. Piras, C.C.; Mahon, C.S.; Genever, P.G.; Smith, D.K. Shaping and Patterning Supramolecular Materials Stem Cell-Compatible Dual-Network Hybrid Gels Loaded with Silver Nanoparticles. *ACS Biomater. Sci. Eng.* **2021**, *8*, 1829–1840. [CrossRef]
71. Zohreband, Z.; Adeli, M.; Zebardasti, A. Self-Healable and Flexible Supramolecular Gelatin/MoS2 Hydrogels with Molecular Recognition Properties. *Int. J. Biol. Macromol.* **2021**, *182*, 2048–2055. [CrossRef]
72. Madl, A.C.; Madl, C.M.; Myung, D. Injectable Cucurbit [8]Uril-Based Supramolecular Gelatin Hydrogels for Cell Encapsulation. *ACS Macro Lett.* **2020**, *9*, 619–626. [CrossRef] [PubMed]
73. Mihajlovic, M.; Fermin, L.; Ito, K.; van Nostrum, C.F.; Vermonden, T. Hyaluronic Acid-Based Supramolecular Hydrogels for Biomedical Applications. *Multifunct. Mater.* **2021**, *4*, 032001. [CrossRef]
74. Jung, H.; Park, J.S.; Yeom, J.; Selvapalam, N.; Park, K.M.; Oh, K.; Yang, J.A.; Park, K.H.; Hahn, S.K.; Kim, K. 3D Tissue Engineered Supramolecular Hydrogels for Controlled Chondrogenesis of Human Mesenchymal Stem Cells. *Biomacromolecules* **2014**, *15*, 707–714. [CrossRef] [PubMed]
75. Fernandes-Cunha, G.M.; Jeong, S.H.; Logan, C.M.; Le, P.; Mundy, D.; Chen, F.; Chen, K.M.; Kim, M.; Lee, G.H.; Na, K.S.; et al. Supramolecular Host-Guest Hyaluronic Acid Hydrogels Enhance Corneal Wound Healing through Dynamic Spatiotemporal Effects. *Ocul. Surf.* **2022**, *23*, 148–161. [CrossRef]
76. Braun, G.A.; Ary, B.E.; Dear, A.J.; Rohn, M.C.H.; Payson, A.M.; Lee, D.S.M.; Parry, R.C.; Friedman, C.; Knowles, T.P.J.; Linse, S.; et al. On the Mechanism of Self-Assembly by a Hydrogel-Forming Peptide. *Biomacromolecules* **2020**, *21*, 4781–4794. [CrossRef]
77. Bhattacharyya, T.; Saha, P.; Dash, J. Guanosine-Derived Supramolecular Hydrogels: Recent Developments and Future Opportunities. *ACS Omega* **2018**, *3*, 2230–2241. [CrossRef]
78. Ding, T.; Tang, F.; Ni, G.; Liu, J.; Zhao, H.; Chen, Q. The Development of Isoguanosine: From Discovery, Synthesis, and Modification to Supramolecular Structures and Potential Applications. *RSC Adv.* **2020**, *10*, 6223–6248. [CrossRef]
79. Ikeda, M. Stimuli-Responsive Supramolecular Systems Guided by Chemical Reactions. *Polym. J.* **2018**, *51*, 371–380. [CrossRef]
80. Zhou, Y.; Yan, D. Supramolecular Self-Assembly of Amphiphilic Hyperbranched Polymers at All Scales and Dimensions: Progress, Characteristics and Perspectives. *Chem. Commun.* **2009**, *10*, 1172–1188. [CrossRef]
81. Jin, H.; Huang, W.; Zhu, X.; Zhou, Y.; Yan, D. Biocompatible or Biodegradable Hyperbranched Polymers: From Self-Assembly to Cytomimetic Applications. *Chem. Soc. Rev.* **2012**, *41*, 5986–5997. [CrossRef]
82. Bodratti, A.M.; Alexandridis, P. Amphiphilic Block Copolymers in Drug Delivery: Advances in Formulation Structure and Performance. *Expert Opin. Drug Deliv.* **2018**, *15*, 1085–1104. [CrossRef]
83. Wang, C.; Wang, Z.; Zhang, X. Amphiphilic Building Blocks for Self-Assembly: From Amphiphiles to Supra-Amphiphiles. *Acc. Chem. Res.* **2012**, *45*, 608–618. [CrossRef]
84. Li, Z.; Lin, Z. Self-Assembly of Block Copolymers for Biological Applications. *Polym. Int.* **2022**, *71*, 366–370. [CrossRef]
85. Dong, Y.; Chen, Y.; Zhu, D.; Shi, K.; Ma, C.; Zhang, W.; Rocchi, P.; Jiang, L.; Liu, X. Self-Assembly of Amphiphilic Phospholipid Peptide Dendrimer-Based Nanovectors for Effective Delivery of SiRNA Therapeutics in Prostate Cancer Therapy. *J. Control. Release* **2020**, *322*, 416–425. [CrossRef]
86. Saunders, L.; Ma, P.X. Self-Healing Supramolecular Hydrogels for Tissue Engineering Applications. *Macromol. Biosci.* **2019**, *19*, 1800313. [CrossRef]
87. Dodero, A.; Alberti, S.; Gaggero, G.; Ferretti, M.; Botter, R.; Vicini, S.; Castellano, M. An Up-to-Date Review on Alginate Nanoparticles and Nanofibers for Biomedical and Pharmaceutical Applications. *Adv. Mater. Interfaces* **2021**, *8*, 2100809. [CrossRef]
88. Nii, T. Strategies Using Gelatin Microparticles for Regenerative Therapy and Drug Screening Applications. *Molecules* **2021**, *26*, 6795. [CrossRef]
89. Mohandoss, S.; Palanisamy, S.; You, S.G.; Shim, J.J.; Lee, Y.R. Supramolecular Nanogels Based on Gelatin–Cyclodextrin-Stabilized Silver Nanocomposites with Antibacterial and Anticancer Properties. *J. Biomater. Sci. Polym. Ed.* **2022**, *33*, 689–704. [CrossRef]
90. Löwenberg, C.; Tripodo, G.; Julich-Gruner, K.K.; Neffe, A.T.; Lendlein, A.; Löwenberg, C.; Tripodo, G.; Julich-Gruner, K.K.; Neffe, A.T.; Lendlein, A. Supramolecular Gelatin Networks Based on Inclusion Complexes. *Macromol. Biosci.* **2020**, *20*, 2000221. [CrossRef]
91. Feng, Q.; Wei, K.; Lin, S.; Xu, Z.; Sun, Y.; Shi, P.; Li, G.; Bian, L. Mechanically Resilient, Injectable, and Bioadhesive Supramolecular Gelatin Hydrogels Crosslinked by Weak Host-Guest Interactions Assist Cell Infiltration and in Situ Tissue Regeneration. *Biomaterials* **2016**, *101*, 217–228. [CrossRef]
92. Akbarzadeh, A.; Rezaei-Sadabady, R.; Davaran, S.; Joo, S.W.; Zarghami, N.; Hanifehpour, Y.; Samiei, M.; Kouhi, M.; Nejati-Koshki, K. Liposome: Classification, Preparation, and Applications. *Nanoscale Res. Lett.* **2013**, *8*, 102. [CrossRef] [PubMed]
93. Has, C.; Sunthar, P. A Comprehensive Review on Recent Preparation Techniques of Liposomes. *J. Liposome Res.* **2019**, *30*, 336–365. [CrossRef] [PubMed]
94. Porfire, A.; Achim, M.; Barbalata, C.; Rus, I.; Tomuta, I.; Cristea, C. Pharmaceutical Development of Liposomes Using the QbD Approach. In *Liposomes—Advances and Perspectives*; IntechOpen: London, UK, 2019.
95. Yıldız, A.; Kara, A.A.; Acartürk, F. Peptide-Protein Based Nanofibers in Pharmaceutical and Biomedical Applications. *Int. J. Biol. Macromol.* **2020**, *148*, 1084–1097. [CrossRef]

96. Chen, S.; Li, R.; Li, X.; Xie, J. Electrospinning: An Enabling Nanotechnology Platform for Drug Delivery and Regenerativ Medicine. *Adv. Drug Deliv. Rev.* **2018**, *132*, 188–213. [CrossRef] [PubMed]
97. Zhang, J.; Liu, K.; Müllen, K.; Yin, M. Self-Assemblies of Amphiphilic Homopolymers: Synthesis, Morphology Studies anc Biomedical Applications. *Chem. Commun.* **2015**, *51*, 11541–11555. [CrossRef] [PubMed]
98. Avsar, S.Y.; Kyropoulou, M.; Leone, S.d.; Schoenenberger, C.A.; Meier, W.P.; Palivan, C.G. Biomolecules Turn Self-Assemblin Amphiphilic Block Co-Polymer Platforms into Biomimetic Interfaces. *Front. Chem.* **2019**, *7*, 645. [CrossRef] [PubMed]
99. Xiong, X.B.; Binkhathlan, Z.; Molavi, O.; Lavasanifar, A. Amphiphilic Block Co-Polymers: Preparation and Application ir Nanodrug and Gene Delivery. *Acta Biomater.* **2012**, *8*, 2017–2033. [CrossRef]
100. Chen, C.; Posocco, P.; Liu, X.; Cheng, Q.; Laurini, E.; Zhou, J.; Liu, C.; Wang, Y.; Tang, J.; Col, V.D.; et al. Mastering Dendrimer Sel Assembly for Efficient SiRNA Delivery: From Conceptual Design to In Vivo Efficient Gene Silencing. *Small* **2016**, *12*, 3667–367 [CrossRef]
101. Cid-Samamed, A.; Rakmai, J.; Mejuto, J.C.; Simal-Gandara, J.; Astray, G. Cyclodextrins Inclusion Complex: Preparation Methods Analytical Techniques and Food Industry Applications. *Food Chem.* **2022**, *384*, 132467. [CrossRef]
102. Verza, B.S.; van den Beucken, J.J.J.P.; Brandt, J.v.; Jafelicci Junior, M.; Barão, V.A.R.; Piazza, R.D.; Tagit, O.; Spolidorio, D.M.P Vergani, C.E.; de Avila, E.D. A Long-Term Controlled Drug-Delivery with Anionic Beta Cyclodextrin Complex in Layer-by-Layer Coating for Percutaneous Implants Devices. *Carbohydr. Polym.* **2021**, *257*, 117604. [CrossRef]
103. Khushbu; Jindal, R. Thermal Stability and Optimization of Graphene Oxide Incorporated Chitosan and Sodium Alginate Based Nanocomposite Containing Inclusion Complexes of Paracetamol and β-Cyclodextrin for Prolonged Drug Delivery Systems *Polym. Bull.* **2022**, 1–22. [CrossRef]
104. Jolly, R.; Furkan, M.; Khan, A.A.; Ahmed, S.S.; Alam, S.; Farooqi, M.A.; Khan, R.H.; Shakir, M. Synthesis and Characterization of β-Cyclodextrin/Carboxymethyl Chitosan/Hydroxyapatite Fused with Date Seed Extract Nanocomposite Scaffolds for Regenerative Bone Tissue Engineering. *Mater. Adv.* **2021**, *2*, 5723–5736. [CrossRef]
105. Chen, X.; Taguchi, T. Bonding a Titanium Plate and Soft Tissue Interface by Using an Adhesive Bone Paste Composed of α-Tricalcium Phosphate and α-Cyclodextrin/Nonanyl Group-Modified Poly(Vinyl Alcohol) Inclusion Complex. *Colloids Surf. B Biointerfaces* **2021**, *203*, 111757. [CrossRef]
106. Riela, S.; Lazzara, G.; lo Meo, P.; Guernelli, S.; D'Anna, F.; Milioto, S.; Noto, R. Microwave-Assisted Synthesis of Novel Cyclodextrin–Cucurbituril Complexes. *Supramol. Chem.* **2012**, *23*, 819–828. [CrossRef]
107. Das, S.; Mohanty, S.; Maharana, J.; Jena, S.R.; Nayak, J.; Subuddhi, U. Microwave-Assisted β-Cyclodextrin/Chrysin Inclusion Complexation: An Economical and Green Strategy for Enhanced Hemocompatibility and Chemosensitivity in Vitro. *J. Mol. Liq.* **2020**, *310*, 113257. [CrossRef]
108. Liu, Y.; Wang, Z.; Zhang, X. Characterization of Supramolecular Polymers. *Chem. Soc. Rev.* **2012**, *41*, 5922–5932. [CrossRef]
109. Janmey, P.A.; Schliwa, M. Rheology. *Curr. Biol.* **2008**, *18*, R639. [CrossRef]
110. Dawn, A.; Kumari, H. Low Molecular Weight Supramolecular Gels Under Shear: Rheology as the Tool for Elucidating Structure–Function Correlation. *Chem. A Eur. J.* **2018**, *24*, 762–776. [CrossRef]
111. Sun, Y.; Li, X.; Zhao, M.; Chen, Y.; Xu, Y.; Wang, K.; Bian, S.; Jiang, Q.; Fan, Y.; Zhang, X. Bioinspired Supramolecular Nanofiber Hydrogel through Self-Assembly of Biphenyl-Tripeptide for Tissue Engineering. *Bioact. Mater.* **2022**, *8*, 396–408. [CrossRef]
112. Khalily, M.A.; Usta, H.; Ozdemir, M.; Bakan, G.; Dikecoglu, F.B.; Edwards-Gayle, C.; Hutchinson, J.A.; Hamley, I.W.; Dana, A.; Guler, M.O. The Design and Fabrication of Supramolecular Semiconductor Nanowires Formed by Benzothienobenzothiophene (BTBT)-Conjugated Peptides. *Nanoscale* **2018**, *10*, 9987–9995. [CrossRef]
113. Tabet, A.; Sokolowski, K.; Shilts, J.; Kamp, M.; Warner, N.; Hoogland, D.; Scherman, O.A. Supramolecular Protein-Mediated Assembly of Brain Extracellular Matrix Glycans. *F1000Res* **2018**, *7*, 1827. [CrossRef] [PubMed]
114. Pal, V.K.; Jain, R.; Roy, S. Tuning the Supramolecular Structure and Function of Collagen Mimetic Ionic Complementary Peptides via Electrostatic Interactions. *Langmuir* **2020**, *36*, 1003–1013. [CrossRef] [PubMed]
115. Radvar, E.; Shi, Y.; Grasso, S.; Edwards-Gayle, C.J.C.; Liu, X.; Mauter, M.S.; Castelletto, V.; Hamley, I.W.; Reece, M.J.; Azevedo, H.S. Magnetic Field-Induced Alignment of Nanofibrous Supramolecular Membranes: A Molecular Design Approach to Create Tissue-like Biomaterials. *ACS Appl. Mater. Interfaces* **2020**, *12*, 22661–22672. [CrossRef] [PubMed]
116. Wankar, J.; Kotla, N.G.; Gera, S.; Rasala, S.; Pandit, A.; Rochev, Y.A.; Wankar, J.; Kotla, N.G.; Rasala, S.; Pandit, A.; et al. Recent Advances in Host–Guest Self-Assembled Cyclodextrin Carriers: Implications for Responsive Drug Delivery and Biomedical Engineering. *Adv. Funct. Mater.* **2020**, *30*, 1909049. [CrossRef]
117. Balavigneswaran, C.K.; Muthuvijayan, V. Nanohybrid-Reinforced Gelatin-Ureidopyrimidinone-Based Self-Healing Injectable Hydrogels for Tissue Engineering Applications. *ACS Appl. Bio Mater.* **2021**, *4*, 5362–5377. [CrossRef]
118. Grimaldi, M.; Santoro, A.; Buonocore, M.; Crivaro, C.; Funicello, N.; Saponetti, M.S.; Ripoli, C.; Rodriquez, M.; de Pasquale, S.; Bobba, F.; et al. A New Approach to Supramolecular Structure Determination in Pharmaceutical Preparation of Self-Assembling Peptides: A Case Study of Lanreotide Autogel. *Pharmaceutics* **2022**, *14*, 681. [CrossRef]
119. Ladiè, R.; Cosentino, C.; Tagliaro, I.; Antonini, C.; Bianchini, G.; Bertini, S. Supramolecular Structuring of Hyaluronan-Lactose-Modified Chitosan Matrix: Towards High-Performance Biopolymers with Excellent Biodegradation. *Biomolecules* **2021**, *11*, 389. [CrossRef]

120. Susapto, H.H.; Alhattab, D.; Abdelrahman, S.; Khan, Z.; Alshehri, S.; Kahin, K.; Ge, R.; Moretti, M.; Emwas, A.H.; Hauser, C.A.E. Ultrashort Peptide Bioinks Support Automated Printing of Large-Scale Constructs Assuring Long-Term Survival of Printed Tissue Constructs. *Nano Lett.* **2021**, *21*, 2719–2729. [CrossRef]
121. Dai, W.; Zhang, L.; Yu, Y.; Yan, W.; Zhao, F.; Fan, Y.; Cao, C.; Cai, Q.; Hu, X.; Ao, Y. 3D Bioprinting of Heterogeneous Constructs Providing Tissue-Specific Microenvironment Based on Host–Guest Modulated Dynamic Hydrogel Bioink for Osteochondral Regeneration. *Adv. Funct. Mater.* **2022**, *32*, 2200710. [CrossRef]
122. Wang, Z.; Ren, Y.; Zhu, Y.; Hao, L.; Chen, Y.; An, G.; Wu, H.; Shi, X.; Mao, C. A Rapidly Self-Healing Host–Guest Supramolecular Hydrogel with High Mechanical Strength and Excellent Biocompatibility. *Angew. Chem.* **2018**, *130*, 9146–9150. [CrossRef]
123. Zhou, Y.; Zhang, Y.; Dai, Z.; Jiang, F.; Tian, J.; Zhang, W. A Super-Stretchable, Self-Healing and Injectable Supramolecular Hydrogel Constructed by a Host–Guest Crosslinker. *Biomater. Sci.* **2020**, *8*, 3359–3369. [CrossRef]
124. Singh, P.; Chen, Y.; Tyagi, D.; Wu, L.; Ren, X.; Feng, J.; Carrier, A.; Luan, T.; Tang, Y.; Zhang, J.; et al. β-Cyclodextrin-Grafted Hyaluronic Acid as a Supramolecular Polysaccharide Carrier for Cell-Targeted Drug Delivery. *Int. J. Pharm.* **2021**, *602*, 120602. [CrossRef]
125. Angelerou, M.G.F.; Frederix, P.W.J.M.; Wallace, M.; Yang, B.; Rodger, A.; Adams, D.J.; Marlow, M.; Zelzer, M. Supramolecular Nucleoside-Based Gel: Molecular Dynamics Simulation and Characterization of Its Nanoarchitecture and Self-Assembly Mechanism. *Langmuir* **2018**, *34*, 6912–6921. [CrossRef]
126. Okesola, B.O.; Wu, Y.; Derkus, B.; Gani, S.; Wu, D.; Knani, D.; Smith, D.K.; Adams, D.J.; Mata, A. Supramolecular Self-Assembly to Control Structural and Biological Properties of Multicomponent Hydrogels. *Chem. Mater.* **2019**, *31*, 7883–7897. [CrossRef]
127. Gu, Z.; Huang, K.; Luo, Y.; Zhang, L.; Kuang, T.; Chen, Z.; Liao, G. Double Network Hydrogel for Tissue Engineering. *Wiley Interdiscip. Rev. Nanomed. Nanobiotechnol.* **2018**, *10*, e1520. [CrossRef]
128. Cheng, J.; Amin, D.; Latona, J.; Heber-Katz, E.; Messersmith, P.B. Supramolecular Polymer Hydrogels for Drug-Induced Tissue Regeneration. *ACS Nano* **2019**, *13*, 5493–5501. [CrossRef]
129. Mousavi, A.; Mashayekhan, S.; Baheiraei, N.; Pourjavadi, A. Biohybrid Oxidized Alginate/Myocardial Extracellular Matrix Injectable Hydrogels with Improved Electromechanical Properties for Cardiac Tissue Engineering. *Int. J. Biol. Macromol.* **2021**, *180*, 692–708. [CrossRef]
130. Park, J.; Oh, Y.; Jeong, S.; Song, H.W.; Choi, E.; Kim, H. Biobased Stimuli-Responsive Hydrogels That Comprise Supramolecular Interpenetrating Networks and Exhibit Programmed Behaviors. *Chem. Mater.* **2021**, *33*, 8124–8132. [CrossRef]
131. Lee, S.Y.; Jeon, S.I.; Sim, S.B.; Byun, Y.; Ahn, C.H. A Supramolecular Host-Guest Interaction-Mediated Injectable Hydrogel System with Enhanced Stability and Sustained Protein Release. *Acta Biomater.* **2021**, *131*, 286–301. [CrossRef]
132. Hwang, I.; Jeon, W.S.; Kim, H.-J.; Kim, D.; Kim, H.; Selvapalam, N.; Fujita, N.; Shinkai, S.; Kim, K. Cucurbit [7]Uril: A Simple Macrocyclic, PH-Triggered Hydrogelator Exhibiting Guest-Induced Stimuli-Responsive Behavior. *Angew. Chem. Int. Ed.* **2007**, *46*, 210–213. [CrossRef]
133. Xia, C.; Ming, P.; Zhou, A.; Zhang, S.; Chen, J.; Huang, X. Supramolecular Self-Assembly of Oligopeptide Hybrid Films with Liquid Crystal Texture: Effects on Cell Behaviour for Vascular Grafts. *Bull. Mater. Sci.* **2021**, *44*, 1–10. [CrossRef]
134. Ursu, E.L.; Rotaru, A.; Ursu, E.L.; Rotaru, A.; Rotaru, A. Supramolecular Guanosine-Quadruplex Hydrogels and Hydrogel Composites for Cell Growth Applications. *New Trends Macromol. Supramol. Chem. Biol. Appl.* **2021**, 331–343. [CrossRef]
135. Miller, B.; Hansrisuk, A.; Highley, C.B.; Caliari, S.R. Guest-Host Supramolecular Assembly of Injectable Hydrogel Nanofibers for Cell Encapsulation. *ACS Biomater. Sci. Eng.* **2021**, *7*, 4164–4174. [CrossRef]
136. Tang, J.D.; Mura, C.; Lampe, K.J. Stimuli-Responsive, Pentapeptide, Nanofiber Hydrogel for Tissue Engineering. *J. Am. Chem. Soc.* **2019**, *141*, 4886–4899. [CrossRef]
137. Chakraborty, P.; Oved, H.; Bychenko, D.; Yao, Y.; Tang, Y.; Zilberzwige-Tal, S.; Wei, G.; Dvir, T.; Gazit, E.; Chakraborty, P.; et al. Nanoengineered Peptide-Based Antimicrobial Conductive Supramolecular Biomaterial for Cardiac Tissue Engineering. *Adv. Mater.* **2021**, *33*, 2008715. [CrossRef]
138. Wang, T.-W.; Chang, K.-C.; Chen, L.-H.; Liao, S.-Y.; Yeh, C.-W.; Chuang, Y.-J. Effects of an Injectable Functionalized Self-Assembling Nanopeptide Hydrogel on Angiogenesis and Neurogenesis for Regeneration of the Central Nervous System. *Nanoscale* **2017**, *9*, 16281–16292. [CrossRef]
139. Ma, X.; Agas, A.; Siddiqui, Z.; Kim, K.K.; Iglesias-Montoro, P.; Kalluru, J.; Kumar, V.; Haorah, J. Angiogenic Peptide Hydrogels for Treatment of Traumatic Brain Injury. *Bioact. Mater.* **2020**, *5*, 124–132. [CrossRef]
140. Yuan, T.; Shao, Y.; Zhou, X.; Liu, Q.; Zhu, Z.; Zhou, B.; Dong, Y.; Stephanopoulos, N.; Gui, S.; Yan, H.; et al. Highly Permeable DNA Supramolecular Hydrogel Promotes Neurogenesis and Functional Recovery after Completely Transected Spinal Cord Injury. *Adv. Mater.* **2021**, *33*, 2102428. [CrossRef]
141. Wang, C.; Yue, H.; Feng, Q.; Xu, B.; Bian, L.; Shi, P. Injectable Nanoreinforced Shape-Memory Hydrogel System for Regenerating Spinal Cord Tissue from Traumatic Injury. *ACS Appl. Mater. Interfaces* **2018**, *10*, 29299–29307. [CrossRef]
142. Guo, W.; Feng, W.; Huang, J.; Zhang, J.; Fan, X.; Ma, S.; Li, M.; Zhan, J.; Cai, Y.; Chen, M. Supramolecular Self-Assembled Nanofibers Efficiently Activate the Precursor of Hepatocyte Growth Factor for Angiogenesis in Myocardial Infarction Therapy. *ACS Appl. Mater. Interfaces* **2021**, *13*, 22131–22141. [CrossRef]
143. Fan, X.; Zhan, J.; Pan, X.; Liao, X.; Guo, W.; Chen, P.; Li, H.; Feng, W.; Cai, Y.; Chen, M. Enzymatic Self-Assembly Nanofibers Anchoring Mesenchymal Stem Cells Induce Cell Spheroids and Amplify Paracrine Function for Myocardial Infarction Therapy. *Chem. Eng. J.* **2022**, *436*, 135224. [CrossRef]

144. Bastings, M.M.C.; Koudstaal, S.; Kieltyka, R.E.; Nakano, Y.; Pape, A.C.H.; Feyen, D.A.M.; van Slochteren, F.J.; Doevendans, P.A.; Sluijter, J.P.G.; Meijer, E.W.; et al. A Fast PH-Switchable and Self-Healing Supramolecular Hydrogel Carrier for Guided, Local Catheter Injection in the Infarcted Myocardium. *Adv. Healthc. Mater.* **2014**, *3*, 70–78. [CrossRef] [PubMed]
145. Bonito, V.; Koch, S.E.; Krebber, M.M.; Carvajal-Berrio, D.A.; Marzi, J.; Duijvelshoff, R.; Lurier, E.B.; Buscone, S.; Dekker, S.; de Jong, S.M.J.; et al. Distinct Effects of Heparin and Interleukin-4 Functionalization on Macrophage Polarization and In Situ Arterial Tissue Regeneration Using Resorbable Supramolecular Vascular Grafts in Rats. *Adv. Healthc. Mater.* **2021**, *10*, 2101103. [CrossRef] [PubMed]
146. Wang, H.; Shang, Y.; Chen, X.; Wang, Z.; Zhu, D.; Liu, Y.; Zhang, C.; Chen, P.; Wu, J.; Wu, L.; et al. Delivery of MSCs with a Hybrid β-Sheet Peptide Hydrogel Consisting IGF-1C Domain and D-Form Peptide for Acute Kidney Injury Therapy. *Int. J. Nanomed.* **2020**, *15*, 4311. [CrossRef]
147. Zhang, C.; Shang, Y.; Chen, X.; Midgley, A.C.; Wang, Z.; Zhu, D.; Wu, J.; Chen, P.; Wu, L.; Wang, X.; et al. Supramolecular Nanofibers Containing Arginine-Glycine-Aspartate (RGD) Peptides Boost Therapeutic Efficacy of Extracellular Vesicles in Kidney Repair. *ACS Nano* **2020**, *14*, 12133–12147. [CrossRef]
148. Han, Q.; Ai, S.; Hong, Q.; Zhang, C.; Song, Y.; Wang, X.; Wang, X.; Cui, S.; Li, Z.; Zhu, H.; et al. A Supramolecular Hydrogel Based on the Combination of YIGSR and RGD Enhances Mesenchymal Stem Cells Paracrine Function via Integrin A2β1 and PI3K/AKT Signaling Pathway for Acute Kidney Injury Therapy. *Chem. Eng. J.* **2022**, *436*, 135088. [CrossRef]
149. Cheng, Y.Q.; Yue, Y.X.; Cao, H.M.; Geng, W.C.; Wang, L.X.; Hu, X.Y.; Li, H.b.; Bian, Q.; Kong, X.L.; Liu, J.F.; et al. Coassembly of Hypoxia-Sensitive Macrocyclic Amphiphiles and Extracellular Vesicles for Targeted Kidney Injury Imaging and Therapy. *J. Nanobiotechnol.* **2021**, *19*, 1–21. [CrossRef]
150. Yao, Q.; Huang, Z.-W.; Zhai, Y.-Y.; Yue, M.; Luo, L.-Z.; Xue, P.-P.; Han, Y.-H.; Xu, H.-L.; Kou, L.; Zhao, Y.-Z. Localized Controlled Release of Bilirubin from β-Cyclodextrin-Conjugated ε-Polylysine to Attenuate Oxidative Stress and Inflammation in Transplanted Islets. *ACS Appl. Mater. Interfaces* **2020**, *12*, 5462–5475. [CrossRef]
151. Wang, W.; Zeng, Z.; Xiang, L.; Liu, C.; Diaz-Dussan, D.; Du, Z.; Asha, A.B.; Yang, W.; Peng, Y.Y.; Pan, M.; et al. Injectable Self-Healing Hydrogel via Biological Environment-Adaptive Supramolecular Assembly for Gastric Perforation Healing. *ACS Nano* **2021**, *15*, 9913–9923. [CrossRef]
152. Eren Cimenci, C.; Uzunalli, G.; Uysal, O.; Yergoz, F.; Karaca Umay, E.; Guler, M.O.; Tekinay, A.B. Laminin Mimetic Peptide Nanofibers Regenerate Acute Muscle Defect. *Acta Biomater.* **2017**, *60*, 190–200. [CrossRef]
153. Shang, Y.; Kuang, M.; Wang, Z.; Huang, Y.; Liu, L.; Zhao, X.; Zhang, R.; Zhao, Y.; Peng, R.; Sun, S.; et al. An Ultrashort Peptide-Based Supramolecular Hydrogel Mimicking IGF-1 to Alleviate Glucocorticoid-Induced Sarcopenia. *ACS Appl. Mater. Interfaces* **2020**, *12*, 34678–34688. [CrossRef]
154. Mori da Cunha, M.G.M.C.; Arts, B.; Hympanova, L.; Rynkevic, R.; Mackova, K.; Bosman, A.W.; Dankers, P.Y.W.; Deprest, J. Functional Supramolecular Bioactivated Electrospun Mesh Improves Tissue Ingrowth in Experimental Abdominal Wall Reconstruction in Rats. *Acta Biomater.* **2020**, *106*, 82–91. [CrossRef]
155. Bairagi, D.; Biswas, P.; Basu, K.; Hazra, S.; Hermida-Merino, D.; Sinha, D.K.; Hamley, I.W.; Banerjee, A. Self-Assembling Peptide-Based Hydrogel: Regulation of Mechanical Stiffness and Thermal Stability and 3D Cell Culture of Fibroblasts. *ACS Appl. Bio Mater.* **2019**, *2*, 5235–5244. [CrossRef]
156. Yan, X.; Yang, B.; Chen, Y.; Song, Y.; Ye, J.; Pan, Y.; Zhou, B.; Wang, Y.; Mao, F.; Dong, Y.; et al. Anti-Friction MSCs Delivery System Improves the Therapy for Severe Osteoarthritis. *Adv. Mater.* **2021**, *33*, 2104758. [CrossRef]
157. Ebada, H.M.; Nasra, M.M.; Nassra, R.A.; Solaiman, A.A.; Abdallah, O.Y. Cationic Nanocarrier of Rhein Based on Hydrophobic Ion Pairing Approach as Intra-Articular Targeted Regenerative Therapy for Osteoarthritis. *Colloids Surf. B Biointerfaces* **2022**, *211*, 112285. [CrossRef]
158. Siddiqui, Z.; Sarkar, B.; Kim, K.K.; Kadincesme, N.; Paul, R.; Kumar, A.; Kobayashi, Y.; Roy, A.; Choudhury, M.; Yang, J.; et al. Angiogenic Hydrogels for Dental Pulp Revascularization. *Acta Biomater.* **2021**, *126*, 109–118. [CrossRef]
159. Tan, J.; Zhang, M.; Hai, Z.; Wu, C.; Lin, J.; Kuang, W.; Tang, H.; Huang, Y.; Chen, X.; Liang, G. Sustained Release of Two Bioactive Factors from Supramolecular Hydrogel Promotes Periodontal Bone Regeneration. *ACS Nano* **2019**, *13*, 5616–5622. [CrossRef]
160. Wang, Z.; Zhang, Y.; Yin, Y.; Liu, J.; Li, P.; Zhao, Y.; Bai, D.; Zhao, H.; Han, X.; Chen, Q.; et al. High-Strength and Injectable Supramolecular Hydrogel Self-Assembled by Monomeric Nucleoside for Tooth-Extraction Wound Healing. *Adv. Mater.* **2022**, *34*, 2108300. [CrossRef]
161. Xiao, M.; Gao, L.; Chandrasekaran, A.R.; Zhao, J.; Tang, Q.; Qu, Z.; Wang, F.; Li, L.; Yang, Y.; Zhang, X.; et al. Bio-Functional G-Molecular Hydrogels for Accelerated Wound Healing. *Mater. Sci. Eng. C* **2019**, *105*, 110067. [CrossRef]
162. Zhou, S.; Hokugo, A.; McClendon, M.; Zhang, Z.; Bakshi, R.; Wang, L.; Segovia, L.A.; Rezzadeh, K.; Stupp, S.I.; Jarrahy, R. Bioactive Peptide Amphiphile Nanofiber Gels Enhance Burn Wound Healing. *Burns* **2019**, *45*, 1112–1121. [CrossRef]
163. Jian, K.; Yang, C.; Li, T.; Wu, X.; Shen, J.; Wei, J.; Yang, Z.; Yuan, D.; Zhao, M.; Shi, J. PDGF-BB-Derived Supramolecular Hydrogel for Promoting Skin Wound Healing. *J. Nanobiotechnol.* **2022**, *20*, 1–9. [CrossRef]
164. Jeong, S.H.; Kim, M.; Kim, T.Y.; Choi, H.; Hahn, S.K. Biomimetic Supramolecular Drug Delivery Hydrogels for Accelerated Skin Tissue Regeneration. *ACS Biomater. Sci. Eng.* **2021**, *7*, 4581–4590. [CrossRef]
165. Hoque, J.; Sangaj, N.; Varghese, S. Stimuli-Responsive Supramolecular Hydrogels and Their Applications in Regenerative Medicine. *Macromol. Biosci.* **2019**, *19*, 1800259. [CrossRef]

166. Municoy, S.; Álvarez Echazú, M.I.; Antezana, P.E.; Galdopórpora, J.M.; Olivetti, C.; Mebert, A.M.; Foglia, M.L.; Tuttolomondo, M.v.; Alvarez, G.S.; Hardy, J.G.; et al. Stimuli-Responsive Materials for Tissue Engineering and Drug Delivery. *Int. J. Mol. Sci.* **2020**, *21*, 4724. [CrossRef]
167. Xian, S.; Webber, M.J. Temperature-Responsive Supramolecular Hydrogels. *J. Mater. Chem. B* **2020**, *8*, 9197–9211. [CrossRef]
168. Hao, L.; Yegin, C.; Talari, J.V.; Oh, J.K.; Zhang, M.; Sari, M.M.; Zhang, L.; Min, Y.; Akbulut, M.; Jiang, B. Thermo-Responsive Gels Based on Supramolecular Assembly of an Amidoamine and Citric Acid. *Soft Matter* **2018**, *14*, 432–439. [CrossRef]
169. Pugliese, R.; Gelain, F. Characterization of Elastic, Thermo-Responsive, Self-Healable Supramolecular Hydrogel Made of Self-Assembly Peptides and Guar Gum. *Mater. Des.* **2020**, *186*, 108370. [CrossRef]
170. Rapp, T.L.; DeForest, C.A. Visible Light-Responsive Dynamic Biomaterials: Going Deeper and Triggering More. *Adv. Healthc. Mater.* **2020**, *9*, 1901553. [CrossRef]
171. Ji, W.; Wu, Q.; Han, X.; Zhang, W.; Wei, W.; Chen, L.; Li, L.; Huang, W. Photosensitive Hydrogels: From Structure, Mechanisms, Design to Bioapplications. *Sci. China Life Sci.* **2020**, *63*, 1813–1828. [CrossRef]
172. Ruskowitz, E.R.; Deforest, C.A. Photoresponsive Biomaterials for Targeted Drug Delivery and 4D Cell Culture. *Nat. Rev. Mater.* **2018**, *3*, 1–17. [CrossRef]
173. Tomatsu, I.; Peng, K.; Kros, A. Photoresponsive Hydrogels for Biomedical Applications. *Adv. Drug Deliv. Rev.* **2011**, *63*, 1257–1266. [CrossRef] [PubMed]
174. Mañas-Torres, M.C.; Gila-Vilchez, C.; Vazquez-Perez, F.J.; Kuzhir, P.; Momier, D.; Scimeca, J.C.; Borderie, A.; Goracci, M.; Burel-Vandenbos, F.; Blanco-Elices, C.; et al. Injectable Magnetic-Responsive Short-Peptide Supramolecular Hydrogels: Ex Vivo and in Vivo Evaluation. *ACS Appl. Mater. Interfaces* **2021**, *13*, 49692–49704. [CrossRef] [PubMed]
175. Carayon, I.; Gaubert, A.; Mousli, Y.; Philippe, B. Electro-Responsive Hydrogels: Macromolecular and Supramolecular Approaches in the Biomedical Field. *Biomater. Sci.* **2020**, *8*, 5589–5600. [CrossRef] [PubMed]
176. Ghosh, G.; Barman, R.; Sarkar, J.; Ghosh, S. PH-Responsive Biocompatible Supramolecular Peptide Hydrogel. *J. Phys. Chem. B* **2019**, *123*, 5909–5915. [CrossRef] [PubMed]
177. Talloj, S.K.; Mohammed, M.; Lin, H.C. Construction of Self-Assembled Nanostructure-Based Tetraphenylethylene Dipeptides: Supramolecular Nanobelts as Biomimetic Hydrogels for Cell Adhesion and Proliferation. *J. Mater. Chem. B* **2020**, *8*, 7483–7493. [CrossRef] [PubMed]
178. Gačanin, J.; Hedrich, J.; Sieste, S.; Glaßer, G.; Lieberwirth, I.; Schilling, C.; Fischer, S.; Barth, H.; Knöll, B.; Synatschke, C.V.; et al. Autonomous Ultrafast Self-Healing Hydrogels by PH-Responsive Functional Nanofiber Gelators as Cell Matrices. *Adv. Mater.* **2019**, *31*, 1805044. [CrossRef]
179. Liu, X.; Zhao, L.; Liu, F.; Astruc, D.; Gu, H. Supramolecular Redox-Responsive Ferrocene Hydrogels and Microgels. *Coord. Chem. Rev.* **2020**, *419*, 213406. [CrossRef]
180. Milcovich, G.; Contessotto, P.; Marsico, G.; Ismail, S.; Pandit, A. Synthetic/ECM-Inspired Hybrid Platform for Hollow Microcarriers with ROS-Triggered Nanoporation Hallmarks. *Sci. Rep.* **2017**, *7*, 13138. [CrossRef]
181. Zuo, C.; Peng, J.; Cong, Y.; Dai, X.; Zhang, X.; Zhao, S.; Zhang, X.; Ma, L.; Wang, B.; Wei, H. Fabrication of Supramolecular Star-Shaped Amphiphilic Copolymers for ROS-Triggered Drug Release. *J. Colloid Interface Sci.* **2018**, *514*, 122–131. [CrossRef]
182. Brouns, J.E.P.; Dankers, P.Y.W. Introduction of Enzyme-Responsivity in Biomaterials to Achieve Dynamic Reciprocity in Cell-Material Interactions. *Biomacromolecules* **2021**, *22*, 4–23. [CrossRef]
183. Wang, M.; Gao, B.; Wang, X.; Li, W.; Feng, Y. Enzyme-Responsive Strategy as a Prospective Cue to Construct Intelligent Biomaterials for Disease Diagnosis and Therapy. *Biomater. Sci.* **2022**. [CrossRef]
184. Vemula, P.K.; Li, J.; John, G. Enzyme Catalysis: Tool to Make and Break Amygdalin Hydrogelators from Renewable Resources: A Delivery Model for Hydrophobic Drugs. *J. Am. Chem. Soc.* **2006**, *128*, 8932–8938. [CrossRef]
185. Yu, C.; Alkekhia, D.; Shukla, A. Lactamase Responsive Supramolecular Hydrogels with Host-Guest Self-Healing Capability. *ACS Appl. Polym. Mater.* **2020**, *2*, 55–65. [CrossRef]
186. Zou, Y.Q.; Hu, B.; Chen, L.; Ji, T.; Yang, M.; Yang, C.A. Novel PH- and Thermoresponsive Supramolecular Dendronized Copolymer. *Iran. Polym. J.* **2021**, *30*, 47–56. [CrossRef]
187. Frederix, P.W.J.M.; Patmanidis, I.; Marrink, S.J. Molecular Simulations of Self-Assembling Bio-Inspired Supramolecular Systems and Their Connection to Experiments. *Chem. Soc. Rev.* **2018**, *47*, 3470–3489. [CrossRef]
188. Moroni, L.; Burdick, J.A.; Highley, C.; Lee, S.J.; Morimoto, Y.; Takeuchi, S.; Yoo, J.J. Biofabrication Strategies for 3D in Vitro Models and Regenerative Medicine. *Nat. Rev. Mater.* **2018**, *3*, 21–37. [CrossRef]
189. Nii, T.; Makino, K.; Tabata, Y. Three-Dimensional Culture System of Cancer Cells Combined with Biomaterials for Drug Screening. *Cancers* **2020**, *12*, 2754. [CrossRef]
190. Kock, A.; Bergqvist, F.; Steinmetz, J.; Elfman, L.H.M.; Korotkova, M.; Johnsen, J.I.; Jakobsson, P.J.; Kogner, P.; Larsson, K. Establishment of an in Vitro 3D Model for Neuroblastoma Enables Preclinical Investigation of Combined Tumor-Stroma Drug Targeting. *FASEB J.* **2020**, *34*, 11101–11114. [CrossRef]
191. Lazzari, G.; Nicolas, V.; Matsusaki, M.; Akashi, M.; Couvreur, P.; Mura, S. Multicellular Spheroid Based on a Triple Co-Culture: A Novel 3D Model to Mimic Pancreatic Tumor Complexity. *Acta Biomater.* **2018**, *78*, 296–307. [CrossRef]
192. Hart, L.R.; Li, S.; Sturgess, C.; Wildman, R.; Jones, J.R.; Hayes, W. 3D Printing of Biocompatible Supramolecular Polymers and Their Composites. *ACS Appl. Mater. Interfaces* **2016**, *8*, 3115–3122. [CrossRef]

193. Sather, N.A.; Sai, H.; Sasselli, I.R.; Sato, K.; Ji, W.; Synatschke, C.v.; Zambrotta, R.T.; Edelbrock, J.F.; Kohlmeyer, R.R Hardin, J.O.; et al. 3D Printing of Supramolecular Polymer Hydrogels with Hierarchical Structure. *Small* **2021**, *17*, 200574 [CrossRef] [PubMed]
194. Rupp, H.; Döhler, D.; Hilgeroth, P.; Mahmood, N.; Beiner, M.; Binder, W.H. 3D Printing of Supramolecular Polymers: Impact o Nanoparticles and Phase Separation on Printability. *Macromol. Rapid Commun.* **2019**, *40*, 1900467. [CrossRef] [PubMed]
195. Ashammakhi, N.; Ahadian, S.; Zengjie, F.; Suthiwanich, K.; Lorestani, F.; Orive, G.; Ostrovidov, S.; Khademhosseini, A. Advance and Future Perspectives in 4D Bioprinting. *Biotechnol. J.* **2018**, *13*, 1800148. [CrossRef] [PubMed]

*pharmaceutics*

MDPI

*Article*

# L-Serine-Modified Poly-L-Lysine as a Biodegradable Kidney-Targeted Drug Carrier for the Efficient Radionuclide Therapy of Renal Cell Carcinoma

**Hidemasa Katsumi [1,*], Sho Kitada [1], Shintaro Yasuoka [1], Rie Takashima [1], Tomoki Imanishi [1], Rina Tanaka [1], Satoru Matsuura [1], Hiroyuki Kimura [2], Hidekazu Kawashima [3], Masaki Morishita [1] and Akira Yamamoto [1]**

[1] Department of Biopharmaceutics, Division of Clinical Pharmaceutical Sciences, Kyoto Pharmaceutical University, Yamashina-ku, Kyoto 607-8414, Japan
[2] Department of Analytical and Bioinorganic Chemistry, Division of Analytical and Physical Sciences, Kyoto Pharmaceutical University, Yamashina-ku, Kyoto 607-8414, Japan
[3] Radioisotope Research Center, Kyoto Pharmaceutical University, Yamashina-ku, Kyoto 607-8414, Japan
* Correspondence: hkatsumi@mb.kyoto-phu.ac.jp; Tel.: +81-75-595-4662; Fax: +81-75-595-4761

**Abstract:** In the present study, L-serine (Ser)-modified poly-L-lysine (PLL) was synthesized to develop a biodegradable, kidney-targeted drug carrier for efficient radionuclide therapy in renal cell carcinoma (RCC). Ser-PLL was labeled with $^{111}$In/$^{90}$Y via diethylenetriaminepentaacetic acid (DTPA) chelation for biodistribution analysis/radionuclide therapy. In mice, approximately 91% of the total dose accumulated in the kidney 3 h after intravenous injection of $^{111}$In-labeled Ser-PLL. Single-photon emission computed tomography/computed tomography (SPECT/CT) imaging showed that $^{111}$In-labeled Ser-PLL accumulated in the renal cortex following intravenous injection. An intrarenal distribution study showed that fluorescein isothiocyanate (FITC)-labeled Ser-PLL accumulated mainly in the renal proximal tubules. This pattern was associated with RCC pathogenesis. Moreover, $^{111}$In-labeled Ser-PLL rapidly degraded and was eluted along with the low-molecular-weight fractions of the renal homogenate in gel filtration chromatography. Continuous Ser-PLL administration over five days had no significant effect on plasma creatinine, blood urea nitrogen (BUN), or renal histology. In a murine RCC model, kidney tumor growth was significantly inhibited by the administration of the beta-emitter $^{90}$Y combined with Ser-PLL. The foregoing results indicate that Ser-PLL is promising as a biodegradable drug carrier for kidney-targeted drug delivery and efficient radionuclide therapy in RCC.

**Keywords:** kidney-targeted delivery; radionuclide therapy; renal cell carcinoma; L-serine; yttrium ($^{90}$Y)

## 1. Introduction

Renal cell carcinoma (RCC) is a kidney cancer originating in the lining of the proximal tubules and is reputed to be the most lethal malignant urological tumor [1]. The current standard treatments for RCC include inhibitors of tyrosine kinase, mTOR, and immune checkpoints. As these therapies have several pharmacokinetic issues, however, their efficacy and safety are questionable [2–4]. It is therefore necessary to develop a drug delivery system (DDS) for the selective transport of therapeutic agents, particularly to the proximal tubule associated with RCC pathogenesis. Nevertheless, it is difficult to develop a drug carrier with high renal selectivity simply by using the conventional kidney-targeted approach of DDS technology. Furthermore, there are few reports of the successful development of renal-targeted DDS with superior efficacy and safety [5–7].

Recently, we observed that after L-serine (Ser)-modified polyamideamine (PAMAM) dendrimer (Ser-PAMAM) was intravenously injected into mice, it accumulated in the proximal tubules of the renal cortex. In Ser-PAMAM, multiple Ser moieties are covalently bound to the PAMAM surface [8–10]. Ser is a biological component and its physicochemical properties are well known. Thus, it is considered superior to conventional kidney-targeted moieties in terms of safety and ease of synthesis. PAMAM is familiar as a novel artificial dendritic macromolecular drug carrier and is anticipated for clinical use [11]. It is unknown, however, whether Ser modification could be applied in a kidney-targeted delivery system using linear macromolecular drug carriers. In addition, little is known about the biocompatibility and biodegradability of the inner core of the drug carrier in this kidney-targeted drug delivery system.

In the present study, we selected linear poly-L-lysine hydrobromide (PLL) as a carrier backbone and modified it with Ser to obtain Ser-modified poly-L-lysine (Ser-PLL). Ser-PLL consists almost exclusively of amino acids. Hence, it is expected to have high biocompatibility and biodegradability.

The indium ($^{111}$In) (imaging)/yttrium ($^{90}$Y) (therapy) combination has been evaluated in cancer radiotheranostics [12–14]. Recently, $^{111}$In/$^{90}$Y-loaded ibritumomab (anti-CD20 antibody) thiuxetane was approval by the United States Food and Drug Administration and has been used to treat CD20-positive relapsed or refractory low-grade B-cell non-Hodgkin's lymphoma and mantle cell lymphoma. In this formulation, ibritumomab is bound to $^{111}$In/$^{90}$Y via the chelating agent (1-(2)-methyl-4-isocyanatobenzyl-diethylenetriamine-N,N,N′,N″,N″-pentaacetic acid (MX-DTPA; thiuxetane) [15,16]. We hypothesized that an imaging/therapy combination involving $^{111}$In/$^{90}$Y may facilitate the development of an innovative RCC treatment modality.

The aims of this study were to develop a biodegradable kidney-targeted drug carrier using the amino acids Ser and Lys and evaluate its efficacy as a radionuclide therapy for RCC. We endeavored to develop a kidney-targeted radiotheranostics system using Ser-PLL with $^{111}$In/$^{90}$Y via the chelating agent diethylenetriaminepentaacetic acid (DTPA). We intravenously injected $^{111}$In-labeled Ser-PLL in mice and analyzed its tissue distribution. We then assessed the efficacy of $^{90}$Y-labeled Ser-PLL at preventing increases in the number of tumor cells in the kidneys of a mouse RCC model.

## 2. Materials and Methods

### 2.1. Chemicals and Reagents

Poly-L-lysine hydrobromide (PLL) (MW range = 4000–15,000) and polyamidoamine (PAMAM) dendrimer with an ethylenediamine core (generation (G) 3) in methanol were purchased from Sigma-Aldrich Corp. (St. Louis, MO, USA). Boc-Ser(tBu)-OH and HOBt were purchased from Watanabe Chemical Industries (Hiroshima, Japan). Hexafluorophosphate benzotriazole tetramethyl uronium (HBTU) was purchased from Merck Millipore (Burlington, MA, USA). Dimethyl sulfoxide (DMSO; super dehydrated grade), N,N-dimethylformamide (DMF; super dehydrated grade), N,N-diisopropylethylamine (DIPEA), piperidine, trifluoroacetic acid (TFA), triisopropylsilane (TIS), Turk's solution, and poly-L-lysine hydrobromide (MW range = 15,000–30,000) were purchased from Fujifilm Wako Pure Chemical Industries Ltd. (Osaka, Japan). PD-10 was purchased from GE Healthcare Japan (Tokyo, Japan). The $^{111}InCl_3$ was supplied by Nihon Medi-Physics (Tokyo, Japan). $^{90}YCl_3$ was purchased from Eckert Radiopharma (Berlin, Germany). DTPA anhydride was purchased from Chemical Dojin Co., Ltd. (Kumamoto, Japan). All other chemicals were of commercial reagent grade.

### 2.2. Animals

Male ddY mice (age 5 wks; average weight 25 g) and male Balb/c mice (age 5 wks; average weight 20 g) were purchased from Japan SLC (Shizuoka, Japan). The animals were maintained under conventional housing conditions. All animal experiments were conducted according to the principles and procedures outlined in the National Institutes of Health Guide for the Care and Use of Laboratory Animals. The Animal Experimentation Committee of the Kyoto Pharmaceutical University approved this experimental protocol.

### 2.3. Synthesis of Ser-Poly-L-Lysine

Ser-PLL was synthesized by reacting Ser with PLL (MW range = 4000–15,000) using the previously published HBTU-HOBt method with slight modifications [8,17] (Scheme S1). Briefly, PLL (MW range = 4000–15,000) was coupled to its surface amino groups with 1.1 eq (equivalent to the surface amino group of PLL) Boc-Ser(t-Bu)-OH in DMF/DMSO (3:1) by mixing it with 1.1 eq HBTU, 1.1 eq HOBt, and DIPEA to adjust the pH to 8−9. The mixture was stirred at room temperature until a ninhydrin test yielded negative results for thin-layer chromatography (TLC) analysis. After the coupling, the reaction mixture was evaporated and the product was dissolved in chloroform. The organic phase was washed three times with 5% $NaHCO_3$ and saturated with sodium chloride thrice. Then, the organic phase was dried over anhydrous $MgSO_4$ and vacuum-filtered and evaporated. The precipitates were then dissolved in a trifluoroacetic acid (TFA) cocktail (95% ($v/v$) TFA, 2.5% ($v/v$) thioanisole (TIS), and 2.5% ($v/v$) purified water) to deprotect the Boc and *t*-Bu groups and protect the Ser oxygen atom. The mixture was then incubated at room temperature for 90 min. After deprotection and evaporation, the crude precipitate was dispersed in ultrapure water. After dialysis with ultrapure water overnight, the solution was lyophilized to obtain Ser-PLL, which was identified using a $^1H$ nuclear magnetic resonance (NMR) spectroscopy (AM-300 FT-NMR spectrometer; Bruker Corp., Billerica, MA, USA) in deuterated water ($D_2O$). In the PLL $^1H$ NMR spectrum, peaks were observed at $\delta$ 4.18 (s, $\alpha$–CH), 2.81 (m, $\varepsilon$–$CH_2$), 1.82–1.05 (s, $\beta$–$CH_2$, $\gamma$–$CH_2$, and $\delta$–$CH_2$) [18]. In the Ser-PLL $^1H$ NMR spectrum, the peaks corresponding to Ser appeared at $\delta$ 3.72–3.85 (m, $CH_2$), and the integral ratio of Ser methylene protons to PLL methylene protons indicated that the desired product had been obtained (the degree of modification of the Ser moiety linked to the amino groups of PLL was approximately 97%) (Figure S1). As the polymerization degree of PLL is estimated to be approximately 19–72 units with a MW range of 4000–15,000, these results indicate that the average composition of Ser units of the obtained Ser-PLL was 45, with an approximate Ser-PLL molar mass of 10 kDa.

Ser-PLL was then dissolved in phosphate-buffered saline (PBS) (pH 7.4), and its mean particle diameter and zeta potential were measured with a Zetasizer PRO Blue Label (Malvern Instruments, Worcestershire, UK). To synthesize high-MW Ser-PLL (Ser-PLL (H)), we reacted PLL (MW = 15,000–30,000) with Boc-Ser(t-Bu)-OH using the preceding methods. Ser-modified polyamidoamine dendrimer (G3) (Ser-PAMAM conjugating ~32 Ser molecules) was synthesized and used as a control according to the previously reported HBTU-HOBt method [8].

### 2.4. Tissue Distribution of $^{111}$In-Labeled Ser-Poly-L-Lysine

Ser-PLL was labeled with $^{111}$In using DTPA according to a previously published method to determine the tissue distribution of Ser-PLL [19,20]. The $^{111}$In-labeled Ser-PLL was intravenously injected at 1 mg/kg dose into the tail vein of each ddY mouse. At appropriate time points after the injection, blood was collected from the abdominal vena cava under isoflurane anesthesia. The liver, kidneys, spleen, heart, and lungs were excised, rinsed with saline, blotted dry, and weighed. The blood was centrifuged at 2000× *g* for 5 min to obtain the plasma. The organ samples and 100 μL plasma were transferred to counter tubes and their radioactivity levels were measured with a gamma counter (1480 WizardTM 3′; PerkinElmer, Boston, MA, USA). The tissue distribution of PLL was determined as previously described, using $^{111}$In-labeled PLL as a control.

### 2.5. In Vivo SPECT/CT Imaging of $^{111}$In-Labeled Ser-Poly-L-Lysine Tissue Distribution

Single-photon emission computed tomography/computed tomography (SPECT/CT) was performed with a NanoSPECT/CT (Bioscan Inc., Washington, DC, USA) according to a previously reported method [10]. Briefly, $^{111}$In-labeled Ser-PLL (15.6 MBq/mouse) was intravenously injected into a ddY mouse. A CT scan of the mouse was performed under isoflurane anesthesia for anatomical reference. Three hours after the injection, a 1-h SPECT scan was obtained under isoflurane anesthesia. The SPECT image was reconstructed and analyzed with VivoQuant v. 5.1 (inviCRO, Hillsboro, OR, USA).

### 2.6. Intrarenal Distribution of FITC-Labeled Ser-Poly-L-Lysine

Ser-PLL was labeled with fluorescein isothiocyanate (FITC), as previously reported [8]. The FITC-labeled Ser-PLL was then injected into the tail vein of each ddY mouse. After 60 min, the kidneys were excised under isoflurane anesthesia, immersed with 30% sucrose solution. After the immersion at 4 °C overnight, the kidneys were fixed with optimal cutting temperature (OCT) compound, and frozen. The frozen kidney sections were stained with 10 μg/mL of 4′,6-diamidino-2-phenylindole (DAPI) (Fujufilm Wako Pure Chemical Industries Ltd.). The stained kidney sections were observed under a laser-scanning confocal microscope (Nikon A1R, Nikon Corp.; Tokyo, Japan).

### 2.7. Biodegradability of Ser-Poly-L-Lysine

Ser-PLL biodegradability was evaluated using a previously published method, with slight modifications [21]. Briefly, $^{111}$In-labeled Ser-PLL, $^{111}$In-labeled PLL (control), $^{111}$In-labeled PAMAM (G3) (control), and $^{111}$In-labeled Ser-PAMAM (G3) (control) were intravenously injected at 1 mg/kg dose into the tail vein of each ddY mouse and the animals were sacrificed 3 h later by abdominal vena cava amputation under isoflurane anesthesia. Residual blood in each kidney was removed by passing saline through the left ventricle. Each kidney was then immediately ice-cooled, combined with 4 mL purified water, and homogenized. Saturated KCl solution (1 mL) was added to each kidney homogenate. The suspension was allowed to stand at 4 °C overnight and then centrifuged. The supernatant (1 mL) was eluted with a PD-10 column and 0.1 M acetate buffer (pH 6.0). The radioactivity levels of each fraction (10 drops, 0.35 mL) were measured. The high- and low-MW fractions were determined based on the elution patterns.

### 2.8. Ser-Poly-L-Lysine Nephrotoxicity in Mice

Ser-PLL (1 mg/kg/d) was continuously injected intravenously into the tail vein of each ddY mouse for 5 d and acute nephrotoxicity was evaluated [8]. Six days after the first intravenous injection, blood was collected from the vena cava, the kidneys were isolated under isoflurane anesthesia, and the mice were sacrificed. Plasma creatinine was measured with a commercially available kit (Lab Assay; Fujifilm Wako Pure Chemical Industries Ltd.). Blood urea nitrogen (BUN) was measured with a commercially available kit (DIUR-100; BioAssay Systems, Hayward, CA, USA). The kidneys were then excised, fixed with 4% (*v*/*v*) buffered paraformaldehyde (PFA), and embedded in paraffin blocks. Then 5-μm sections were cut with a microtome from the paraffin blocks. The kidney sections were stained with hematoxylin and eosin (H&E), and hepatic injury was evaluated under a light microscope (Biozero; KEYENCE, Osaka, Japan). $HgCl_2$ was subcutaneously injected at a dose of 8 mg/kg, and the mouse group bred for 2 d served as a positive control.

### 2.9. Effects of $^{90}$Y-Labeled Ser-Poly-L-Lysine on Tumor Growth in a Mouse Renal Cell Carcinoma Model

Ser-PLL was labeled with $^{90}$Y using DTPA and the method applied for $^{111}$In-labeling [14,19]. The RCC model was established using a previously published method with slight modifications [22]. Briefly, the RCC model was produced by injecting $2.5 \times 10^5$ firefly luciferase gene-labeled Colon/26 (Colon26/Luc) cells along with Matrigel® matrix (Corning, NY, USA) into the right renal cortex of each Balb/c mouse under isoflurane anesthesia. Then PBS, free $^{90}$Y and $^{90}$Y-labeled Ser-PLL was immediately injected into the tail vein at a dose of 0.3 MBq/mouse. After 14 d, blood was collected from each vena cava and the kidneys were isolated under isoflurane anesthesia. The right kidney was homogenized in lysis buffer and its luciferase activity was measured with a luminometer (Lumat LB9507; EG&G Berthold, Württemberg, Germany). The cancer cells in each kidney were enumerated based on the luciferase activity and by using a regression line, as previously reported [23,24].

Blood was transferred to a microtube containing ethylenediamine-N,N,N′,N′-tetraacetic acid dipotassium salt dihydrate (EDTA-2K) and diluted tenfold with Turk's solution (Fujifilm Wako Pure Chemical Industries Ltd.). The white blood cells were then enumerated on a counting plate (Improved NEUBAUER; Elma Sales Co., Ltd., Saitama, Japan) under a microscope [25]. Sections of the untreated left kidneys were examined, and plasma creatinine was measured according to previously described methods.

### 2.10. Statistical Analysis

Statistical significance was analyzed using Student's $t$-test for two independent groups at a significance level of $p < 0.05$ and Dunnett's test for multiple comparisons with $p < 0.05$ as the minimum level of significance.

## 3. Results

### 3.1. Physicochemical Properties of Ser-Poly-L-Lysine

Table 1 shows the physicochemical properties of Ser-PLL and PLL. The mean particle diameters of PLL and Ser-PLL were 3.3 ± 0.5 and 4.1 ± 0.9 nm, respectively. The zeta potentials of PLL and Ser-PLL were 8.9 ± 1.6 and 6.6 ± 3.7 mV, respectively.

**Table 1.** Physicochemical properties of poly-L-lysine and Ser-poly-L-lysine.

| Compound | Diameter (nm) | Zeta Potential (mV) |
|---|---|---|
| Poly-L-lysine | 3.3 ± 0.5 | 8.9 ± 1.6 |
| Ser-poly-L-lysine | 4.1 ± 0.9 | 6.6 ± 3.7 |

### 3.2. Tissue Distribution of $^{111}$In-Labeled Ser-Poly-L-Lysine

Figure 1 shows the tissue distribution of $^{111}$In-labeled Ser-PLL following intravenous injection. Unmodified $^{111}$In-labeled PLL quickly disappeared from the plasma and was distributed to the liver and kidneys to levels of ~39% and ~23% of the dose, respectively, after 3 h. By contrast, $^{111}$In-labeled Ser-PLL accumulated mainly in the kidneys and ~91% of the original dose was retained there. Kidney accumulation was inversely proportional to the MW of Ser-PLL (Figures 1 and S2B). Ser-PAMAM accumulated mainly in the kidneys to levels of ~84% after 3 h in a similar manner to our previous study (Figure S2A) [8].

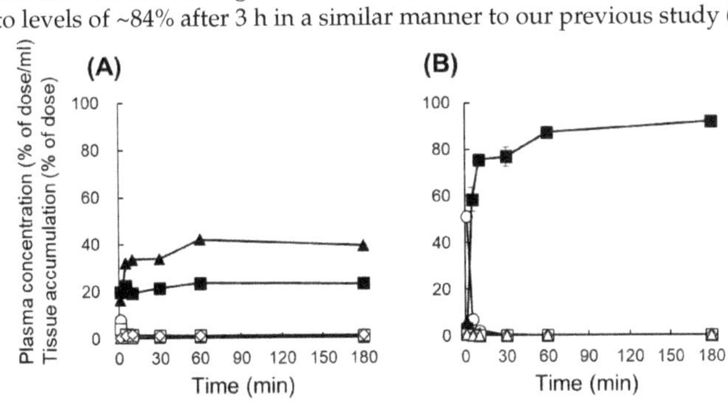


**Figure 1.** Plasma concentrations and tissue distributions of $^{111}$In-labeled poly-L-lysine (PLL) (**A**) and $^{111}$In-labeled Ser-poly-L-lysine (Ser-PLL) (**B**) after intravenous injection into mice. Data are means ± SE for three mice. ○, plasma; ▲, liver; ■, kidney; ◇, spleen; △, heart; □, lung.

### 3.3. Biodistribution Imaging of $^{111}$In-Labeled Ser-Poly-L-Lysine

Figure 2 shows SPECT/CT images of tissue distribution of $^{111}$In-labeled Ser-PLL after intravenous injection. The $^{111}$In-labeled Ser-PLL accumulated mainly in the renal cortex.

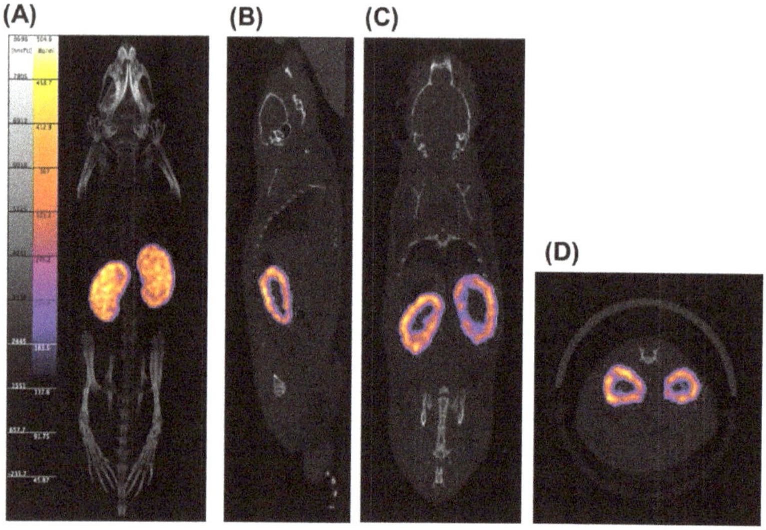

**Figure 2.** SPECT/CT imaging 180 min after intravenous injection of $^{111}$In-labeled Ser-poly-L-lysine (Ser-PLL) in mice. (**A**) 3D imaging; (**B**) sagittal plane; (**C**) coronal plane; (**D**) transverse plane.

### *3.4. Intrarenal Distribution of FITC-Labeled Ser-Poly-L-Lysine*

An evaluation of the intrarenal accumulation by FITC labeling clearly displayed fluorescence intensity derived from FITC-labeled Ser-PLL in the renal cortex (Figure 3A) but none in the renal medulla (data not shown). Enlarged microscopic images of the renal cortex exhibited high fluorescence intensity derived from FITC-labeled Ser-PLL in the proximal tubules (Figure 3B).

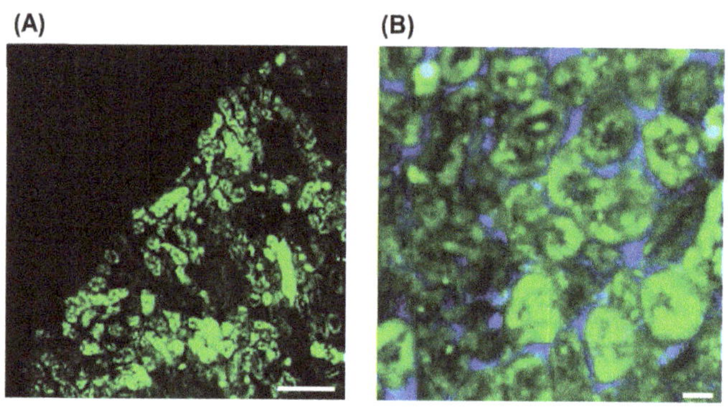

**Figure 3.** Intrarenal distribution of FITC-labeled Ser-poly-L-lysine (Ser-PLL) in tissue sections 60 min after intravenous injection into mice. (**A**) Renal cortex (scale bar = 200 μm) and (**B**) magnified image of cortex (scale bar = 25 μm). Fluorescence intensity was observed under a laser-scanning confocal microscope.

### *3.5. Ser-Poly-L-Lysine Biodegradability*

The biodegradability of $^{111}$In-labeled Ser-PLL was evaluated using the elution profiles of $^{111}$In-radioactivity recovered from the kidney homogenates (Figure 4). Relatively high $^{111}$In-radioactivity was detected in the high-MW fractions after the elution of intact $^{111}$In -labeled Ser-PLL, PLL, Ser-PAMAM, and PAMAM. The $^{111}$In-radioactivity partially shifted to the low-MW fraction. Nonetheless, it remained in the high-MW fraction after the elution of the kidney homogenates derived from mice injected with $^{111}$In-labeled Ser-PAMM and PAMAM (Figure 4A,B). In contrast, the $^{111}$In-radioactivity shifted to the low-MW fraction after the elution of the kidney homogenates derived from the mice injected with $^{111}$In-labeled Ser-PLL and PLL (Figure 4C,D).

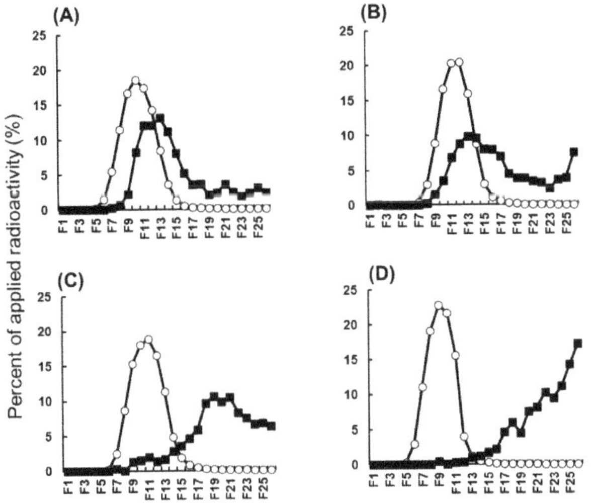


**Figure 4.** Gel filtration patterns of $^{111}$In-radioacticity in kidney homogenates from mice injected with $^{111}$In-labeled polyamidoamine (PAMAM) (**A**), $^{111}$In-labeled Ser-PAMAM (**B**), $^{111}$In-labeled poly-L-lysine (PLL) (**C**), and $^{111}$In-labeled Ser-poly-L-lysine (Ser-PLL) (**D**). ○, pre-injection (intact compounds); ■, 180 min post-injection.

### 3.6. Ser-Poly-L-Lysine Nephrotoxicity

Figure 5 shows the renal toxicity of Ser-PLL after continuous intravenous injection in mice. $HgCl_2$ administration significantly increased the nephrotoxicity indicators plasma creatine and BUN. By contrast, Ser-PLL did not increase the foregoing biomarkers after continuous intravenous injection for 5 d (Figure 5A,B). The kidney sections disclosed severe gap junction damage and necrosis (arrows) after the $HgCl_2$ treatment. However, Ser-PLL had negligible adverse effects on renal structure, and the tissue from Ser-PLL-treated mice was similar to that from PBS-treated and naïve mice (Figure 5C).

### 3.7. Therapeutic Potential and Safety of $^{90}$Y-Labeled Ser-Poly-L-Lysine in Mouse Model of Renal Cell Carcinoma (RCC)

Figure 6 shows the therapeutic potential of $^{90}$Y-labeled Ser-PLL in a mouse RCC model. Intravenously injected free $^{90}$Y had a negligible effect on kidney tumor growth. By contrast, intravenously injected $^{90}$Y-labeled Ser-PLL significantly suppressed any increase in the number of kidney tumor cells.

Intravenously injected free $^{90}$Y had a negligible effect on the white blood cell counts but significantly increased plasma creatine. In contrast, intravenously injected $^{90}$Y-labeled Ser-PLL had a negligible effect on plasma creatine or the white blood cell counts (Figure 7A,B). Partial glomerular damage and necrosis (arrow) was observed in the kidney sections of the free $^{90}$Y group. By contrast, no severe damage was detected in the kidney sections of the $^{90}$Y-labeled Ser-PLL group (Figure 7C).

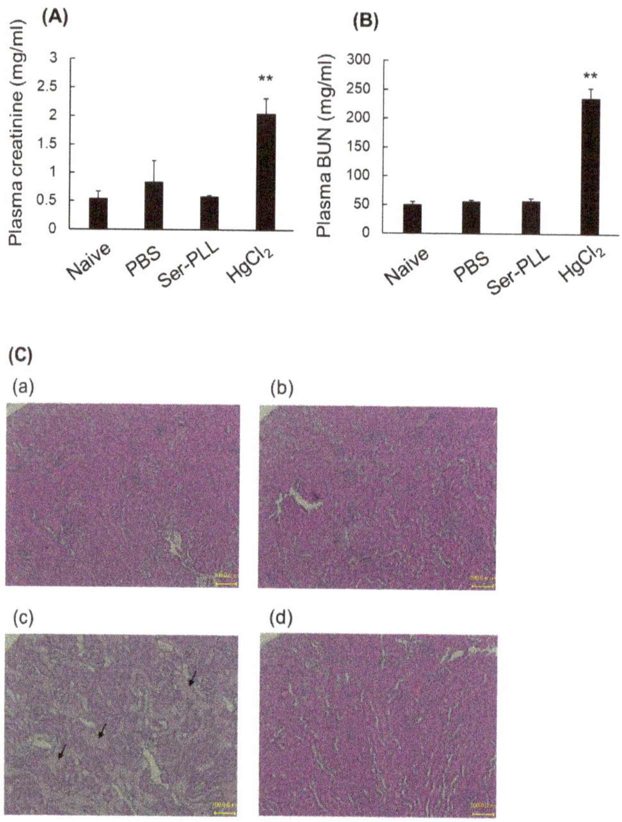


**Figure 5.** Plasma creatinine (**A**) and BUN (**B**) levels after continuous intravenous Ser-poly-L-lysine (Ser-PLL) injection for 5 d. Data are means ± SE for ≥ three mice. ** statistically significant difference compared with the naïve group ($p < 0.01$). (**C**) Histological examination of kidneys of mice in the naïve group (**a**), PBS (**b**), $HgCl_2$ (**c**), and Ser-poly-L-lysine (Ser-PLL) (**d**). (scale bar = 100 μm).

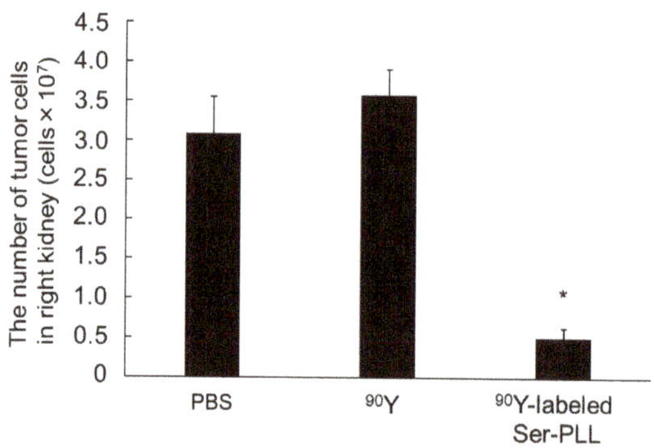


**Figure 6.** Effects of $^{90}$Y-labeled Ser-poly-L-lysine (Ser-PLL) on kidney tumor growth after tumor induction and intravenous injections. Number of Colon26/Luc cells in kidneys of mice intravenously injected either with free $^{90}$Y or with $^{90}$Y-labeled Ser-poly-L-lysine (Ser-PLL). Mice were sacrificed 14 d after tumor inoculation. Data are means ± SE for seven mice. * statistically significant difference compared with PBS group ($p < 0.05$).

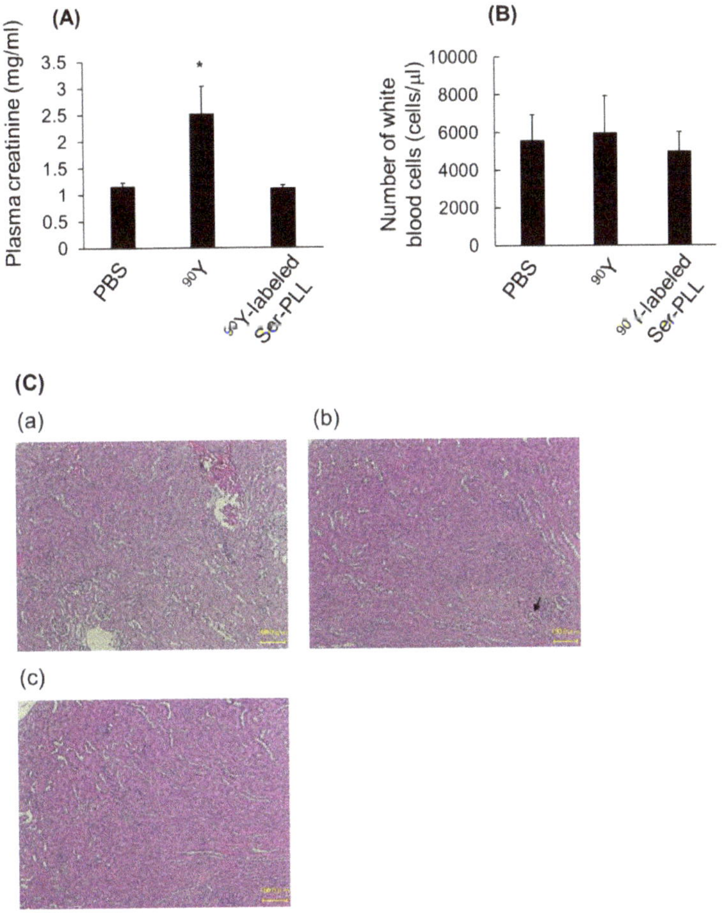


**Figure 7.** Plasma creatinine (**A**) and white blood cell counts (**B**) after intravenous injection of $^{90}$Y-labeled Ser-poly-L-lysine (Ser-PLL) at 0.3 MBq/mouse into mice inoculated with Colon26/Luc cells in right kidney cortex. (**C**) Histological examination of left kidneys of mice injected with $^{90}$Y-labeled Ser-poly-L-lysine (Ser-PLL) at 0.3 MBq/mouse and inoculated with Colon26/Luc cells in right kidney cortex. PBS (**a**), free $^{90}$Y (**b**), $^{90}$Y-labeled Ser-poly-L-lysine (Ser-PLL) (**c**). (scale bar = 100 μm) Mice were sacrificed 14 d after tumor induction. Data are means ± SE of ≥ three mice. * statistically significant difference compared with PBS group ($p < 0.05$).

## 4. Discussion

In the present study, we successfully developed and evaluated Ser-PLL as a biodegradable kidney-targeted drug carrier to be administered as radionuclide therapy for renal cell carcinoma (RCC). We previously reported that Ser-PAMAM accumulated mainly in the kidneys, and the hydroxyl and amino groups of Ser play important roles in kidney targeting [8]. For this reason, we coupled the amino groups of PLL with the carboxyl groups of Ser to form Ser-PLL, which bears both hydroxyl and amino groups. Ser-PLL had slightly greater kidney accumulation than Ser-PAMAM (Figure S2A), possibly because the estimated average number of conjugated Ser residues was 45 in Ser-PLL, whereas Ser-PAMAM conjugated only 32. The number of conjugated Ser residues is proportional to renal affinity [8]. These results indicate that Ser modification could be applied in a kidney-targeted delivery system using linear macromolecular drug carriers in addition to branched macromolecular drug carriers.

Kidney targeting is challenging because most drug nanocarriers are trapped in the hepatic and splenic reticuloendothelial systems. It is essential to maintain the balance between target site affinity and non-target site elimination [26,27]. Here, the hydroxyl groups of Ser might have eluded recognition by the hepatic and splenic reticuloendothelial systems as they are readily hydrated and induce a cage effect against the reticuloendothelial system [28]. In our previous study, we demonstrated that Ser-PAMAM was distributed in the proximal tubules via glomerular filtration. Micropinocytosis and caveola-mediated endocytosis have been implicated in the affinity of Ser-PAMAM for proximal tubules [8]. Therefore, we postulate that Ser-PLL is distributed in the proximal tubules in the same manner as Ser-PAMAM, due to the size of Ser-PLL (~5 nm), which is smaller than the glomerular filtration size cutoff (10 nm) [29–31]. Moreover, both Ser-PLL and Ser-PAMAM have the same surface functional groups. The foregoing results of Ser-PLL (PLL MW = 4000–15,000) (Figure 1) and the low renal accumulation of Ser-PLL (H) (PLL MW range = 15,000–30,000) (Figure S2B) suggest that Ser-PLL (PLL MW = 4000–15,000) is the optimal size for kidney-targeted delivery mediated by glomerular filtration.

Post-elution $^{111}$In radioactivity detection by gel filtration chromatography was established as a method to assess the biodegradability of macromolecular drug carriers [21]. Akamatsu et al. (1998) evaluated the biodegradability of poly-L-glutamic acid (PLGA) and PLL using the aforementioned system and demonstrated that PLGA and PLL were degraded and eluted in the low-MW fractions of gel filtration chromatography [21]. This finding was in good agreement with the results for unmodified PLL in the present study (Figure 4C). Ser-PLL is a polymeric bilayer with two different types of amino acids. Its surface Ser layer was released into the kidneys at 3 h after intravenous injection (Figure 4D). Gel filtration chromatography of unmodified PLL and Ser-PLL, together with the results of quick kidney distribution (Figure 1), indicated that both substances were digested in the kidneys within 3 h after their distribution. Ser-PAMAM was synthesized by coupling Ser with PAMAM via the same amido linkage as Ser-PLL. Nevertheless, these two conjugates differed in terms of the release rates of their surface Ser layers. Ser-PLL released its surface Ser layer faster than Ser-PAMAM (Figure 4B,D) possibly because the dendritic structure of Ser-PAMAM partially blocked peptidase access and, by extension, conjugate digestion in the kidneys. These discoveries, along with the fact that unmodified PAMAM is more slowly biodegradable than unmodified PLL (Figure 4A,C), indicate that Ser-PLL has superior biodegradability to dendritic Ser conjugates.

The $^{90}$Y isotope is a β-emitter with a high endpoint energy. It is classified as a first-order unique forbidden emitter and is expected to be suitable for radionuclide therapy against various tumor cells [12–14]. As $^{90}$Y beta rays do not penetrate from outside the body, however, it is impossible to confirm their tissue distribution by imaging. Therefore, $^{111}$In was selected for the tissue distribution analysis as it is a gamma-nucleus species with high penetrating power, imageable gamma rays, and a physical half-life near that of $^{90}$Y. It was confirmed from the results of the animal experiments that there was no significant difference between $^{111}$In and $^{90}$Y [12,13] in terms of their in vivo tissue distributions. Hence, both $^{90}$Y-labeled Ser-PLL and $^{111}$In-labeled Ser-PLL would be similar in this respect. In the mouse RCC model, cancer cells were inoculated into the proximal tubules and their vicinity in the renal cortex as these structures are associated with RCC pathogenesis. Here, specific kidney renal cortex distributions of $^{111}$In-labeled Ser-PLL were observed. According to the intrarenal distribution study, FITC-labeled Ser-PLL accumulated mainly in the proximal tubules. Thus, we postulate that $^{90}$Y-labeled Ser-PLL would also accumulate in the proximal tubules, where the tumor localizes. Furthermore, beta-rays suppressed kidney tumor growth.

It was reported that $^{90}$Y readily induces bone marrow depression (BMD) [14]. However, neither free $^{90}$Y nor $^{90}$Y-labeled Ser-PLL affected the white blood cell counts here.

Therefore, the beta ray energy derived from $^{90}Y$ fell below the BMD threshold. Moreover, the selective renal distribution of Ser-PLL also avoided inducing BMD.

It was previously reported that glomerular capillary endothelial and mesangial cells play important roles in the pathogenesis of radiation-induced nephropathy. In addition, $^{90}Y$ caused radiation damage mostly in the glomeruli [32]. Based on the tissue and intrarenal distribution analyses performed here, Ser-PLL should pass through the glomeruli after intravenous injection. Hence, we suggest that the glomerular distribution and radiation nephrotoxicity of $^{90}Y$ could be avoided by using Ser-PLL. Detailed toxicological studies on $^{90}Y$-Ser-PLL are required before it can be clinically applied. Notwithstanding, the results of this work indicated that $^{90}Y$-labeled Ser-PLL effectively suppresses renal tumor growth while attenuating $^{90}Y$ nephrotoxicity. To the best of our knowledge, this is the first study to demonstrate suppression of renal tumor growth by kidney-targeting of $^{90}Y$ after intravenous injection.

## 5. Conclusions

The present study demonstrated that Ser modification was effective in kidney-targeted drug delivery using a linear PLL as the drug carrier core. Ser-PLL selectively accumulated in the renal proximal tubules which are the sites of renal cell carcinoma (RCC) pathogenesis. Ser-PLL had higher biodegradability than the dendritic Ser conjugate. Renal tumor growth was effectively suppressed by $^{90}Y$-mediated kidney targeting via Ser-PLL. The foregoing findings indicate that Ser-PLL is promising as a biodegradable kidney-targeted drug carrier for radionuclide therapy against RCC.

**Supplementary Materials:** The following supporting information can be downloaded at: https://www.mdpi.com/article/10.3390/pharmaceutics14091946/s1. Scheme S1: Ser-poly-L-lysine (Ser-PLL) synthesis; Figure S1: $^{1}H$-NMR spectra for Ser (A), poly-L-lysine (PLL) (B), and Ser-poly-L-lysine (Ser-PLL) (C,D) in deuterated water.; Figure S2: (A) Kidney accumulation of $^{111}In$-labeled Ser-polyamidoamine (PAMAM) dendrimer (G3) and $^{111}In$-labeled Ser-poly-L-lysine (Ser-PLL) after intravenous injection in mice. (B) Plasma concentration and tissue accumulation of $^{111}In$-labeled high-MW Ser-poly-L-lysine (Ser-PLL(H)) wherein poly-L-lysine (MW range = 15,000–30,000) was conjugated with Ser after intravenous injection into mice. Data are means ± SE for three mice. ○, plasma; ▲, liver; ■, kidney; ◇, spleen; △, heart; □, lung. * statistically significant difference compared with Ser-PAMAM group ($p < 0.05$).

**Author Contributions:** Conceptualization, H.K. (Hidemasa Katsumi); methodology, H.K. (Hidemasa Katsumi), H.K. (Hiroyuki Kimura) and H.K. (Hidekazu Kawashima); validation, H.K. (Hidemasa Katsumi), M.M. and A.Y.; formal analysis, H.K. (Hidemasa Katsumi); investigation, H.K. (Hidemasa Katsumi), S.K., S.Y., R.T. (Rie Takashima), T.I., R.T. (Rina Tanaka), S.M. and H.K. (Hiroyuki Kimura); resources, H.K. (Hidemasa Katsumi) and A.Y.; data curation, H.K. (Hidemasa Katsumi); writing—original draft preparation, H.K. (Hidemasa Katsumi); writing—review and editing, M.M. and A.Y.; visualization, H.K. (Hidemasa Katsumi); supervision, H.K. (Hidemasa Katsumi) and A.Y.; and project administration, H.K. (Hidemasa Katsumi). All authors have read and agreed to the published version of the manuscript.

**Funding:** This work was partially supported by The Canon Foundation (H. Katsumi) and JSPS KAKENHI Grant No. 19K22982.

**Institutional Review Board Statement:** The animal study protocol was approved by the Animal Experimentation Committee of Kyoto Pharmaceutical University under Protocol Code Nos. 17-029 and 17-024 approved in April 2017 and under Protocol Code No. BIOP-20-002 approved in April 2020 and under Protocol Code No. A22-020 and A22-022 approved in April 2022.

**Informed Consent Statement:** Not applicable.

**Data Availability Statement:** Not applicable.

**Conflicts of Interest:** The authors have no conflict of interest to declare.

## References


1. Muglia, V.F.; Prando, A. Renal Cell Carcinoma: Histological Classification and Correlation With Imaging Findings. *Radiol. Bras* **2015**, *48*, 166–174. [CrossRef]
2. Wood, L.S. Management of Vascular Endothelial Growth Factor and Multikinase Inhibitor Side Effects. *Clin. J. Oncol. Nurs.* **2009** *13* (Suppl. 1), 13–18. [CrossRef]
3. Battelli, C.; Cho, D.C. mTOR Inhibitors in Renal Cell Carcinoma. *Therapy* **2011**, *8*, 359–367. [CrossRef]
4. Jung, K.; Zeng, X.; Bilusic, M. Nivolumab-Associated Acute Glomerulonephritis: A Case Report and Literature Review. *BMC Nephrol.* **2016**, *17*, 188. [CrossRef]
5. Huang, X.; Ma, Y.; Li, Y.; Han, F.; Lin, W. Targeted Drug Delivery Systems for Kidney Diseases. *Front. Bioeng. Biotechnol.* **2021**, *9*, 683247 [CrossRef]
6. Liu, D.; Du, Y.; Jin, F.Y.; Xu, X.L.; Du, Y.Z. Renal Cell-Targeted Drug Delivery Strategy for Acute Kidney Injury and Chronic Kidney Disease: A Mini-Review. *Mol. Pharm.* **2021**, *18*, 3206–3222. [CrossRef]
7. Yuan, Z.X.; Shang, Z.; Gu, J.; He, L. Renal Targeting Delivery Systems. *Future Med. Chem.* **2019**, *11*, 2237–2240. [CrossRef]
8. Matsuura, S.; Katsumi, H.; Suzuki, H.; Hirai, N.; Hayashi, H.; Koshino, K.; Higuchi, T.; Yagi, Y.; Kimura, H.; Sakane, T.; et al. l-Serine-Modified Polyamidoamine Dendrimer as a Highly Potent Renal Targeting Drug Carrier. *Proc. Natl. Acad. Sci. USA* **2018** *115*, 10511–10516. [CrossRef]
9. Matsuura, S.; Katsumi, H.; Suzuki, H.; Hirai, N.; Takashima, R.; Morishita, M.; Sakane, T.; Yamamoto, A. l-Cysteine and l-Serine Modified Dendrimer with Multiple Reduced Thiols as a Kidney-Targeting Reactive Oxygen Species Scavenger to Prevent Renal Ischemia/Reperfusion Injury. *Pharmaceutics* **2018**, *10*, 251. [CrossRef]
10. Katsumi, H.; Takashima, R.; Suzuki, H.; Hirai, N.; Matsuura, S.; Kimura, H.; Morishita, M.; Yamamoto, A. S-nitrosylated l-Serine-Modified Dendrimer as a Kidney-Targeting Nitric Oxide Donor for Prevention of Renal Ischaemia/Reperfusion Injury. *Free Radic. Res.* **2020**, *54*, 841–847. [CrossRef]
11. Roberts, J.C.; Bhalgat, M.K.; Zera, R.T. Preliminary Biological Evaluation of Polyamidoamine (PAMAM) Starburst Dendrimers. *J. Biomed. Mater. Res.* **1996**, *30*, 53–65. [CrossRef]
12. Sugyo, A.; Tsuji, A.B.; Sudo, H.; Okada, M.; Koizumi, M.; Satoh, H.; Kurosawa, G.; Kurosawa, Y.; Saga, T. Evaluation of Efficacy of Radioimmunotherapy With 90Y-Labeled Fully Human Anti-transferrin Receptor Monoclonal Antibody in Pancreatic Cancer Mouse Models. *PLoS ONE* **2015**, *10*, e0123761. [CrossRef]
13. Fujiwara, K.; Koyama, K.; Suga, K.; Ikemura, M.; Saito, Y.; Hino, A.; Iwanari, H.; Kusano-Arai, O.; Mitsui, K.; Kasahara, H.; et al. 90Y-Labeled Anti-ROBO1 Monoclonal Antibody Exhibits Antitumor Activity Against Small Cell Lung Cancer Xenografts. *PLoS ONE* **2015**, *10*, e0125468. [CrossRef]
14. Aung, W.; Tsuji, A.B.; Sudo, H.; Sugyo, A.; Ukai, Y.; Kouda, K.; Kurosawa, Y.; Furukawa, T.; Saga, T. Radioimmunotherapy of Pancreatic Cancer Xenografts in Nude Mice Using 90Y-Labeled Anti-α6β4 Integrin Antibody. *Oncotarget* **2016**, *7*, 38835–38844. [CrossRef]
15. Knox, S.J.; Goris, M.L.; Trisler, K.; Negrin, R.; Davis, T.; Liles, T.M.; Grillo-López, A.; Chinn, P.; Varns, C.; Ning, S.C.; et al. Yttrium-90-Labeled Anti-CD20 Monoclonal Antibody Therapy of Recurrent B-Cell Lymphoma. *Clin. Cancer Res.* **1996**, *2*, 457–470.
16. Spies, S.M. Imaging and Dosing in Radioimmunotherapy with Yttrium 90 Ibritumomab Tiuxetan (Zevalin). *Semin. Nucl. Med.* **2004**, *34* (Suppl. 1), 10–13. [CrossRef]
17. Okuda, T.; Sugiyama, A.; Niidome, T.; Aoyagi, H. Characters of dendritic poly(L-lysine) analogues with the terminal lysines replaced with arginines and histidines as gene carriers in vitro. *Biomaterials* **2004**, *25*, 537–544. [CrossRef]
18. Katsuraya, K.; Jeon, K.J.; Nakashima, H.; Uryu, T. NMR Studies on Structure and Action Mechanism of Sulfated Dodecyl Laminaripentaoside with High Anti-Human Immunodeficiency Virus Activity. *Polym. J.* **1999**, *31*, 924–928. [CrossRef]
19. Hnatowich, D.J.; Layne, W.W.; Childs, R.L. The Preparation and Labeling of DTPA-Coupled Albumin. *Int. J. Appl. Radiat. Isot.* **1982**, *33*, 327–332. [CrossRef]
20. Katsumi, H.; Nishikawa, M.; Ma, S.F.; Yamashita, F.; Hashida, M. Physicochemical, Tissue Distribution, and Vasodilation Characteristics of Nitrosated Serum Albumin: Delivery of Nitric Oxide In Vivo. *J. Pharm. Sci.* **2004**, *93*, 2343–2352. [CrossRef]
21. Akamatsu, K.; Imai, M.; Yamasaki, Y.; Nishikawa, M.; Takakura, Y.; Hashida, M. Disposition Characteristics of Glycosylated Poly(Amino Acids) as Liver Cell-Specific Drug Carrier. *J. Drug Target.* **1998**, *6*, 229–239. [CrossRef]
22. Norian, L.A.; Kresowik, T.P.; Rosevear, H.M.; James, B.R.; Rosean, T.R.; Lightfoot, A.J.; Kucaba, T.A.; Schwarz, C.; Weydert, C.J.; Henry, M.D.; et al. Eradication of metastatic renal cell carcinoma after adenovirus-encoded TNF-related apoptosis-inducing ligand (TRAIL)/CpG immunotherapy. *PLoS ONE* **2012**, *7*, e31085. [CrossRef]
23. Hyoudou, K.; Nishikawa, M.; Umeyama, Y.; Kobayashi, Y.; Yamashita, F.; Hashida, M. Inhibition of Metastatic Tumor Growth in Mouse Lung by Repeated Administration of Polyethylene Glycol-Conjugated Catalase: Quantitative Analysis with Firefly Luciferase-Expressing Melanoma Cells. *Clin. Cancer Res.* **2004**, *10*, 7685–7691. [CrossRef]
24. Katsumi, H.; Sano, J.; Nishikawa, M.; Hanzawa, K.; Sakane, T.; Yamamoto, A. Molecular Design of Bisphosphonate-Modified Proteins for Efficient Bone Targeting In Vivo. *PLoS ONE* **2015**, *10*, e0135966. [CrossRef]
25. Bayrami, G.; Boskabady, M.H. The Potential Effect of the Extract of Crocus sativus and Safranal on the Total and Differential White Blood Cells of Ovalbumin-Sensitized Guinea Pigs. *Res. Pharm. Sci.* **2012**, *7*, 249–255.
26. Takakura, Y.; Hashida, M. Macromolecular Carrier Systems for Targeted Drug Delivery: Pharmacokinetic Considerations on Biodistribution. *Pharm. Res.* **1996**, *13*, 820–831. [CrossRef]

27. Hashida, M. Role of Pharmacokinetic Consideration for the Development of Drug Delivery Systems: A Historical Overview. *Adv. Drug Deliv. Rev.* **2020**, *157*, 71–82. [CrossRef]
28. Zhang, Z.; Lin, Y.A.; Kim, S.Y.; Su, L.; Liu, J.; Kannan, R.M.; Kannan, S. Systemic Dendrimer-Drug Nanomedicines for Long-Term Treatment of Mild-Moderate Cerebral Palsy in a Rabbit Model. *J. Neuroinflammation* **2020**, *17*, 319. [CrossRef]
29. Williams, R.M.; Shah, J.; Tian, H.S.; Chen, X.; Geissmann, F.; Jaimes, E.A.; Heller, D.A. Selective Nanoparticle Targeting of the Renal Tubules. *Hypertension* **2018**, *71*, 87–94. [CrossRef]
30. Williams, R.M.; Jaimes, E.A.; Heller, D.A. Nanomedicines for Kidney Diseases. *Kidney Int.* **2016**, *90*, 740–745. [CrossRef]
31. Zuckerman, J.E.; Davis, M.E. Targeting Therapeutics to the Glomerulus with Nanoparticles. *Adv. Chronic Kidney Dis.* **2013**, *20*, 500–507. [CrossRef] [PubMed]
32. Rolleman, E.J.; Melis, M.; Valkema, R.; Boerman, O.C.; Krenning, E.P.; de Jong, M. Kidney Protection During Peptide Receptor Radionuclide Therapy with Somatostatin Analogues. *Eur. J. Nucl. Med. Mol. Imaging* **2010**, *37*, 1018–1031. [CrossRef] [PubMed]

*pharmaceutics*

MDPI

*Article*

# Single -and Multi-Walled Carbon Nanotubes as Nanocarriers for the Delivery of 7-Hydroxyflavone

**Cecilia Espíndola [1], Alejandro Javier Correa [1], Manuel López-López [2,*], Pilar López-Cornejo [1,*], Eva Bernal [1], José Antonio Lebrón [1], Francisco José Ostos [1,3,4], Mohammed Rafii-El-Idrissi Benhnia [3,4] and María Luisa Moyá [1,*]**

1 Department of Physical Chemistry, University of Seville, C/Profesor García González 1, 41012 Seville, Spain
2 Department of Chemical Engineering, Physical Chemistry and Material Sciences, Campus de El Carmen, Avda. de las Fuerzas Armadas s/n, 21071 Huelva, Spain
3 Clinical Unit of Infectious Diseases, Microbiology and Parasitology, Institute of Biomedicine of Seville (IBiS), Virgen del Rocío University Hospital, CSIC, University of Seville, 41013 Seville, Spain
4 Department of Medical Biochemistry, Molecular Biology, and Immunology, School of Medicine, University of Seville, 41009 Seville, Spain
* Correspondence: manuel.lopez@diq.uhu.es (M.L.-L.); pcornejo@us.es (P.L.-C.); moya@us.es (M.L.M.); Tel.: +34-954557175 (M.L.M.)

**Abstract:** The research on flavonoids has exponentially grown since their first therapeutic evidence, in 1937. They are effective in vitro in a wide range of human diseases, particularly those mediated by free radicals, such as cancer, atherosclerosis, AIDS, or neuronal diseases. However, their applications have been reduced due to their low solubility, poor absorption, and rapid metabolism. Flavonoid encapsulation in nanocarriers significantly improves their oral absorption, protects the drug against degradation, decreases the first-pass hepatic effect, and makes absorption through the lymphatic system easier. In this work, carbon nanotubes were used as nanocarriers of 7-hydroxyflavone, 7-HF. The encapsulation of 7-HF into pristine single- and multi-walled carbon nanotubes, and into -COOH functionalized single-walled carbon nanotubes has been investigated. The equilibrium association constants were estimated. The structural backbone of 7-HF, two benzene rings linked through three carbon atoms that form a pyran heterocyclic ring containing a keto group, seems to play a key role in the 7-HF/CNT interactions, although other types of interactions are also at work. The in vitro release of 7-HF was studied at three pHs, 2.0, 7.4, and 9.2, mimicking the different biological barriers of the human organism.

**Keywords:** 7-Hydroxyflavone; single-walled carbon nanotubes; multi-walled carbon nanotubes; encapsulation; equilibrium binding constants; drug release

## 1. Introduction

Flavonoids are polyphenolic phytochemicals, formed from the secondary metabolism of plants. They present a wide range of structures and contribute to the nutritional and organoleptic properties of edible plants, vegetables, fruits, and some beverages, such as coffee, tea, beer, or wine [1–3]. Flavonoids can be classified into various groups: flavones, flavanones, flavonoids glycosides, flavonolignans, flavanas, isoflavones, anthocyanidins, aurones, leucoanthocyanidines, neoflavonoids, and chalcones [4]. All flavonoid groups have several therapeutic activities [5], but among them, flavones have been extensively studied due to their anti-inflammatory [4], antimicrobial [6], antioxidant [7], or antitumor activities [8,9]; being used in the treatment of a wide range of human diseases, such as atherosclerosis, diabetes, cancer, Alzheimer's disease, etc.

7-Hydroxyflavone, 7-HF, has the structure shown in Figure 1. Its basic structural feature is the benzo-c-pyrone (C6–C3–C6) skeleton. This C6–C3–C6 skeleton consists of two aromatic rings (rings A and C) linked through a linear three-carbon chain which formed a closed pyran ring (ring B), where a keto group is present. A hydroxyl group can be found in position 7. Despite 7-HF having a low antioxidant activity measured through methods such as DPPH, 7-hydroxyflavone has been shown to be effective against nicotine-associated oxidative stress [10]. This is so because, although the most frequent mechanism of flavones' antioxidant activity involves the scavenging of reactive oxygen species (ROS) and peroxynitrite, they can exert an indirect antioxidant activity through the transcriptional induction of genes with antioxidant properties. 7-HF has been found to inhibit lipopolysaccharides-induced inflammation via attenuating the production of NO, prostaglandin E2, PGE2, tumor necrosis factor α, TNF-α, and interleukin 6, IL-6, which are mediators in the inflammatory processes accompanying several diseases such as arthritis [11,12]. 7-HF also exerts a cytotoxic and antiproliferative effect on leukemia H60 cells [13] and inhibits the replication of the enterovirus 71, which causes the hand, foot, and mouth disease, an infection affecting many children in Asia [14]. The neuroprotectant activity of 7-HF, important in relation to aging-associated neurological diseases, has also been investigated [15]. Notwithstanding the therapeutic properties, 7-HF has a low solubility in water, which limits its applications due to poor absorption and rapid metabolism. The encapsulation of this flavone in suitable nanocarriers can substantially increase its solubility, thus improving oral absorption, protecting 7-HF from degradation, and enhancing its therapeutic effects.

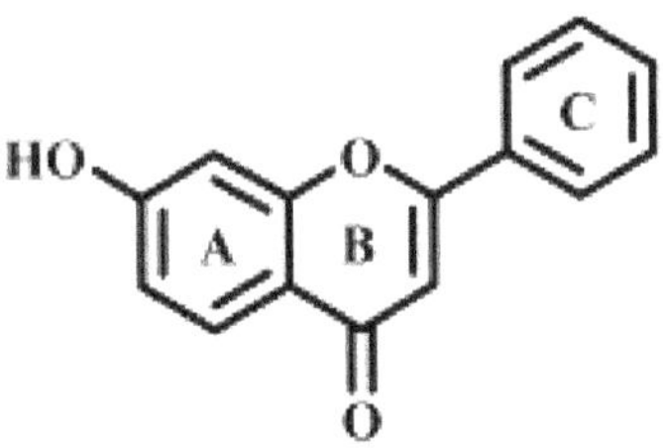


**Figure 1.** Structure of 7-hydroxyflavone, 7-HF.

Several types of nanocarriers had been used to encapsulate and, subsequently, release drugs in the therapeutic target [16–19]. One of those types are carbon nanotubes, CNTs. They are constituted by pure carbon atoms, present in a repetitive hexagonal pattern for cylindrical tubes. They were discovered by Ijima [20] as an allotropic form of carbon by the electric arc discharge of graphitic materials at a high temperature. CNTs can be described as folded forms of graphenes, which are single-layered graphitic sheets. CNTs can be classified into single-walled carbon nanotubes, SWCNTs, double-walled carbon nanotubes, DWCNTs, multi-walled carbon nanotubes, MWCNT, and functionalized carbon nanotubes, f-CNTs [21]. SWCNTs are formed by the folding of one single graphene sheet; in the case of DWCNTs, two sheets of graphene are folded upon each other; and, for MWCNTs, 2 to 10 sheets of graphene are folded into each other or a single sheet is rolled to produce a multi-walled structure (see Figure 2). The functionalization of the CNTs is achieved by a synthetic process with the goal of changing some properties of pristine CNTs, such as water solubility.

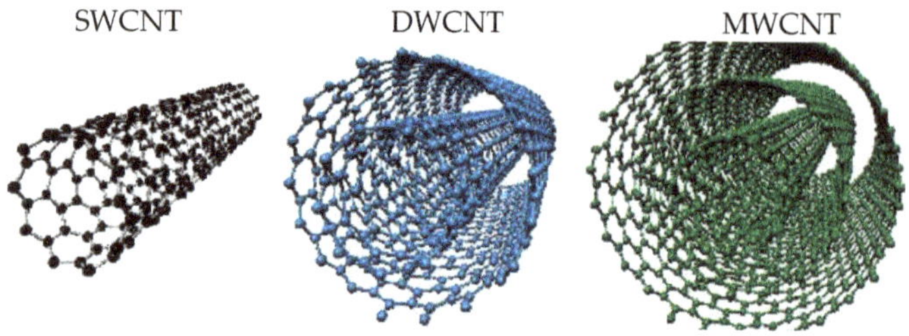


**Figure 2.** Structure of carbon nanotubes, CNTs.

CNTs have several characteristics which make them interesting for their use in drug delivery applications: high inner volume, ability for the immobilization of many species, and excellent functionalization ability, accompanied by their biocompatibility [21]. In fact, they have been used in cancer treatment, theranostic applications, and the delivery of therapeutic molecules, such as proteins, peptides, RNA, DNA, siRNA, etc. [22–26]. With this in mind, and with the goal of improving the bioavailability of 7-HF, in this work, the binding of 7-hydroxyflavone to single- and multi-walled carbon nanotubes has been investigated. It is important to point out that, as was mentioned above in the Introduction, 7-HF has important therapeutic properties, which make its encapsulation in adequate nanocarriers an issue worth investigating. The equilibrium association constants were estimated by considering the changes in the flavone emission fluorescence intensity upon increasing the CNTs' concentration. Pristine MWCNTs and SWCNTs were used, as well as the functionalized SWCNTCOOH. Subsequently, the in vitro release of 7-HF from the CNTs was studied at pHs 2.0, 7.4, and 9.2, mimicking the different biological barriers in a human organism.

## 2. Materials and Methods

### 2.1. Materials

7-Hydroxyflavone (purity > 98%), the organic solvents (purity > 99.9%) used, as well as all the components of the buffer solutions prepared (with the highest purity available), were purchased from Sigma (Darmstadt, Germany). Pristine and functionalized SWCNTs were obtained from NanoLab Inc. (Waltham, MA, USA), both of them with a 1–5 μm length and 1.5 nm diameter. MWCNTs were supplied by Dropsens S.L. (Oviedo, Spain), with a 1.5 μm length and 10 nm diameter.

### 2.2. Preparation of Buffer Solutions

The buffer solution at pH = 9.2 was prepared with $NaH_2PO_4$ and $Na_2HPO_4$, at concentrations of 3.7 mM and 96.3 mM, respectively. The pH was adjusted using a pH-meter Basic 20+ from Crison (Barcelona, Spain).

The neutral buffer solution Tris/HCl, pH = 7.4, was 22.7 mM in tris(hydroxymethyl) aminomethane and 9.8 mM in HCl. The pH was adjusted with the above-mentioned pH-meter.

The acid buffer solution NaCl/HCl, pH = 2.0, was 8.06 mM in NaCl and 1.9 mM in HCl. The pH was adjusted with the above-mentioned pH-meter.

All solutions were prepared with deionized water (from a Millipore Milli-Q system, Darmstadt, Germany), with a conductivity < $10^{-6}$ S $m^{-1}$.

### 2.3. In vitro Cytotoxicity Assays

The cytotoxicity of the CNTs, at different concentration values, was estimated in vitro using the CyQUANT™ LDH cytotoxicity assay [27]. Several cell lines from a commercial supplier (ATCC®, Manassas, VA, USA) were used, Vero E6 (normal monkey kidney epithelial cells), HeLa (human cervical carcinoma epithelial cells), U937 (human leukemia monocytic cells), THP-1 (human leukemia monocytic cells), and Jurkat (human T leukaemia cells). Each cell line was seeded at $10 \times 10^4$ cells/well into Nunc flat-bottomed 96-well plates (ThermoFisher Scientific, Waltham, MA, USA), using complete D-10 or R-10 (Dulbecco's modified Eagle medium (DMEM) or Roswell Park Memorial Institute (RPMI) supplemented with 10% of fetal bovine serum (FBS), and penicillin, streptomycin, and L-glutamine), incubated at 37 °C in 5% $CO_2$, and used the following day (75 to 90% confluence). The FBS used in all experiments was heat inactivated (56 °C, 30 min) prior to use to eliminate complement activity. CNT solutions at different concentration values were added to each well and the plates were incubated for 36 h at 37 °C in 5% $CO_2$. Controls D-10 or R-10 medium alone were used as the negative control. An amount of 10 µL of 10X Lysis Buffer, and 10 µL of sterile ultrapure water were added to each set of triplicate wells, and used as the Maximum LDH Activity and Spontaneous LDH activity, respectively. Later, the medium from each well was collected by centrifugation of the plate and used to test the cytotoxicity of the CNT solutions using the CyQUANT™ LDH Cytotoxicity Assay Kit according to the manufacturer's instructions (Invitrogen™ from Thermo Fisher Scientific, Waltham, MA, USA). The cytotoxicity was measured by fluorescence in a CLARIOstar® (BMG LABTECH, Allmendgrün, Ortenberg, Germany). Each CNT concentration was measured in triplicate and the tests were repeated thrice independently. The cell viability was calculated by using Equation (1):

$$\%\ \text{Cell viability} = 100 - \left(\left[\frac{\text{Compound} - \text{treated LDH activity} - \text{Spontaneous LDH activity}}{\text{Maximum LDH activity} - \text{Spontaneous LDH activity}}\right] \times 100\right) \quad (1)$$

Cell viability values were also checked by trypan blue method [28] and no significant differences were observed.

### 2.4. *Fluorescence Measurements*

Fluorescence emission spectra of 7-HF were registered in a Hitachi 2500 spectrofluorimeter, connected to a Lauda water flow thermostat to keep the temperature constant at $298.0 \pm 0.1$ K. A quartz cell of 10 mm path length was used.

The excitation wavelength was λ = 350 nm and the spectra were recorded from λ = 400 to λ = 650 nm. The maximum fluorescence emission intensity was measured at λ = 526.nm. The excitation and emission slits were 2.5 and 5 nm, respectively.

#### 2.4.1. Fluorescence Emission Intensity Calibration Curves

A concentrated 7-HF solution, $5.04 \cdot 10^{-4}$ M, in ethanol was prepared. This solution was kept at 4 °C in the dark in order to avoid the flavone degradation. Three calibration curves were obtained, each one for the three different pH conditions. 7-HF solutions of known concentrations, within the range $2.52 \cdot 10^{-7}$–$2.02 \cdot 10^{-5}$ M, were prepared as follows. An adequate aliquot of the ethanolic concentrated 7-HF solution was added to a 10 mL flask. The organic solvent was evaporated with an air flow and, subsequently, the buffer was added up to the calibration mark. The flask was then introduced in a sonicator for 20 min, in darkness. In this way, the flavone is totally dissolved in the buffer solution. Once the fluorescence emission intensity of each solution is measured at λ = 526 nm, the calibration curve is obtained. Temperature was kept at $298.0 \pm 0.1$ K.

### 2.5. *Encapsulation of 7-HF in the CNTs*

The encapsulation of 7-HF in the different CNTs investigated was carried out at pH = 7.4 (buffer Tris/HCl), keeping the flavone concentration constant at $1.50 \cdot 10^{-5}$ M and varying the CNT concentration within the range 0–0.35 g/L for the SWCNTs, 0–0.22 g/L for the MWCNTs, and 0–0.10 g/L for the SWCNT-COOH. First, an adequate aliquot of the ethanolic flavone solution was added to an Eppendorf tube of 2 mL. After evaporating the organic solvent with an air flow, 2 mL of a CNT solution of a known concentration, in a Tris/HCl buffer, was added to the Eppendorf tube. Afterwards, the tube was sonicated for 20 min in darkness. Finally, the tube was centrifuged at 13,500 rpm for 30 min. Once the supernatant was separated, the fluorescence emission intensity was measured, at

298.0 ± 0.1 K, under the working conditions indicated in Section 2.4. In this way, the amount of 7-HF not bound to the CNTs can be known by using the calibration curve at pH = 7.4.

*2.6. Encapsulation Efficiency*

The encapsulation efficiency was calculated by using the following equation:

$$\%7 - HF_{encapsulated} = \left(1 - \frac{m_{7-HF}^{supernatant}}{m_{7-HF}^{total}}\right)\cdot 100 \quad (2)$$

where $m_{7-HF}^{supernatant}$ is the amount of the flavone left in the supernatant when the 7-HF bound to the CNTs was removed, and $m_{7-HF}^{total}$ is the total amount of flavone initially added in the Eppendorf tube. $m_{7-HF}^{supernatant}$ was estimated by measuring the fluorescence emission intensity at $\lambda$ = 526 nm and 298.0 ± 0.1 K, as was mentioned above.

*2.7. Zeta Potential Measurements*

The zeta potential, ξ, was determined by using a Zetasizer Nano ZS Malvern Instrument Ltd. (UK). The samples were diluted with filtered water to an adequate concentration. A scattering angle of 90° was used in the size distribution analysis. All measurements were carried out at 298.0 K. At least six measurements were obtained for each sample and the average value (standard deviation) was considered.

*2.8. In Vitro 7-HF Release*

With the goal of studying the 7-HF release from the CNTs, a method described elsewhere was used [29]. An adequate aliquot of the 7-HF ethanolic solution was added to a 2 mL flask. The organic solvent was evaporated with an air flow. Afterwards, a buffer solution was added up to the calibration mark. Then, the flask, in darkness, was sonicated for 20 min to make sure all the flavone was dissolved in the buffer solution. The 7-HF concentration in the buffer solution was $2.52\cdot10^{-4}$ M. This flavone solution will be called solution A.

In a 2 mL Eppendorf tube, 2 mg of CNTs were weighted and then, 2 mL of solution A were added to the tube, which was sonicated for 30 min in darkness and, subsequently, it was centrifuged at 13,500 rpm for 30 min. The supernatant was separated and the CNTs with the bound 7-HF were dried under vacuum by using an Eppendorf Concentrator Plus from Eppendorf Ibérica (Madrid, Spain) for 45 min. The 7-HF concentration in the supernatant was estimated measuring the fluorescence emission intensity of the solution at $\lambda$ = 526 nm and using the corresponding calibration curve, depending on the pH of the medium. In this way, the amount of 7-HF not bound to the CNTs can be estimated and, therefore, that of the CNTs' associated 7-HF (7-HF/CNT). Finally, 1.8 mL of the buffer solution was added to 10 mg of the dried 7-HF/CNT complexes within the Eppendorf tube, which was maintained under continuous magnetic stirring (200 rpm) in darkness. At determined time intervals, approximately 24 h, the tube was centrifuged at 13,500 rpm for 30 min. Subsequently, 1 mL of supernatant was removed, and the same volume of the corresponding buffer replaced in the Eppendorf tube. This is a way of mimicking the in vivo removal into the systemic circulation. The Eppendorf tube was put under continuous magnetic stirring, always in darkness, to avoid 7-HF photodegradation. The emission fluorescence intensity of the supernatant sample was measured at 526 nm in order to calculate the flavone concentration using the corresponding calibration curve.

Each experiment was conducted by triplicate. In addition, the release was studied at pHs 2.0, 7.4, and 9.2, simulating the different biological barriers in our organism.

### 2.9. Statistical Analysis

Values are expressed as the mean ± standard errors of separate experiments. Statistical analysis was performed with Student's *t*-test and One-way analysis of variance (ANOVA). When $p < 0.05$ (95% confidence), the differences were considered as significant.

## 3. Results and Discussion

### 3.1. Fluorescence Emission Intensity Calibration Curves for 7-HF at Different pHs

The fluorescence emission intensity calibration curves at different pHs were obtained as detailed in Section 2.4.1. They are shown in Figure 3. In all cases, straight lines with good correlation coefficients were observed.

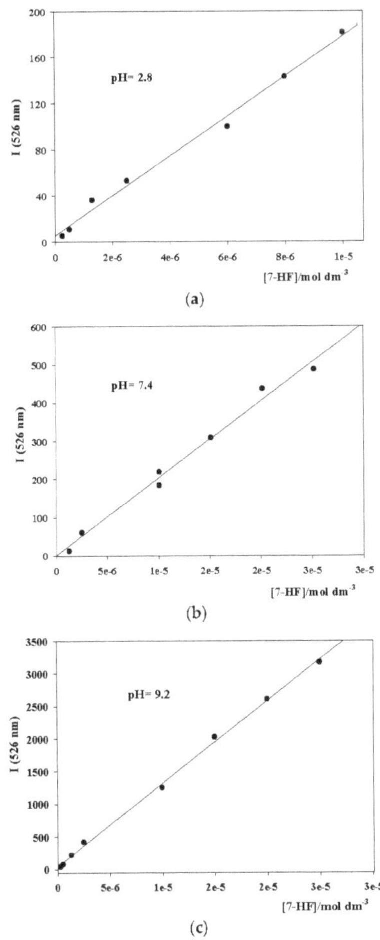


**Figure 3.** Fluorescence emission intensity calibration straight lines for 7-HF at different pHs. (**a**) pH = 2.0; (**b**) pH = 7.4; (**c**) pH = 9.2. T = 298.0 ± 0.1 K.

### 3.2. Cytotoxicity of CNTs

It is important to have information about the toxic character of any nanosystem being used as a drug carrier. Bearing this in mind, the cytotoxicity measurements of the SWCNT, MWCNT, and MWCNT were investigated using the cell lines Vero E6 (normal monkey kidney epithelial cells), HeLa (human cervical carcinoma epithelial cells), U937 (human leukemia monocytic cells), THP-1 (human leukemia monocytic cells), and Jurkat (human T leukaemia cells). The results are shown in Figure 4.

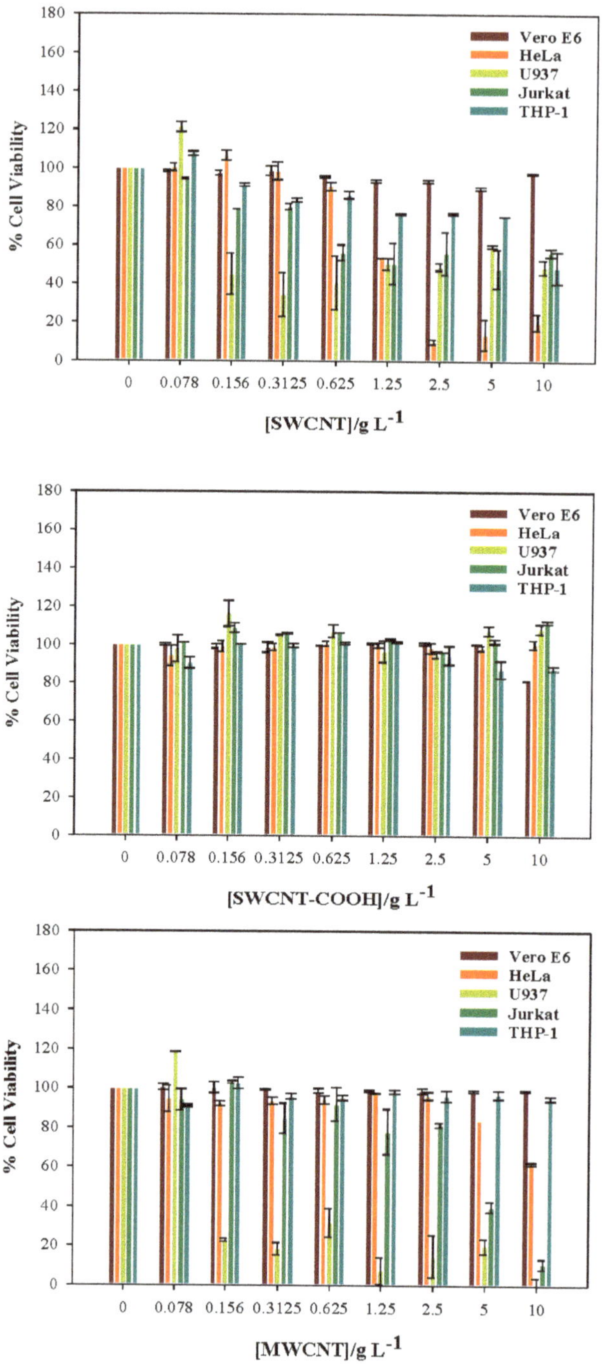


**Figure 4.** Cell viability of different carbon nanotubes in normal and cancer cell lines.

Figure 4 shows that the CNTs are non-toxic for the normal cell line Vero E6, even for concentrations well above those used in this work. The SWCNTs begin to be toxic for the U937 and Jurkat lines for [SWCNT] > 0.156 g $L^{-1}$, although at higher concentrations the toxicity is highest for the HeLa cancer line. The THP-1 cancer cell line is not much affected by the presence of these carbon nanotubes. The MWCNTs are non-toxic for the normal cell lines within the concentration range studied, as in the case of the SWCNTs. The former are particularly toxic for the U937 cell line for [MWCNT] > 0.156 g $L^{-1}$. For subsequent increases in [MWCNT], they are also toxic for the Jurkat cell lines and, only at high MWCNT concentrations, the CNTs are toxic for the HeLa cell line. As in the case of the SWCNT, the THP-1 is practically not affected for the MWCNTs. With regard to the SWCNTCOOH, these carbon nanotubes are non-toxic, within a wide concentration range, for all the cell lines investigated.

### *3.3. Encapsulation of 7-HF in CNTs*

Following the methodology described in Section 2.4 and using Equation (2), it is possible to calculate the amount of flavone encapsulated for each CNT concentration at pH = 7.4. Figure 5 shows the dependence of $I/I_o$ on the CNT concentration, where I and $I_o$ are the emission fluorescence intensities at $\lambda$ = 526 nm of the 7-HF solutions in the presence and in the absence of the CNTs, respectively. Since the encapsulation percentage of 7-HF bound to the CNTs is proportional to $I/I_o$, the data in Figure 4 indicate that the amount of 7-HF associated depends on [CNTs], following a sigmoidal function for the three types of CNTs investigated. The sigmoidal dependence of $I/I_o$ on the CNT concentration indicates that the association between 7-HF and the CNTs is cooperative. This means that the binding of one 7-HF molecule favors the association of a new flavone molecule to the CNTs and so on [30]. Table 1 summarizes the CNT concentrations for which a complete encapsulation of 7-HF is reached. At this point, it is worth noting that the interaction is expected to occur between the aromatic rings of the flavone and the cloud of $\pi$ electrons at the CNT surfaces. However, since these interactions would be operative in all the CNTs studied, the differences observed point out that other interactions should be at work. This issue will be considered below.

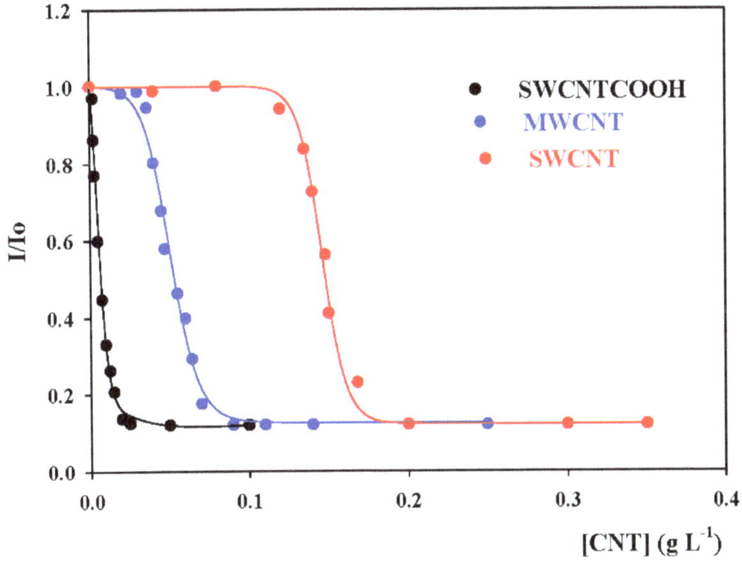


**Figure 5.** Dependence of $I/I_o$ (526 nm) on CNT concentration at pH = 7.4. Solid lines are the result of fitting the experimental data to Equations (4) and (5). T = 298.0 $\pm$ 0.1 K.

**Table 1.** CNT concentration necessary to completely encapsulate the 7-HF at pH = 7.4.

| | | **100% 7-HF$_{encapsulated}$** | |
|---|---|---|---|
| pH = 7.4 | [SWNCTs]/g·L$^{-1}$ | [SWCNT-COOH]/g·L$^{-1}$ | [MWNCTs]/g·L$^{-1}$ |
| [7-HF] = 1.51·10$^{-5}$ M | 0.20 | 0.025 | 0.090 |

With the goal of quantifying the 7-HF/CNT interactions, the equilibrium binding constant of 7-HF to the three types of CNTs, K, was calculated. The equilibrium can be written as:

$$7-\mathrm{HF}+\mathrm{CNTs} \rightleftharpoons 7-\mathrm{HF/CNT} \tag{3}$$

Therefore:

$$K=\frac{[7-\mathrm{HF/CNT}]}{[7-\mathrm{HF}][\mathrm{CNT}]} \tag{4}$$

The dependence of I/I$_o$, on [CNTs] can be expressed, considering the Pseudophase Model, as follows [31]:

$$I/I_o=\frac{(I)_f+(I)_b K[CNT]}{1+K[CNT]} \tag{5}$$

where $(I)_f$ and $(I)_b$ are the fluorescence emission intensity of 7-HF free in the solution and bound to the CNTs, respectively. In a cooperative interaction, K depends on [CNT], increasing upon augmenting the CNT concentration, until reaching a maximum value, the limiting value $K_{max}$. Taking this into account, K can be written as [31]:

$$K=\frac{K_{max}\cdot e^t}{1+e^t} \tag{6}$$

where t is given by Equation (6):

$$t=\frac{[\mathrm{CNT}]-h}{j} \tag{7}$$

In this equation, $K_{max}$ is the maximum value reached by K, h is the CNT concentration, for which K = $K_{max}$, and j is an adjustable parameter.

The dependence of I/I$_o$ on the CNT concentration shown in Figure 4 was fitted by using Equations (5)–(7). The result of the fittings is represented by the solid lines in this Figure. One can see that the agreement between the experimental and the theoretical data is good. The limit $K_{max}$ values obtained from the fittings are listed in Table 2.

**Table 2.** Values of $K_{max}$ obtained by fitting the I/I$_p$ data shown in Figure 4 using Equations (5)–(7). T = 298.0 ± 0.1 K.

| **CNTs** | **$K_{max}$/g$^{-1}$ L** |
|---|---|
| SWCNT | (1.5 ± 0.3)·10$^3$ |
| MWCNT | (1.2 ± 0.2)·10$^3$ |
| SWCNT-COOH | (1.5 ± 0.3)·10$^3$ |

The estimated $K_{max}$ values are similar, within experimental errors, for the three CNTs investigated. The fact that K is different, at the same CNT concentration, for the different carbon nanotubes investigated, explained the observed trend $[\mathrm{SWNCT}]_{100\ 7\%\text{-HFencapsulated}}$ > $[\mathrm{MWNCT}]_{100\%\ 7\text{-HFencapsulated}}$ > $[\mathrm{SWNCTCOOH}]_{100\ 7\%\text{-HFencapsulated}}$ (Figure 5 and Table 1). A plausible explanation to rationalize the differences observed between pristine single- and multi-CNTs, could be related to the length and diameter of both types of nanotubes. The SWCNTs have a length of 1–5 µm and a diameter of 1.5 nm, whereas the MWCNTs have a length of 1.5 µm and a diameter of 10 nm. In addition, the latter have multiple inner layers. Taking this into account, a higher number of 7-HF molecules would be expected to be bound to one MWCNT molecule than to an SWCNT one. As a consequence, $[SWNCT]_{100\ 7\%\text{-}HFencapsulated}$ would be higher than $[MWNCT]_{100\%\ 7\text{-}HFencapsulated}$, in agreement with the observations. In relation to the high affinity shown by the flavone for the SWCNTCOOH carbon nanotubes, at pH 7.4, most of the COOH groups would be ionized [32]. Therefore, these CNTs would be negatively charged. On the other hand, the 7-HF molecules are expected to be mainly non-ionic in water at pH 7.4 [33], although some anionic form is present. Maybe, the increase in the charge density at the CNT surface will favor the interactions with the aromatic rings of 7-HF, thus explaining the low SWCNT-COOH concentration necessary to completely bind the 7-HF. Additionally, the functionalization of the nanotube with carboxylic groups favors the formation of hydrogen bonds with the –OH groups of 7-HF, increasing the affinity of the flavone for the nanotubes.

The stability of the 7-HF/CNT complexes was checked using zeta potential measurements. The results were $\xi = -10 \pm 3$ for the 7-HF/SWCNT complexes, $\xi = -15 \pm 5$ for the 7-HF/MWCNT complexes, and $\xi = -31 \pm 7$ for the 7-HF/SWCNTCOOH complexes. These values did not change, within experimental errors, for various days.

### 3.4. Study of the In Vitro 7-HF Release

The in vitro release of 7-HF from the 7-HF/CNT complexes was studied following the procedure described in Section 2.3. Since most flavonoids, and 7-HF in particular, are orally administered to patients, the 7-HF release was investigated at different pHs, mimicking the conditions of the stomach, large intestine, and small intestine; that is, pHs 2.0, 7.4, and 9.2, respectively. In addition, pH 7.4 is also the physiological pH, which is that which the 7-HF/CNT complexes will encounter after its absorption in the small intestine.

From the fluorescence emission intensity values, the amount of 7-HF released from the 7-HF/CNT complexes can be calculated as:

$$\%7 - HF_{released} = \frac{[7 - HF]^{t}_{accumulated}}{[7 - HF]_{total}} \cdot 100 \tag{8}$$

where $[7 - HF]^{t}_{accumulated}$ is the flavone concentration released after a time t and $[7 - HF]_{total}$ is the total flavone concentration initially present in the Eppendorf tube (containing 10 mg of the 7-HF/CNT complex and 1.8 mL of buffer). Figure 6 shows the release profiles at the three pHs for the 7-HF/SWCNT complexes; that is, the dependence of the percentage of the flavone, initially encapsulated, which has been released, $\%7\text{-}HF_{released}$, against time.

In all the buffer solutions used, the release of 7-HF was followed for at least 400 h. After this time, the flavone release in neutral and basic media is really slow. However, after 400 h, in acid medium, $\%7\text{-}HF_{released}$ continues increasing with time. Taking the acid-based properties of 7-HF into account [33], at pH 2.0, all the flavone molecules are in their non-ionic form. At pH 7.4, most of the flavone is in its non-ionic form, but the anionic form is also present. At pH 9.2, the 7-HF anionic form concentration is twice or three times higher than that of the non-ionic form. At first, different interactions between the non-ionic and anionic forms of the flavone with the CNTs would be expected, thus resulting in different release rates for the two flavone forms [33]. Therefore, a one-phase release profile was expected in acid medium, whereas a two-phase release profile should be observed in neutral and basic media. Figure 6b,c show a two-phase release profile, in agreement with the expectations. Not enough data were available in acid medium. Even so, in order to further investigate this issue, a kinetic analysis of the release profiles has been performed. Data in Figure 5a, acid medium, were fitted using Equation (9) and data in Figure 5b,c, neutral and basic media, were fitted by using Equation (10).

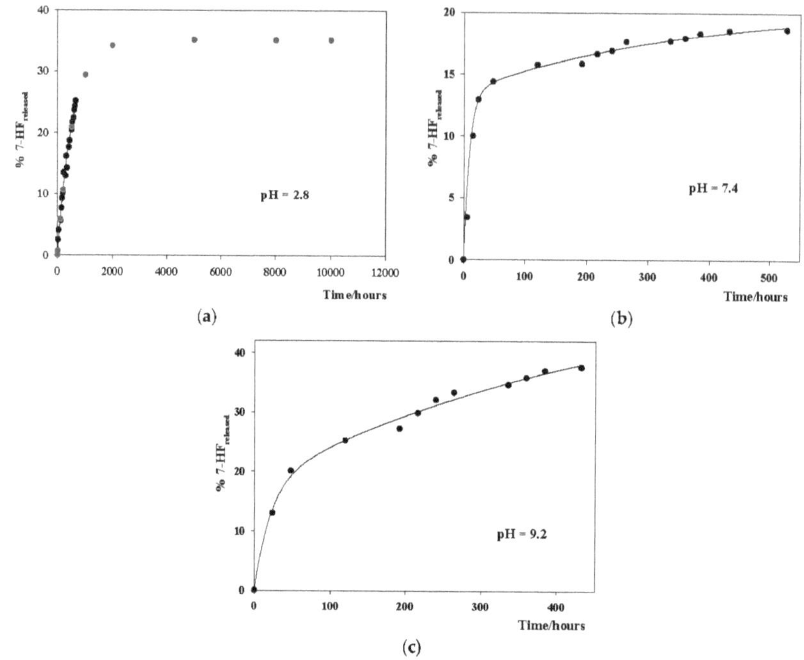


**Figure 6.** In vitro release profiles of 7-HF from 7-HF/SWCNT complexes at different pHs. (**a**) pH = 2.0; (**b**) pH = 7.4; (**c**) pH = 9.2. Solid lines correspond to the fitting of the experimental data using Equation (8), for pH = 2.0, and Equations (8) and (9), for pHs 7.4 and 9.2. The red dots are the predicted values for the complete release profile at pH = 2.0. These values were obtained by using Equation (8).

$$\%7 - HF_{released} = a \cdot (1 - exp(-k_n \cdot t)) \quad (9)$$

$$\%7 - HF_{released} = a \cdot (1 - exp(-k_n \cdot t)) + b \cdot (1 - exp(-k_a \cdot t)) \quad (10)$$

Here, $k_n$ and $k_a$ are the first order rate constants corresponding to the release of the non-ionic 7-HF and anionic 7-HF forms, respectively. *a* and *b* are two adjustable parameters related to the released 7-HF in its non-ionic and anionic forms, respectively. The first order rate constants obtained from the fittings are listed in Table 3. The solid lines in Figure 5 are the result of the fittings. The agreement between the experimental and the theoretical values was good. The red dots in Figure 6a were calculated by using the adjustable parameters estimated from the fitting by using Equation (9).

Table 3 shows that the estimated $k_n$ and $k_a$ values are the same in the different buffer solutions, within experimental errors, as was expected. One can see that $k_n < k_a$; that is, the release rate of the anionic form from the 7-HF/SWCNT complexes is faster than that of the non-ionic form. This could explain the results shown in Figure 6. In acid medium, only non-ionic 7-HF molecules are present. After their association with the CNTs, the subsequent release follows a one-phase profile. This release is really slow. In fact, the estimated time to reach the maximum value of %7-$HF_{released}$ would be longer than 2000 h. In neutral and basic media, the non-ionic and anionic flavone forms are present in the solution. Once they are bound to the CNTs, the release presents a two-phase profile. Taking into account the percentages of flavone anionic form present in the solution at pH 7.4 and 9.2, the amount of flavone released, within the same period of time, would be expected to be larger in basic medium than in neutral medium since $k_a > k_n$.

**Table 3.** First order rate constants obtained from the fittings of the dependence of %7-$HF_{released}$ on time, using Equation (9) for the data in acid medium, and Equation (10) for the data in neutral and basic media. The data correspond to the release of 7-HF from the SWCNT/7-HF complex. T = 310.0 ± 0.1 K.

| 7-HF/SWCNT | | |
|---|---|---|
| **pH** | | $10^3$ $k_n$/$h^{-1}$ |
| 2.0 | | 1.7 ± 0.4 |
| **pH** | $10^3$ $k_n$/$h^{-1}$ | $10^3$ $k_a$/$h^{-1}$ |
| 7.4 | 1.8 ± 0.5 | 68 ± 10 |
| 9.2 | 1.9 ± 0.7 | 50 ± 14 |

In relation to the flavone release from the 7-HF/MWCNT complexes, after following the release for more than 400 h, negligible amounts of %7-$HF_{released}$ were found, at the three pHs investigated. The same result was found for the SWCNT-COOH carbon nanotubes. This would point out that the release rate constants, for both the non-ionic and the anionic flavone forms, $k_n$ and $k_a$, would be slower in pristine MWCNTs and functionalized single-walled carbon nanotubes, SWCNT-COOH, in spite of the $K_{max}$ being similar for the three CNTs investigated.

## 4. Conclusions

In the present work, the encapsulation of 7-hydroxyflavone, 7-HF, within pristine single- and multi-walled carbon nanotubes, SWCNTs and MWCNTs, respectively, and within functionalized single-walled carbon nanotubes, SWCNT-COOH, has been investigated. The results show that the binding was cooperative and that 100% of the flavone was encapsulated by the CNTs. In addition, the $K_{max}$ values estimated for the binding of 7-HF to the three CNTs studied were similar, within experimental errors. However, the CNT concentration necessary to completely bind the flavone is different for the three carbon nanotubes, following the trend $[SWNCT]_{100\ 7\%\text{-HFencapsulated}}$ > $[MWNCT]_{100\%\ 7\text{-HFencapsulated}}$ > $[SWNCTCOOH]_{100\ 7\%\text{-HFencapsulated}}$.

A plausible explanation for rationalizing that $[SWNCT]_{100\ 7\%\text{-HFencapsulated}}$ > $[MWNCT]_{100\%\ 7\text{-HFencapsulated}}$ could be that the MWCNTs present a larger binding surface than the SWCNTs. Therefore, a larger number of 7-HF molecules would be associated to one pristine neutral multi-walled CNT molecule than to an SWCNT one. The experimental observation that the lower CNT concentration necessary to bind 100% of the flavone molecules corresponds to the SWCNT-COOH could be related to a more favorable 7-HF/CNT association when the negative charge density at the CNT surface increases. One has to consider that, at pH 7.4, most of the functionalized CNTs are negatively charged, but the majority of the 7-HF molecules are non-ionic. In addition, the functionalization of the nanotube with carboxylic groups favors the formation of hydrogen bonds with the –OH groups of 7-HF, increasing the affinity of the flavone for the nanotubes.

All the CNTs used as nanocarriers in this work are non-toxic for normal cell lines within a wide concentration range.

The in vitro release of 7-HF from the 7-HF/CNT complexes was followed for a long period of time at three different pHs, 2.0, 7.4, and 9.2. These pH values were chosen for mimicking the biological barriers those complexes will encounter when they are orally administered, which is the usual way of flavonoid administration.

The release of the flavone from the 7-HF/SWCNT complexes shows a biphasic profile in neutral and basic media, whereas in acid medium, a monophasic one was found. This was explained by considering that, in acid medium, only the non-ionic 7-HF form was present in the solution, while the non-ionic and anionic flavone forms are present in neutral and basic media. After a kinetic analysis, the first order rate constants corresponding to the non-ionic and anionic flavone forms release, $k_n$ and $k_a$, were estimated by fitting the experimental data to the appropriate equations. It was found that $k_n < k_a$. This result explains that the maximum %7-HF$_{released}$ was found in basic pH, since at this pH the highest amount of anionic flavone form is present.

In the case of the MWCNTs and SWCNT-COOHs, a negligible amount of flavone was released after more than 400 h. This could be due to the first order rate constants $k_n$ and $k_a$ being lower in these CNTs than in the SWCNTs.

From the results mentioned above, one can conclude that SWCNTs can be used as nanocarriers for the oral administration of 7-HF.

**Author Contributions:** Methodology, C.E., A.J.C., M.L.-L., F.J.O., J.A.L., M.L.M. and E.B.; writing-original draft preparation, M.L.M., M.L.-L. and P.L.-C.; supervision, M.L.-L., M.L.M. and P.L.-C.; funding acquisition, M.L.M., P.L.-C. and M.R.-E.-I.B.; administration, M.L.M., P.L.-C. and M.R.-E.-I.B. All authors have read and agreed to the published version of the manuscript.

**Funding:** This research was funded by the Consejería de Educación y Ciencia de la Junta de Andalucía (FQM-206 and FQM-274), the VI Plan Propio Universidad de Sevilla (2018/500) and the European Union (Feder Funds), and the Project PAIDI P20-01234.

**Institutional Review Board Statement:** Not applicable.

**Informed Consent Statement:** Not applicable.

**Data Availability Statement:** Data is contained within de article.

**Acknowledgments:** The authors thank the University of Seville for the grant VPPI-US. F.J. Ostos thanks the Consejeria de Economía, Conocimiento, Empresas y Universidades for the European Social Fund (DOC_00963) for his postdoctoral grant Talento Doctores, PAIDI 2020.

**Conflicts of Interest:** The authors declare no conflict of interest.

## References


1. Es-Safi, N.E.; Ghidouche, S.; Ducrot, P.H. Flavonoids: Hemysinthesis, reactivity, characterization and free radical scavenging activity. *Molecules* **2007**, *12*, 2228–2258. [CrossRef] [PubMed]
2. Shen, N.; Wang, T.; Gan, Q.; Liu, S.; Wang, L.; Jin, B. Plant flavonoids: Classification, distribution, biosynthesis, and antioxidant activity. *Food Chem.* **2022**, *383*, 132531. [CrossRef] [PubMed]
3. Sabino, R.K.; Ranjit, A.; Sharma, K.; Prada's, P.; Shang, X. Bio active compounds of citrus fruits: A review of composition and health benefits of carotenoids, flavonoids, limonoida, and terpenes. *Antioxidants* **2022**, *11*, 239. [CrossRef]
4. Singh, N.; Kaufman, M.; Silakari, O. Flavones: An important scaffold for medicinal chemistry. *Eur. J. Med. Chem.* **2014**, *12*, 206–239. [CrossRef] [PubMed]
5. Kali, A.E.; Habila, J.D. Flavonoids: Isolation, characterization, and health benefits. *J. Basic Appl. Sci.* **2020**, *9*, 45. [CrossRef]
6. Cushnie, T.P.T.; Lamb, A.J. Antimicrobial activity of flavonoids. *Int. J. Antimicrob. Agents* **2005**, *26*, 343–356. [CrossRef]
7. Havsteen, B. Flavonoids, a class of natural products of high pharmacological potency. *Biochem. Pharmacol.* **1983**, *32*, 1141–1148. [CrossRef]
8. Middleton, E.; Chithan, K. The impact of plant flavonoids on mammalian biology: Implications for immunity, inflammation and cancer. In *The Flavonoids: Advances in Research Since 1986*; Harborne, J.B., Ed.; Chapman and Hall: London, UK, 1993; pp. 145–166.
9. Liang, Y.; Xie, M.; Li, J.; Liu, L.; Cao, Y. Influence of 3-Hydroxyflavone on Colloidal Stability and Internationalization of Ag Nanomaterials Into THP-1 Macrophages. *Dose Response* **2019**, *17*, 1–9. [CrossRef]
10. Se Gupta, N.; Sahihi, M.; Dehkhodaei, M.; Kelly, D.; Arany, I. Differential role of 3-hydroxyflavone and 7-hydroxyflavone against nicotine-induced oxidative stress in rat renal proximal tubule cells. *PLoS ONE* **2017**, *12*, e0179777. [CrossRef]
11. Jin, Z.; Yang, Y.Z.; Chen, J.X.; Tang, Y.Z. Inhibition of pro-inflammatory mediators in RAW264.7 cells by 7-hydroxyflavone and 7,8-dihydroxyflavone. *J. Pharm. Pharmacol.* **2017**, *69*, 865–894. [CrossRef]
12. Ferraz, C.R.; Carvalho, T.T.; Manchope, M.F.; Atero, N.A.; Rásquele-Oliveira, F.S.; Fattori, V.; Casageande, R.; Verri, W.A. Therapeutic potential of flavonoids in pain and inflammation: Mechanisms of action, pre-clinicall and clonical data, and pharmaceutical development. *Molecules* **2020**, *25*, 762. [CrossRef] [PubMed]
13. Kawaii, S.; Ishikawa, Y.; Yoshizawa, Y. Relationship between the structure of methoxylated and hydroxylated flavones and their antiproliferative activitty in HL60 cells. *Anticancer Res.* **2018**, *38*, 5679–5684. [CrossRef] [PubMed]
14. Wang, J.; Su, H.; Zhang, T.; Du, J.; Cui, S.; Yang, F.; Jin, Q. Inhibition of enterovirus 71 replication by 7-hydroxyflavone and diidopropyl-flavones-7-yl phosphate. *PLoS ONE* **2014**, *9*, e92565. [CrossRef]
15. Ayaz, M.; Sadiq, A.; Junaid, M.; Ullah, F.; Ovais, M.; Ullah, I.; Ahmed, J.; Shahid, M. Flavonoids as prospective neuroprotectant and their therapeutic propensity in aging associated neurological disorders. *Front. Aging Neurosci.* **2019**, *11*, 155. [CrossRef] [PubMed]

6. Ganguly, S.; Das, P.; Margel, S. Containers for drug delivery. In *Composite Sciences and Technology*; Book Series; Available online: https://link.springer.com/chapter/10.1007/978-981-16-8146-2_6 (accessed on 11 February 2022).
7. Shah, A.; Aftab, S.; Anisad, J.; Ashiq, M.N.; Iftikhar, F.J. Nanocarriers for targeted drug delivery. *J. Drug Deliv. Sci. Technol.* **2021**, *63*, 102426. [CrossRef]
8. Ganguly, S.; Margel, S. Design of magnetic hydrogels for hyperthermia and drug delivery. *Polymers* **2021**, *13*, 4259. [CrossRef]
9. Iacob, A.T.; Lupascu, F.G.; Apotrosoaei, M.; Vasincu, I.M.; Tauser, R.G.; Lupascu, D.; Giusca, S.E.; Caruntu, I.-D.; Profire, L. Recent biomedical approaches.for quitosano based materials as drug delivery nanocarriersBiomedical. *Pharmaceutics* **2021**, *13*, 587. [CrossRef]
20. Ijima, S. Helical microtubules of graphitic carbon. *Nature* **1991**, *354*, 56–58. [CrossRef]
21. Beg, S.; Rahman, M.; Jain, A.; Sabino, S.; Hasnain, M.S.; Swain, S.; Imam, S.; Kazmi, I.; Akhter, S. Emergence in the 4 functionalized carbon nanotubes as smart nanocarriers for drug delivery applications. In *Fullernenes, Graphemes and Nanotubes: A Pharmaceutical Approach*; Frumezescu, A.M., Ed.; Elsevier Inc.: Amsterdam, The Netherlands, 2018; Chapter 4; pp. 105–133. [CrossRef]
22. Gholozadeh, H.; Ghorbani-HasanSaraei, A.; Tahermansouri, H.; Shaidi, S.A. The simultaneous adsorption and desorption of flavonoids from bitter orange peel by the carboxylared multi-walled carbon nanotubes. *Carbon Lett.* **2019**, *29*, 273–279. [CrossRef]
23. Daneshmehr, S. Carbon nanotubes for delivery of quercetin as anticancer drug: Theoretical study. *Procedia Mater. Sci.* **2015**, *11*, 131–136. [CrossRef]
24. Murjani, B.O.; Kadu, P.S.; Bansod, M.; Vaisya, S.S.; Yadav, M.D. Carbon nanotubes in biomedical applications: Current status, promises, and challenges. *Carbon Lett.* **2022**, *32*, 1207–1226. [CrossRef]
25. Hassani, M.; Tahghighi, A.; Rohani, M.; Ekmati, M.; Ahmadian, M.; Ahmavvand, H. Robust *antibacterial* activity of functionalized carbon nanotube-levofloxacine conjugate based on in vitro and in vivo studies. *Sci. Rep.* **2022**, *12*, 10064. [CrossRef] [PubMed]
26. Tang, L.; Xiao, Q.; Mei, Y.; He, S.; Zhang, Z.; Wang, R.; Wang, W. Insights on functionalized carbon nanotubes for cancer theranostics. *J. Nanobiotechnol.* **2021**, *19*, 423. [CrossRef] [PubMed]
27. Pranantyo, D.; Kang, E.; Chan-Park, M.B. Smart nanomicelles with bacterial infection-responsive disassembly for selective antimicrobial applications. *Biomater. Sci.* **2021**, *9*, 1627–1638. [CrossRef] [PubMed]
28. Strober, W. Trypan Blue Exclusion Test of Cell Viability. *Curr. Protoc. Immunol.* **2015**, *111*, A3.B.1–A3.B.3. [CrossRef]
29. Molina-Velázquez, S. Final Master's Project. 2021.
30. Moyá, M.L.; Ostos, F.J.; Moreno, I.; García, D.; Moreno-Gordillo, P.; Rosado, I.V.; López-Cornejo, P. Metallo-Liposomes Derived from the $[Ru(bpy)_3]^{2+}$ complex as nanocarriers of therapeutic agents. *Chemosensors* **2021**, *9*, 90. [CrossRef]
31. López-López, M.; Bernal, E.; Moyá, M.L.; Sánchez, F.; López-Cornejo, P. Study of ionic surfactants interactions with carboxylated single-walled carbon nanotubes by using ion-selective electrodes? *Electrochem. Commun.* **2016**, *67*, 31–34. [CrossRef]
32. Serdiuk, I.E.; Varenikov, A.S.; Roshal, A.D. 7-Hydroxyflavone revisited: Spectral, acid–base properties, and interplay of the protolytic forms in the ground and excited states. *J. Phys. Chem. A* **2014**, *118*, 3068–3080. [CrossRef]
33. Fredenberg, S.; Wahlgren, M.; Reslow, M.; Axelsson, A. The mechanisms of drug release in poly(lactic-co-glycolic acid)-based drug delivery systems—A review. *Int. J. Pharm.* **2011**, *415*, 34–52. [CrossRef]

pharmaceutics

MDPI

Review

# The Human Dermis as a Target of Nanoparticles for Treating Skin Conditions

Javier Salazar [1,2,3], Thais Carmona [1,3,4,5], Flavia C. Zacconi [2,6,7], Diego Venegas-Yazigi [3,5], Claudio Cabello-Verrugio [3,8,9], Won Il Choi [10] and Cristian Vilos [1,3,7,*]

1 Laboratory of Nanomedicine and Targeted Delivery, School of Medicine, Universidad de Talca, Talca 3460000, Chile
2 Departamento de Química Orgánica, Facultad de Química y de Farmacia, Pontificia Universidad Católica de Chile, Av. Vicuña Mackenna 4860, Macul, Santiago 7820436, Chile
3 Center for The Development of Nanoscience & Nanotechnology (CEDENNA), Universidad de Santiago de Chile, Santiago 8350709, Chile
4 Departamento de Química Analítica, Química Física e Ingeniería Química and Instituto de Investigación Química "Andrés M. Del Rio" (IQAR), Universidad de Alcalá, 28805 Alcalá de Henares, Madrid, Spain
5 Materials Chemistry Department, Faculty of Chemistry and Biology, University of Santiago of Chile (USACH), Santiago 9170022, Chile
6 Institute for Biological and Medical Engineering, Schools of Engineering, Medicine and Biological Sciences, Pontificia Universidad Católica de Chile, Av. Vicuña Mackenna 4860, Macul, Santiago 7820436, Chile
7 Center for Nanomedicine, Diagnostic & Drug Development (cND3), Universidad de Talca, Talca 3460000, Chile
8 Laboratory of Muscle Pathology, Fragility and Aging, Faculty of Life Sciences, Universidad Andres Bello, Santiago 8370035, Chile
9 Millennium Institute on Immunology and Immunotherapy, Faculty of Life Sciences, Universidad Andres Bello, Santiago 8370035, Chile
10 Center for Bio-Healthcare Materials, Bio-Convergence Materials R&D Division, Korea Institute of Ceramic Engineering and Technology, 202, Osongsaengmyeong 1-ro, Osong-eup, Heungdeok-gu, Cheongju 28160, Chungbuk, Republic of Korea
* Correspondence: cristian.vilos@utaca.cl

**Abstract:** Skin has a preventive role against any damage raised by harmful microorganisms and physical and chemical assaults from the external environment that could affect the body's internal organs. Dermis represents the main section of the skin, and its contribution to skin physiology is critical due to its diverse cellularity, vasculature, and release of molecular mediators involved in the extracellular matrix maintenance and modulation of the immune response. Skin structure and complexity limit the transport of substances, promoting the study of different types of nanoparticles that penetrate the skin layers under different mechanisms intended for skin illness treatments and dermo-cosmetic applications. In this work, we present a detailed morphological description of the dermis in terms of its structures and resident cells. Furthermore, we analyze the role of the dermis in regulating skin homeostasis and its alterations in pathophysiological conditions, highlighting its potential as a therapeutic target. Additionally, we describe the use of nanoparticles for skin illness treatments focused on dermis release and promote the use of metal-organic frameworks (MOFs) as an integrative strategy for skin treatments.

**Keywords:** skin; dermis; nanoparticles; drug delivery; metal-organic frameworks (MOFs)

## 1. Skin Function and Composition

The skin is the human body's largest organ, and its primary function is to prevent any damage raised by harmful microbes, UV radiation, weather, pollution, or other assaults from the external environment that could affect the body's internal organs [1]. The skin also has a social role because its appearance can determine how people feel towards or judge each other socio-economically, as sexual partners, or even to get a job [2]. Skin affections represent the fourth of global, not lethal, disease burdens [3], and skin-related diseases have prevalence and cost equivalent to other significant public health concerns, such as cardiovascular disease and diabetes [4].

The histological analyses of the skin show the dermis as the more extensive section localized between an outer layer named the epidermis and a deep section called the hypodermis. The dermis is composed mainly of fibrous tissue, such as collagen, elastic fibers, and glycosaminoglycans that, together with diverse structures such as the nerve terminals, glands, blood vessels, and follicles, provide sensorial and protective properties to the skin, as shown Figure 1 [5,6].

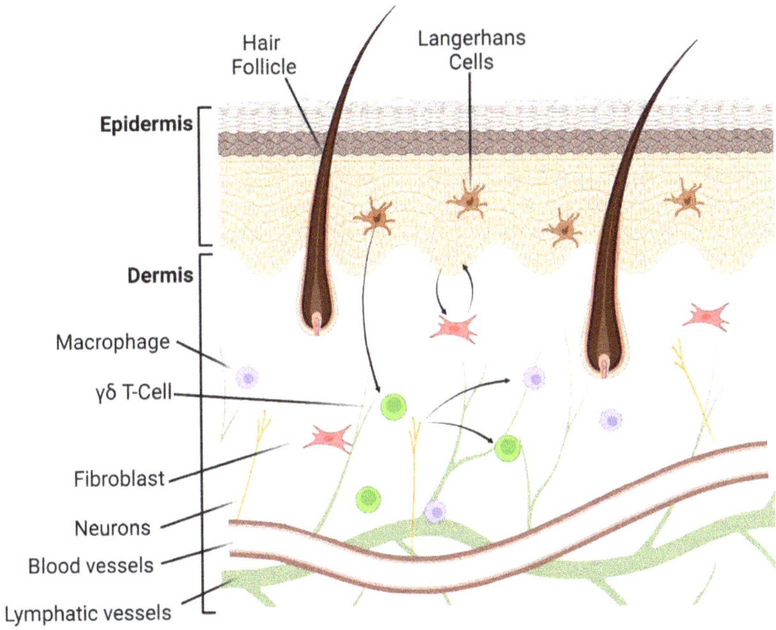


**Figure 1.** Illustration of skin components and their cell distribution.

The skin is exposed daily to countless factors that undermine its protective and structural properties as a peripheral organ. Those unique factors for each individual, such as metabolism, genetics, and epigenetics, can be classified as intrinsic factors; in contrast, those standard elements that affect the group of individuals like environmental conditions (UV exposure, pollution, or weather) or lifestyle (nutrition, smoking, stress or lack of sleep) can be categorized as extrinsic factors [7]. Both intrinsic and extrinsic factors and aging impair keratinocyte and fibroblast's ability to maintain the skin's homeostasis, and some complications, such as inflammation-related illness, autoimmune pathologies, structural disorders, and cancer, can arise [8].

## 2. Dermis

The dermis represents the main section of the skin. The dermis can be classified into papillary and reticular dermis based on the components and morphology of each section [9]. The papillary dermis is the thinner area of the dermis and exhibits an intertwining with the epidermis [5]. Compared to the reticular dermis, the papillary dermis presents a distribution of less compact fibrous components, which allow the presence of blood vessels that nourish the epidermis [10,11]. Furthermore, the Schwann cells on the papillary dermis project their dendrite to the epidermis, making sense through the skin [12]. Conversely, the compact distribution of fibrous content on the reticular dermis gives the stretching and resilience resistant properties to resist the deformation forces applied to the skin [13]. The contribution of the dermis to skin physiology is significant; therefore, deep knowledge about the composition and distribution of their components is critical, as well as the interaction of the cellular population and how they are affected under diverse pathologies that affect the skin. In this sense, it is critical to evaluate the role and relation between each key component of the dermis to generate novel nanotechnology-based systems for treating skin conditions.

## 3. The Cellular Population of the Dermis

Those cellular types on the dermis hold crosstalk that coordinate protection against injury, physical stimuli, or pathogen assault. The cellular population of the dermis also coordinates skin appendage formation, such as hair follicles, sebaceous glands, and sweat glands, that contribute to the protection and thermoregulation of the body. Furthermore, the specialized cells on the dermis as the nervous terminals sense temperature, pain, and mechanics' force. The crosstalk between the different cell types depends on the distribution and maintenance of the fibrillar scaffold in the dermis. The fibroblast is mainly responsible for their synthesis and restructuration [14].

### 3.1. *Fibroblast*

Fibroblasts are mesenchymal cells with different origins, locations, and functions that synthesize and maintain the extracellular components [15]. The dermal fibroblasts can be divided into subtypes, such as papillary fibroblast, reticular fibroblast, dermal papilla (DP), and dermal white adipose tissue (DWAT) [15–17]. The cellular markers that allow for classifying the fibroblast subpopulations fluctuate through embryo development. However, some features remain specific to papillary, reticular, or DWAT. Studies on homologous models such as mice demonstrate that fibroblast on the skin can be isolated through the surface marker FAP and CD90 [18,19].

Interestingly, different from the mouse model, the human skin presents a fibroblast population gradient where FAP and CD90 expression change depending on the dermis section. In the human skin, the papillary fibroblast can be identified as FAP+ CD90−, the reticular fibroblast as FAP+ CD90+, and FAP− CD90+ pre-adipose reticular fibroblast [20]. The difference in these fibroblast populations is not exclusively on cellular markers that describe their anatomical locations. The fibroblast subpopulation presents a different gene and protein expression that determines how the fibroblast responds to environmental stimuli [21]. Under specific signals such as adipogenesis-induced medium reticular fibroblast, FAP− CD90+ can differentiate to adipocyte, whereas papillary fibroblast FAP+ CD90− cannot be differentiated. Sequencing studies also show that papillary fibroblast has enhanced collagen type VII and type III expressions related to papillary dermis formation, blood vessels, and dermo-epidermal junction (DEJ). In contrast, reticular fibroblast presents an enhanced expression of extracellular matrix (ECM)-related genes such as LOXL3, a lysyl oxidase related to elastin and collagen synthesis [21]. The difficult task of studying the fibroblast subpopulation on dermal skin arises because fibroblast changes their surface markers and protein expression profile under cell culture conditions [22].

When the skin's integrity is compromised, as in a wound, the fibroblast and immune cells are recruited by specific cytokines TGFβ-1, IL-1, IL-6, and chemokines secreted by damaged keratinocyte and platelets [23] to produce ECM components and guide the healing process. In some cases, the fibroblast response is overregulated, leading to an aberrant scarring process such as hypertrophic scarring or keloid [23]. The difference between both fibrotic processes is that keloid expands beyond the limits of the original wound, and the amount of fibrillar content increases over time [24]. Nevertheless, both fibrotic processes present an increased presence of activated fibroblast, denominated myofibroblast, that remodel and secrete an increased amount of collagen type I [25]. Furthermore, the conversion to myofibroblast could be mechanical regulation related to collagen fiber contraction [26] and the presence of cytokines TGFβ-1 and IL-11 secreted by papillary fibroblast CD39+ [27]. A recent study demonstrates that the conversion to myofibroblast by TGFβ-1 signaling is mediated by the expression of the Engrailed 1 (EN1) transcription factor [28]. Moreover, the indirect inhibition of EN1 through the inhibition of yes-associated protein (YAP) by verteporfin prevents fibroblast activation and conduces to a scarless wound repair [29].

Together with the wound repair process, the fibroblast function is related to the skin's homeostasis. Skin homeostasis is affected by aging, a complex multifactorial process involving all human beings. Skin aging is affected by extrinsic and intrinsic factors and is characterized by a loss of skin functions such as impaired barrier function, loss of stiffness, the impaired healing process, and altered immunological response [7]. On the fibroblast, the aging process is characterized by the increased production of reactive oxygen species (ROS) generated by ultraviolet radiation overexposure through life [30]. The increased ROS content promotes mutations related to desoxyribonucleic acid (DNA) damage on the fibroblast [31]. Furthermore, the aged fibroblast produces IL-6 and IL-8 cytokines, which are involved in chronic inflammation [32]. Moreover, the aged fibroblast increased the secretion of matrix metalloproteinase-1 (MMP-1), which degrades the collagen content of the dermis, decreasing the stiffness of the skin [33]. The loss of rigidity on the dermis alters the proliferation of keratinocytes on the epidermis [34] and reinforces the aged phenotype on fibroblast, promoting the secretion of MMP-1 [35,36]. These antecedents demonstrate that the fibroblast is present as a critical cell in the dermis physiology, and their misfunction could enhance pathological processes such as fibrosis, keloid, impaired barrier function, and dermatoporosis [37].

### 3.2. Immune Cells

The primordial function of the skin is a barrier achieved through the stratum corneum (SC) of the epidermis and the immune cells on all skin. The heterogeneous presence of immune cells on the skin has been reviewed [38]. However, the dermis remains in other heterogenic populations of immune cells that complement epidermal immune cells' function. The population present on the dermis have linfoid or myeloid origin; some are mast cells, dendritic cells (DC), T CD4+, T CD8+, $\gamma\delta$ T cell, and memory-resident T cells (Trm) [6].

The interaction of sphingosine-1-phosphate (S1P) and the sphingosine-1-phosphate receptor 1 (S1PR1) present on the membrane of immune cells are the primary signal for the migration of resident immune cells to the lymphatic nodule (LN) present on skin [39]. Otherwise, the interaction of S1PR2 and CD 69 is responsible for the lymphatic $\gamma\delta$ T cell resident on the dermis. The interactions of S1PR2 with its ligand inhibit the migratory signal given by S1PR1, whereas CD 69 down-regulates the expression of S1PR1 on the lymphocyte membrane [40]. That mechanism suggests a close regulation between the cells that reside on the dermis and those populations of cells that migrate on the lymphatic nodule. Under this mechanism, diverse lymphocytes, such as Trm CD 8+, patrol the dermis and the epidermis regularly [41]. Trm CD8+ have a dendritic-like shape that lets them search for antigens between the tight interaction of keratinocytes on the epidermis. Upon recognizing an antigen, Trm CD8+ shift their form to a spheric-like. Additionally, they began the synthesis and secretion of interferon $\gamma$ (INF-$\gamma$) that mediate the recruiting of other immune cells, starting a local immune response [42]. Another lymphocyte that mediates the inflammatory response against environmental allergens is $\gamma\delta$T cells, which are present on the dermis from three days after born and could be residents of Dermis (V$\gamma$ 5+ subtype) or surveillance the skin-surrounded environment (V$\gamma$ 4+ subtype) such as skin LN. The IL-17A secreted by $\gamma\delta$ T cells are essential in the inflammatory response, and their dysregulated secretion is a common factor in inflammatory diseases, such as psoriasis, atopic dermatitis, and contact allergies [43].

Dendritic cells (DC) and mast cells are myeloid-derived immune cells that are found to be closely related to neuronal terminals and blood vessels of the dermis [44]. Nerve terminals secrete neuropeptide that stimulates the secretion of IL-23 from DC, and its secretion stimulates the production of IL-17A on $\gamma\delta$ T cells, which mediates a neuronal immune response against viruses such as herpes simplex [45]. However, mast cells form a physical synapse with unmyelinated C-fibers, and they have bidirectional communication with neurons in the skin [46]. Mast cells-derived TNF and nerve growth factor (NGF) stimulate neuronal elongation on the dermis. The crosstalk between mast cells and DC mediates the transition between innate and adaptative immune responses. DC can recognize nickel (Ni) with solid affinity and then migrate to the closed LN for beginning the antigen presentation, and it has been speculated that this interaction is responsible for the allergic response to Ni [47].

In some cases, the skin's immune response can be altered and lead to disorders like omenn syndrome, vitiligo, psoriasis, atopic dermatitis, or allergic contact dermatitis. In immune deficiency syndrome as omen syndrome, where a lack of T or B cells occur, a penetration into the Dermis by Langerhans cells exists. This immune deregulation generates some skin conditions such as erythema and alopecia; the last one is caused by an immune attack over the hair follicle on skin [48–50].

## 4. Dermis as a Target for Nanotechnology-Based Treatments

Nanotechnology intended for dermatology is a domain of research in constant progress. However, less than 1% of the nanoparticles under clinical trials focus on skin conditions, which include skin illness treatment, dermo-cosmetic, and wound care devices [51,52]. Moreover, transdermal applications for vaccination or systemic pathology treatment have been developed due to the vascular distribution of the dermis [53,54]. Those initiatives bypass the hepatic passage of drugs through oral administration or avoid utilizing needles during vaccination, which improves patients' adherence to the different treatments. Indeed, the dermis represents a robust administration route to develop nanoparticles for medical applications, improving immunization through the activations of the dendritic cells and as a pathway to deliver drugs or nutrients to improve systemic or localized diseases.

### *4.1. Skin Penetration of Nanoparticles*

Regardless of the nanoparticle employed, the first obstacle is to penetrate across the skin layers, particularly the stratum corneum. The nanoparticles can penetrate the skin by following one of these routes: (1) The intracellular (transcellular) route, (2) the intercellular route, or (3) the appendage route, as displayed in Figure 2 [55]. On intact skin, the transcellular and intercellular routes can be reached using permeation enhancers that disrupt the integrity of the stratum corneum [56]. An example of the effect of an enhancer was illustrated in a study that analyzed the impact of the surface charge of nanoparticles on skin penetration prepared using different solvents. Despite the surface charge, the particles formulated in water were staked on the SC, whereas the particles prepared with ethanol/water crossed the SC and reached the dermis. The effect on the penetration of nanoparticles was not enhanced when ethanol was applied before the nanoparticles [57]. These researchers hypothesized that the ethanol drags the nanoparticles across the SC, reaching the viable epidermis where the nanoparticle can defund depending on their surface charge. The penetration of particles in the skin increases when skin integrity is compromised, such as through photodamage, atopic dermatitis, psoriasis, and dryness. Skin damaged by UVA radiation presents an increased skin permeation of nanoparticles [58,59].

The skin appendages are the sweat gland and the pilosebaceous unit, including the sebaceous gland and hair follicle [60]. The hair follicles act like ducts that connect the outer environment with the dermis. The dermal papilla in the deepest section of the hair follicle is associated with capillary loops and lymphatic vessels [61–63]. The high content of vessels associated with the dermal papilla transforms the trans appendage route into a critical target to reach systemic drug delivery or immunization through the skin. Nanoparticle penetration through hair follicles depends on the size of nanoparticles, the medium's viscosity, and the hair's movement [64,65]. The theoretical model denominated Ratchet effect explains the influence of these physicochemical properties. Based on the theoretical model, the ideal size of nanoparticles to reach the deepest part of the hair follicle is 600 nm. These theoretical sizes concord with the results obtained by other research where the nanoparticles with size between 400–600 nm present the deepest penetration on hair follicles [66,67].

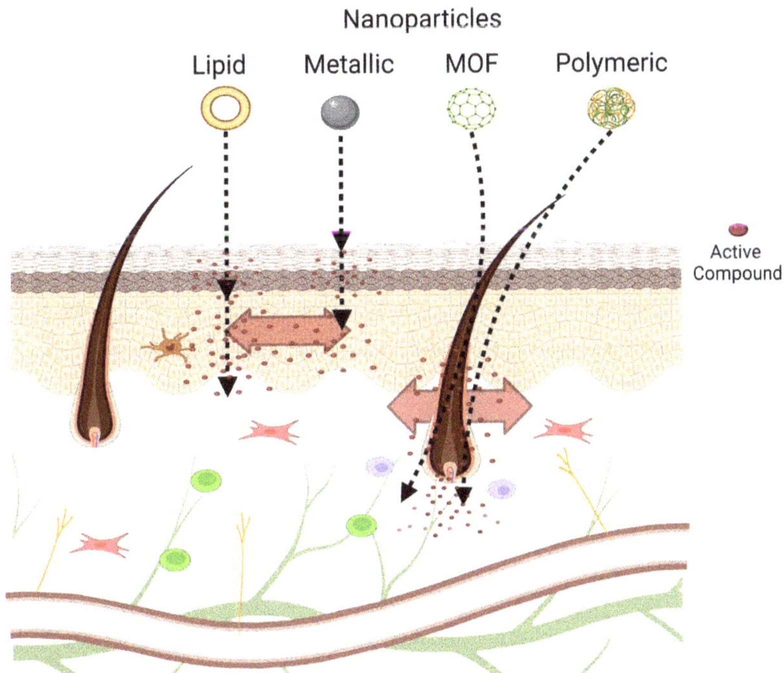


**Figure 2.** Scheme of potential skin penetration routes of different types of nanoparticles.

### 4.2. *Effect of Nanoparticles over the Dermis*

The literature reports numerous works describing nanoparticle formulation intended for topical applications [51,68–70]. Compared to topical treatments, transdermal represents an effective transport from the intact skin into the systemic circulation to treat various chronic diseases. Transdermal treatments offer better patient compliance than more invasive alternative routes avoiding liver metabolic. However, only a limited number of drugs are enough small and lipophilic to pass the skin barrier [71]. Nanocarriers made of lipids, metals, or polymers have been developed to increase the penetration of drugs or vaccines and control drug release by targeting specific areas of the skin [72]. Numerous nanoparticles have been developed, some of which are covered in Table 1.

**Table 1.** Applications of different types of nanoparticles for pathophysiological skin conditions based on dermis strategies.

| Type of Nanoparticle | Formulation | Aims | Reference |
|---|---|---|---|
| Inorganic | SiO/peptide | Reduce the inflammatory response liberating the natural compound from the nanoparticle mesoporous. | [73] |
| Inorganic | ZnO | Prevent microbial infection and decrease the ROS level on the skin. | [74] |
| Inorganic | Nanocomposite of zinc and silver nanocomposite | Promotes the healing of skin wounds | [75] |

**Table 1.** *Cont.*

| Type of Nanoparticle | Formulation | Aims | Reference |
|---|---|---|---|
| Inorganic | Super paramagnetic Iron Oxide/polyethelyimine | Skin penetration via follicular pathways | [76] |
| Polymeric | Polycaprolactone/gum arabic/ ZnO nanocomposite | Promote the regeneration of skin tissue and treat difficult healing skin wounds. | [77] |
| Polymeric | Dexamethasone loaded dentritic nanoparticle | Reduce the inflammatory response of atopic dermatitis. | [78] |
| Polymeric | SIlibilin encapsulated in gellan gum | Platform for skin delivery. | [79] |
| Lipidic | Raloxifene-loaded cubosomes | Transdermal delivery | [80] |
| Lipidic | Cyproterone encapsulated into nanostructure lipid carriers | Promote penetration via follicular appendages. | [81] |

#### 4.2.1. Inorganic Nanoparticles

Inorganic nanoparticles in dermatology comprise metal/metal oxide particles, carbon nanotubes, silica-based nanoparticles, and quantum dots, among others. Those types of nanoparticles are focused on treating cutaneous wounds, particularly in preventing and treating bacterial and fungal infections, and against the harmful effects of the sun as UV blockers. Additionally, they present chemical and thermal stability in the delivery systems; moreover, it can be exploited for simultaneous imaging and treatment. Tak et al. demonstrated shape-dependent skin penetration of Ag-NPs through different layers of the skin, indicating skin penetration of AgNPs through intercellular pathways [82]. Inorganic nanoparticles can be used alone, or in combination with polymers as composites [83] Muchova et al. aimed to provide an antibacterial effect using selenium nanoparticle (SeNP) adsorbed into a scaffold composed of chitosan, collagen, and thermostable fibroblast growth factor 2 (FGF2-STAB®). Those scaffold applications demonstrated a controlled release of SeNP in the dermis, lowering the ROS level and promoting wound regeneration [84]. Over the years, the application of gold nanoparticles as a drug carrier for skin drug delivery has attracted increasing attention because of their unique properties and versatility [85]. For example, Niu et al. synthesized gold nanoparticles conjugated with a peptide and cationic polymer (polyethelyimine, PEI) conjugated (AuPT) that could interact with a pDNAs encoding the miRNA-221 inhibitor gene into cationic nanocomplexes and penetrate through the intact stratum corneum [86]. Some of the inherent properties of metals or metallic oxides, such as magnetism, can be exploited. Yue-feng Rao et al. demonstrated that epirubicin covalently modified SPIONs (superparamagnetic iron-oxide nanoparticles) could be used as transdermal vectors as they could circumvent the stratum corneum via follicular pathways and reach the reticular dermis [76]. Ramadan et al. presented a different approach [87]. They used a photothermal ablation-enhanced transdermal drug delivery methodology on hollow copper sulfide nanoparticles (HCuSNPs). This technique induces skin perforations by a modulated laser that can induce localized thermal ablation of the SC, facilitating the penetration of the particles to the deeper skin layers. This skin disruption by HCuSNP-mediated photothermal ablation significantly increases the permeability of human growth hormone. Carbon nanodots are emerging as potential delivery systems because of their water solubility, chemical inertness, low toxicity, ease of functionalization, and resistance to photobleaching [88]. Bankoti and col. used carbon nanodots adsorbed into decellularized dermis to reduce the local ROS and to promote cellular recruitment and regeneration of wounds [89].

#### 4.2.2. Polymeric-Based Nanoparticles

Polymeric nanoparticles are one of the most attractive topics of research to be used as potential topical transdermal nanocarriers. Polymers have the advantages of low toxicity, biocompatibility, and biodegradability. Popular polymer materials used for delivery purposes are collagen, chitosan, poly(-lactic-co-glycolic) acid (PLGA), polycaprolactone (PCL), and dextran [90].

Chitosan-coated PLGA and bare PLGA with similar-sized but opposite surface charges have been studied by Mittal et al. [91]. They used ovoalbumin (OVA) to evaluate delivery efficacy. They found two–three times higher follicular penetration of NPs than pure OVA solution. These results paved the way for using polymer nanoparticles in formulations used in vaccines. They emphasized the potential of the trans follicular route to the administration of the drug to reach most internal layers of the skin. The application of nanoparticles synthesized with human recombinant keratin has promoted collagen synthesis and angiogenesis and improved wound healing mechanisms [92]. Other researchers have used a multifactorial approach using a polysaccharide-based hydrogel containing exosomes charged with interfering microRNA (miRNA); that complex formulation effectively relieves wound skin from UV damage, promoting the angiogenesis and regeneration of the skin appendages [93]. When the skin's barrier function is compromised, different pathogens such as *Candida* spp., *Pseudomonas* spp., or *Staphylococcus* spp. can promote a permanent infection when they reach the dermis. An alternative to face this infection generated by candida spp. was to improve the biodistribution of the antimycotic itraconazole using absorbable microneedles charged with nanocrystal [94]. Furthermore, nanocrystal of azithromycin has been developed to treat Lyme disease generated by tick bite infection [95]. Recently, Kim et al. studied pH- and temperature-sensitive double cross-linked hydrogels consisting of poly(N-Isopropylacrylamide (PNIPAM) and Hyaluronic Acid (HA) as a transdermal drug delivery carrier of luteolin for its applicability to alleviate psoriasis. The in vitro skin permeation experiments showed that hydrogel effectively delivers luteolin to the epidermis and dermis. Jeong et al. evaluated the applicability of Carboxymethyl Chitosan/2-Hydroxyethyl Acrylate (CmCHT-g-pHEA) hydrogels as a transdermal delivery system. In addition, they confirmed that the CmCHT-g-pHEA hydrogels temporarily interferes with skin barrier function through skin hydration improving the skin penetration to lower layers of skin of nobiletin loaded into the hydrogel matrix [96]. Other researchers, using a multifactorial approach based on polysaccharide-based hydrogel containing exosomes charged with interfering microRNA (miRNA), demonstrated an effectively relieves of wound skin caused by UV damage, thus promoting angiogenesis and improving the regeneration of the skin appendages. Moreover, silver nanoparticles have been used to improve the performance of wound healing matrix composed of biopolymers such as polyvinyl alcohol (PVA), collagen, and hyaluronic acid [97]. From another perspective, towards the control of the fibrosis process, the use of nanoparticles of PLGA charged with pioglitazone decreases the TGF-β signal produced during skin fibrosis in scleroderma patients [98]. The immune cells in the dermis are essential in developing inflammatory diseases. It has been reported that a nanogel composed of hyaluronic acid and β-glucan efficiently activates the dendritic cells when incorporating an immunomodulator such as ovalbumin (OVA) [99]. Additionally, silibinin, a flavonoid that presents antioxidant and anti-inflammatory actions, has been delivered into the dermis using nanocapsules supported in a polymeric matrix to treat dermatitis [79]. Furthermore, nanoparticles of silica functionalized with PDMA (poly(2-(dimethylamine) ethyl methacrylate) were used to scavenge the cellular free DNA present in psoriasis, improving the symptoms in a murine model [100]. In addition, the neuronal component in the dermis has been targeted to improve the treatment of peripheral neuropathic pain using nanoparticles loaded with capsaicinoid and supported into hydrogel based on chitosan. This system's probe has increased permeability and a higher biodistribution of capsaicinoids into the dermis [101]. Another application of the polymeric system was researched by Sanad et al., who prepared a chitosan-HA/Andrographolide nanocomposite scaffold. When applied to second-degree burn wounds, this scaffold enhanced wound healing with no scaring and improved tissue quality [102].

### 4.2.3. Lipid-Based Nanoparticles

Lipid nanoparticles include similar structures such as micelles, reverse micelles, emulsions, microemulsions, transferosomes, ethosomes liposomes, and solid lipid nanoparticles (SLN). These structured systems have been broadly used to release several active compounds, including chemotherapeutic drugs [103], antibiotics [104], and genetic material [105,106]; however, in the last years' diverse studies have described that SLN present an improved capacity to reach the dermis [107]. Different lipidic systems have been used to deliver a plethora of compound to the dermis; in this work, we describe a few applications in which lipid nanoparticle has been utilized to deliver compound with pharmaceutical potential into the dermis. Nanostructured lipid carriers (NLC) have been applied to deliver capsaicin to the dermis with the intent of reducing the irritation associated with the application of raw formulations [108]. Furthermore, Ghasemiyeh et al. loaded cyproterone acetate (CPA) in nanostructure lipid carriers with different sized (100–600 nm). They demonstrated that encapsulated CPA into lipid carriers presented a better penetration than free CPA. The optimal penetration to epidermis-dermis layers via follicular appendage was found for lipids with a 300 nm size [81].

However, in treating immunologically related pathologies, SLN has been used to encapsulate atorvastatin, generating a system that prevents the systemic absorption of this drug and prolongs the anti-inflammatory effect in the treatment of scalp seborrheic dermatitis [109]. Additionally, metformin's anti-inflammatory and ROS reduction capacity, a drug commonly prescribed to treat diabetes, has been studied to improve the treatment of skin inflammatory pathologies. SLN load with metformin particles has shown the capacity to reach the deeper section of the dermis, increasing the dermal concentration of metformin [110]. Another anti-inflammatory application of SLN has been reported with cyclosporine A (CsA), the SLN@CsA particles present an improved retention and penetration into the dermis in comparison to the application of a suspension of CsA [111]. The traditional non-steroidal anti-inflammatory drug (NSAIDs) ibuprofen has been encapsulated using SLN. Those SLN@Ibuprofen particles showed an improved performance in treating skin inflammation in a murine model compared with the topical application of gel-based ibuprofen; additionally, this formulation presents a release profile related to the pH showing an increased liberation rate at pH 7.4, which is the pH present in the dermis [105,112,113]. Other applications of lipid-based nanoparticles oriented toward the cosmetic field have been explored [114], where SLN loaded with vitamin A (Vit-A) has been studied for dermal application, showing that SLN presents a higher load capacity of Vit-A and an increased penetration of the particle and distribution of Vit-A compared to a Vit-A suspension gel [115].

## 5. Metal-Organic Frameworks as an Integrative Tool for Skin Treatments

Metal–organic frameworks (MOFs) are well-defined three-dimensional porous solids assembled from inorganic metal nodes connected by multitopic organic ligands. They present structural flexibility, large surface areas, and pore sizes that can be tailored by a combination of metals, ligands, and synthesis conditions for a given application [116]. Numerous applications in many fields are being developed, such as gas storage [117], separation [118], chemical sensing [119], catalysis [120], and potential biomedical applications, including drug storage and delivery [121,122], biomedical gas storage [123], biosensing [124,125], or molecular imaging [126]. Figure 3 describes a morphological structure of MIL100 acquired by transmission electronic microscopy and illustrates some skin applications of metal–organic frameworks (MOFs).

The first obstacle to using MOFs in skin treatments based on dermis therapeutic targets is penetrating across the epidermal layer by some of the routes mentioned above. As a combination of inorganic and organic materials, MOFs allow the incorporation as primary building blocks of cations ($Au^+$, $Ag^+$, $Cu^{2+}$, or $Zn^{2+}$) involved in diverse biological processes and bioactive ligands as organic connectors. Thus, the progressive degradation of the MOF framework can be an effective therapy for human pathogenic bacteria causing various infections and syndromes in the skin. A completely bioactive MOF constructed with $Zn^{2+}$ and azelaic acid (Az) coordinated to the metallic centers (BioMIL-5) presented interesting antibacterial and dermatological properties for treating several skin disorders [127]. Recently, BioMOFs based on an alkaline element ($K^+$) and Az showed superior antibacterial activity against *Staphylococcus epidermidis* and *Staphylococcus aureus* than azelaic acid [128]. Antibiotic Carbenicillin (Car) was coordinated with $Ga^{3+}$ to form a pH-sensitive MOF and used to coat hollow $TiO_2$ nanoshells. Under an acidic microenvironment at infected sites, the MOF gradually degrades, releasing Car and $Ga^{3+}$ in combination with the ROS (Reactive Oxygen Species) generator $TiO_2$ exhibiting an effective simultaneous inhibition of *Pseudomonas aeruginosa* (PA) and methicillin-resistant *Staphylococcus aureus* (MRSA), supporting that strategy as a potential antibacterial alternative to fight against these relevant pathogens [129]. A pH-responsive core-shell nano assembly has been developed using core mesoporous silica nanoparticles (MSN) loaded with $\beta$-lactamase inhibitor (sulbactam) coated with a pH-responsive MOF based on the antibiotic Car and $Fe^{3+}$. This nano assembly was stable under physiological conditions; however, at lower pH, the MOF on the MSN surfaces degrades gradually, releasing their components and unblocking the MSN pores, which led to the release of the trapped inhibitor [130]. However, an excess of metal ions released may also be dangerous as it can negatively affect the biological processes where they are involved, in addition to bacteria. The in-situ incorporation of folate inside the pores of the Cu-based MOFs HKUST-1 framework increases the hydrophobicity of HKUST-1 pores, which prevents proteins and water molecules diffuse to the $Cu^{2+}$ sites from hampering the break of Cu-carboxylate linkages [131]. Additionally, the presence of the vitamin reduced the cytotoxicity towards human dermal fibroblasts.

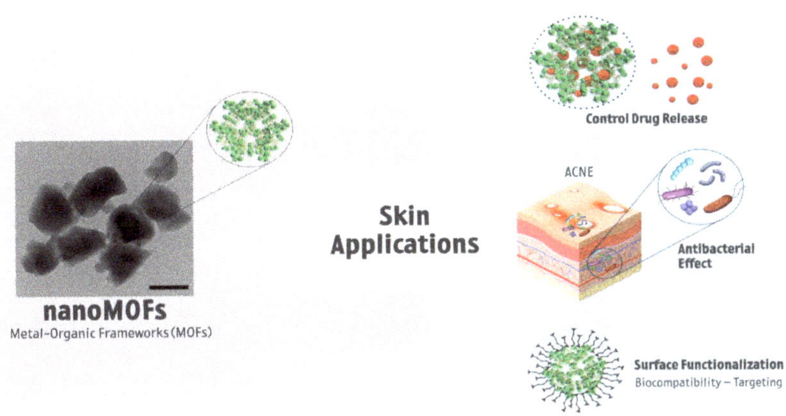


**Figure 3.** Morphological structure of MIL100 metal-organic frameworks (MOFs) acquired by electronic transmission microscopy (TEM), and some schematic representations of MOFs applications on the skin.

An alternative route to creating effective antibacterial agents based on MOFs is the possibility of attaching additional organic fragments by covalent post-synthetic modifications in the organic ligands. A series of MOF/Ce-based nanozymes have been developed using a peroxidase-like activity of Au-doped MIL-88B(Fe) MOFs. The ligands located at the external surfaces were modified with Ce-NTA ((1S)-N-(5-amino-1-carboxypentyl)iminodiacetic acid) complexes that presented DNase-mimetic activity to catalyze the hydrolysis of extracellular DNA. In vivo tests revealed that cumulative effects of dual enzyme-like MOFs on treated subcutaneous abscesses demonstrated a significant reduction of inflammatory cells and improved wound healing [132]. On the other hand, MIL-88B(Fe)-based nanozymes presented a relatively lower catalytic activity. A strategy to increase their therapeutic activity was modifying the MOF's external surfaces with a COF (Covalent Organic Framework), creating a MOF @COF hybrid. The COF proportionated an external morphology proper to catch bacteria and presented a microenvironment close to the MOF catalytic sites capable of activating the substrates via non-covalent interactions [133].

The presence of unsaturated metal nodes at the external MOFs surfaces provides opportunities for their surface engineering. This surface modification of MOFs improves their colloidal stability, permits the control of the release of the ions, guests, or ligands, and tunes the hydrophobic/hydrophilic character of their external surfaces, improving their applicability. It can form composites in which MOF particles are embedded into functional (co)polymers with intrinsic bactericidal properties that protect MOFs from a fast degradation in physiological fluids. Additionally, as a strategy, the inherent properties of those polymers can be exploited. Studies based on films as crosslinking agents from HKUST-1 and CS exhibited a relatively slow release of copper ions, efficient antibacterial activity to *Staphylococcus aureus*, and negligible biotoxicity [134]. The incorporation of HKUST-1 within citrate-based hydrogels enables a sustainable copper ions release to maintain antioxidant and thermoresponsive hydrogel properties [135]. Studies of ZIF8@PVA (polyvinylalcohol) hydrogel omniphobic membranes also allow the controllabe release of Zinc ions [136].

Efficient wound dressing can be created by the sustained release of non-toxic amounts of calcium, copper, and zinc ions from a combination of $Zn^{2+}$ and $Cu^{2+}$ ions in MOFs-niacin and MOFs encapsulated in alginate microcapsules [137]. The photothermal properties of MOFs (Prussian Blue) embedded into CS-based hydrogels can be exploited as an antibacterial agent through the synergistic effect of heat and the electropositive surface from hydrogel [138]. Ag-based MOF composites with CS can act as barriers to the permeation of bacteria to wounds due to their antibacterial activities and can also release trace amounts of $Ag^{+}$ to reduce inflammation and accelerate wound healing [139]. In addition to the release of their primary components due to their progressive degradation MOFs provide sites to be loaded with biologically active substances such as gases, organic molecules, ions, enzymes, or nanoparticles [140].

Nitric oxide (NO) is an essential molecule with well-recognized therapeutic properties [141]. Pinto et al., developed novel vitamin B3 MOFs with Ni and Co as metal centers and titanium carboxylate MIP-177 for NO storage and demonstrated possible therapeutic applications of the NO release [142,143]. The liporeductor cosmetic caffeine (Caf) was loaded into MIL100, and nanoparticles were embedded into biocompatible polymers (PVA) and gelatin. Caf was progressively released from the composite and could permeate through the skin, reaching the targeted adipocyte region, paving the way for the topical administration of MOF polymer-based devices for the cutaneous or transdermal administration [144].

Photosensitive properties of MOFs also can be exploited. Zirconium-based PCN-224 MOFs loaded with $Ag^{+}$ ions and coated with HA were tested with MRSA bacteria. The combination of ROS from PCN-224 organic ligands and the release of Ag ions-Ag showed a much higher antibacterial activity effect than separated PCN-224Ag and silver ions. MFM-300(Sc) MOFs can be excellent drug carriers for the transdermal administration of natural antioxidant ferulic acid (FA), which has a protective role for the main skin structures such as collagen, fibroblasts, keratinocytes, and elastin [145]. Recently, Taherzade et al. [146], created topical patches based on water-stable and biosafe Fe carboxylate MOFs (MIL-100 and MIL-127), the biopolymer polyvinyl alcohol (PVA), and the selective adsorption of two co-encapsulated drugs used in skin disorders (azelaic acid (Az) as antibiotic, and nicotinamide (Nic) as anti-inflammatory), to develop an advanced cutaneous combined therapy. MOFs for cutaneous applications can be further optimized for combined treatments using both progressive framework degradation and slow delivery of active substances. A dual cooperative controllable release system has been designed by incorporating small molecular drugs (dimethyloxalylglycine, DMOG) into ZIF-67 nanoparticles. The strategy used to perform a controlled release of DMOG and $Co^{2+}$ ions included the nanoparticles in a micro-patterned poly (L-lactic acid) PLLA/Gellatin nanofibrous scaffolds. Synergistic effects that promoted accelerated healing in diabetic chronic wounds were found [147]. HKUST-1 MOFs have been utilized in the design of multifunctional antimicrobial agents through the delivery of antibacterial gases, antibiotic molecules, and antibacterial metal ions at different rates as a strategy that permits both fast and long-lived bactericidal action [148].

## 6. Conclusions and Future Perspectives

The progression of pathologies and symptoms, such as inflammation, allergies, psoriasis, and dermatitis, are directly related to alteration in the dermis' cellular communication and maintenance of matrix components. However, most literature based on nanoparticle formulations to treat skin conditions is commonly targeted to trespass de SC and reach the epidermis, the external layer of the skin. Our revision aims to illustrate how the integrity of the dermis is essential to maintain the skin's protective functions and to attain a significant improvement in treating pathologies. The diverse works summarized in this article prove that targeting the dermis is essential to produce a promising treatment based on nanotechnology. Indeed, the main challenge for dermis drug delivery is the stratum corneum as a physical barrier. Several types of nanoparticles (inorganic, polymeric, or lipidic) have been developed in recent years to circumvent this issue. Those nanoparticles are selected depending on the route chosen to cross the epidermis or considering the chemical properties of the cargo molecule being studied. However, the nanoparticle composition must be considered in the rational strategy to reach an adequate therapeutical effect in the targeted region. Some components, such as metals, can control microbial growth on damaged skin or reduce ROS production. Likewise, some polymers can stimulate the fibroblast to produce extracellular matrix components, contributing considerably to improving the dermis function.

In this context, MOF appears with unique characteristic of inorganic/organic composition that integrate the properties of metals and organic compounds in a unique system; MOFs also have a clear structure, adjustable pore size and shape, excellent surface area and porosity, easy chemical functionalization and can be prepared in large amounts. Despite the numerous articles published on (nano)MOFs, the development of the new (nano)MOFs centered on the dermis as a therapeutic target has not reached their maturity because the full potential of (nano)MOFs has not been exploited yet. MOFs present some drawbacks: They present some degree of matrix degradation, which induces premature drug leakage before reaching the target; their syntheses are often rigorous with high pressures and/or temperatures or involve toxic solvents. Another obstacle is the intrinsic toxicity of the MOF primary components. All these issues reduce their applicability in biomedical applications. Thus, the near future challenge passes from creating MOFs-based nanoparticles whose characteristics permit precise control of the target and drug release without loss of sturdiness. Additionally, it is necessary to carefully investigate the toxicity of the primary building blocks and metals and the biocompatibility issues. However, the most ambitious future approach is the creation of totally bioactive (nano)MOFs in which both metal and organics have an active role.

**Author Contributions:** Conceptualization C.V., D.V.-Y. and C.C.-V.; writing—original draft preparation J.S. and T.C.; figure preparation J.S., T.C. and C.V.; writing—review and editing C.V., F.C.Z. and W.I.C.; funding acquisition C.V., F.C.Z., D.V.-Y. and C.C.-V. All authors have read and agreed to the published version of the manuscript.

**Funding:** The design of the study, the collection, analysis, interpretation of data, and the writing of the manuscript were supported by research grants from the National Fund for Science & Technology Development, [FONDECYT 1201147 (C.V.), 1200944 (C.C.-V.), 1210763 (F.C.Z.), FONDECYT 1201249 (D.V.-Y.)] and BASAL Grant: CEDENNA from the National Research and Development Agency (ANID), Government of Chile (AFB180001 [C.V., C.C.-V., and D.V.-Y.]). Millennium Science Initiative Program—ICN09_016/ICN 2021_045: Millennium Institute on Immunology and Immunotherapy (ICN09_016/ICN 2021_045; former P09/016-F) [C.C.-V.]). Research Associate of European Union's Horizon 2020 Research and Innovation Program under the Marie Sklodowsks-Curie Grant Agreement No. 734801 (C.V.). J.S. Acknowledge to CONICYT-PFCHA/Doctorado Nacional/2017-21171302, and ANID/ACT210057. T.C. Acknowledge the Postdoctoral Program from Universidad de Talca.

**Conflicts of Interest:** The authors declare no conflict of interest. The authors have no other relevant affiliations or financial involvement with any organization or entity with a financial interest in or financial conflict with the subject matter or materials discussed in the manuscript apart from those disclosed.

## References

1. Gonzales, K.A.U.; Fuchs, E. Skin and Its Regenerative Powers: An Alliance between Stem Cells and Their Niche. *Dev. Cell* **2017**, *43*, 387–401. [CrossRef] [PubMed]
2. Foo, Y.Z.; Simmons, L.W.; Rhodes, G. Predictors of facial attractiveness and health in humans. *Sci. Rep.* **2017**, *7*, 39731. [CrossRef] [PubMed]
3. Seth, D.; Cheldize, K.; Brown, D.; Freeman, E.F. Global Burden of Skin Disease: Inequities and Innovations. *Curr. Derm. Rep.* **2017**, *6*, 204–210. [CrossRef] [PubMed]
4. Lim, H.W.; Collins, S.A.B.; Resneck, J.S., Jr.; Bolognia, J.L.; Hodge, J.A.; Rohrer, T.A.; Van Beek, M.J.; Margolis, D.J.; Sober, A.J.; Weinstock, M.A.; et al. The burden of skin disease in the United States. *J. Am. Acad. Derm.* **2017**, *76*, 958–972.e952. [CrossRef] [PubMed]
5. Haydont, V.; Bernard, B.A.; Fortunel, N.O. Age-related evolutions of the dermis: Clinical signs, fibroblast and extracellular matrix dynamics. *Mech. Ageing Dev.* **2019**, *177*, 150–156. [CrossRef]
6. Eyerich, S.; Eyerich, K.; Traidl-Hoffmann, C.; Biedermann, T. Cutaneous Barriers and Skin Immunity: Differentiating A Connected Network. *Trends Immunol.* **2018**, *39*, 315–327. [CrossRef]
7. Krutmann, J.; Bouloc, A.; Sore, G.; Bernard, B.A.; Passeron, T. The skin aging exposome. *J. Derm. Sci.* **2017**, *85*, 152–161. [CrossRef]
8. Horsley, V. Skin in the Game: Stem Cells in Repair, Cancer, and Homeostasis. *Cell* **2020**, *181*, 492–494. [CrossRef]
9. Fisher, G.J.; Shao, Y.; He, T.; Qin, Z.; Perry, D.; Voorhees, J.J.; Quan, T. Reduction of fibroblast size/mechanical force down-regulates TGF-beta type II receptor: Implications for human skin aging. *Aging Cell* **2016**, *15*, 67–76. [CrossRef]
10. Janson, D.G.; Saintigny, G.; van Adrichem, A.; Mahe, C.; El Ghalbzouri, A. Different gene expression patterns in human papillary and reticular fibroblasts. *J. Investig. Derm.* **2012**, *132*, 2565–2572. [CrossRef]
11. Dengjel, J.; Bruckner-Tuderman, L.; Nystrom, A. Skin proteomics—Analysis of the extracellular matrix in health and disease. *Expert Rev. Proteom.* **2020**, *17*, 377–391. [CrossRef] [PubMed]
12. Abdo, H.; Calvo-Enrique, L.; Lopez, J.M.; Song, J.; Zhang, M.D.; Usoskin, D.; El Manira, A.; Adameyko, I.; Hjerling-Leffler, J.; Ernfors, P. Specialized cutaneous Schwann cells initiate pain sensation. *Science* **2019**, *365*, 695–699. [CrossRef] [PubMed]
13. Jansen, K.A.; Licup, A.J.; Sharma, A.; Rens, R.; MacKintosh, F.C.; Koenderink, G.H. The Role of Network Architecture in Collagen Mechanics. *Biophys. J.* **2018**, *114*, 2665–2678. [CrossRef] [PubMed]
14. Rippa, A.L.; Kalabusheva, E.P.; Vorotelyak, E.A. Regeneration of Dermis: Scarring and Cells Involved. *Cells* **2019**, *8*, 607. [CrossRef]
15. Thulabandu, V.; Chen, D.; Atit, R.P. Dermal fibroblast in cutaneous development and healing. *Wiley Interdiscip. Rev. Dev. Biol.* **2018**, *7*, e307. [CrossRef]
16. Griffin, M.F.; desJardins-Park, H.E.; Mascharak, S.; Borrelli, M.R.; Longaker, M.T. Understanding the impact of fibroblast heterogeneity on skin fibrosis. *Dis. Model. Mech.* **2020**, *13*, dmm044164. [CrossRef]
17. Driskell, R.R.; Watt, F.M. Understanding fibroblast heterogeneity in the skin. *Trends Cell Biol.* **2015**, *25*, 92–99. [CrossRef]
18. Hu, M.S.; Moore, A.L.; Longaker, M.T. A Fibroblast Is Not a Fibroblast Is Not a Fibroblast. *J. Investig. Derm.* **2018**, *138*, 729–730. [CrossRef]
19. Philippeos, C.; Telerman, S.B.; Oules, B.; Pisco, A.O.; Shaw, T.J.; Elgueta, R.; Lombardi, G.; Driskell, R.R.; Soldin, M.; Lynch, M.D.; et al. Spatial and Single-Cell Transcriptional Profiling Identifies Functionally Distinct Human Dermal Fibroblast Subpopulations. *J. Investig. Derm.* **2018**, *138*, 811–825. [CrossRef]
20. Korosec, A.; Frech, S.; Gesslbauer, B.; Vierhapper, M.; Radtke, C.; Petzelbauer, P.; Lichtenberger, B.M. Lineage Identity and Location within the Dermis Determine the Function of Papillary and Reticular Fibroblasts in Human Skin. *J. Investig. Derm.* **2019**, *139*, 342–351. [CrossRef]
21. Nauroy, P.; Barruche, V.; Marchand, L.; Nindorera-Badara, S.; Bordes, S.; Closs, B.; Ruggiero, F. Human Dermal Fibroblast Subpopulations Display Distinct Gene Signatures Related to Cell Behaviors and Matrisome. *J. Investig. Derm.* **2017**, *137*, 1787–1789. [CrossRef] [PubMed]
22. Korosec, A.; Frech, S.; Lichtenberger, B.M. Isolation of Papillary and Reticular Fibroblasts from Human Skin by Fluorescence-activated Cell Sorting. *J. Vis. Exp.* **2019**, *147*, e59372. [CrossRef] [PubMed]
23. Karppinen, S.M.; Heljasvaara, R.; Gullberg, D.; Tasanen, K.; Pihlajaniemi, T. Toward understanding scarless skin wound healing and pathological scarring. *F1000Research* **2019**, *8*, 787. [CrossRef] [PubMed]
24. Jiao, H.; Zhang, T.; Fan, J.; Xiao, R. The Superficial Dermis May Initiate Keloid Formation: Histological Analysis of the Keloid Dermis at Different Depths. *Front. Physiol.* **2017**, *8*, 885. [CrossRef] [PubMed]
25. Deng, C.C.; Hu, Y.F.; Zhu, D.H.; Cheng, Q.; Gu, J.J.; Feng, Q.L.; Zhang, L.X.; Xu, Y.P.; Wang, D.; Rong, Z.; et al. Single-cell RNA-seq reveals fibroblast heterogeneity and increased mesenchymal fibroblasts in human fibrotic skin diseases. *Nat. Commun.* **2021**, *12*, 3709. [CrossRef] [PubMed]

26. Hinz, B.; McCulloch, C.A.; Coelho, N.M. Mechanical regulation of myofibroblast phenoconversion and collagen contraction. *Exp. Cell Res.* **2019**, *379*, 119–128. [CrossRef]
27. Huang, X.; Gu, S.; Liu, C.; Zhang, L.; Zhang, Z.; Zhao, Y.; Khoong, Y.; Li, H.; Gao, Y.; Liu, Y.; et al. CD39(+) Fibroblasts Enhance Myofibroblast Activation by Promoting IL-11 Secretion in Hypertrophic Scars. *J. Investig. Derm.* **2022**, *142*, 1065–1076.e1019. [CrossRef]
28. Gyorfi, A.H.; Matei, A.E.; Fuchs, M.; Liang, C.; Rigau, A.R.; Hong, X.; Zhu, H.; Luber, M.; Bergmann, C.; Dees, C.; et al. Engrailed 1 coordinates cytoskeletal reorganization to induce myofibroblast differentiation. *J. Exp. Med.* **2021**, *218*, e20201916. [CrossRef]
29. Mascharak, S.; desJardins-Park, H.E.; Davitt, M.F.; Griffin, M.; Borrelli, M.R.; Moore, A.L.; Chen, K.; Duoto, B.; Chinta, M.; Foster, D.S.; et al. Preventing Engrailed-1 activation in fibroblasts yields wound regeneration without scarring. *Science* **2021**, *372*, eaba2374. [CrossRef]
30. Montoni, A.; George, K.M.; Soeur, J.; Tran, C.; Marrot, L.; Rochette, P.J. Chronic UVA1 Irradiation of Human Dermal Fibroblasts: Persistence of DNA Damage and Validation of a Cell Cultured-Based Model of Photoaging. *J. Investig. Derm.* **2019**, *139*, 1821–1824.e1823. [CrossRef]
31. Birch-Machin, M.A.; Russell, E.V.; Latimer, J.A. Mitochondrial DNA damage as a biomarker for ultraviolet radiation exposure and oxidative stress. *Br. J. Derm.* **2013**, *169* (Suppl. S2), 9–14. [CrossRef] [PubMed]
32. Wolf, J.; Weinberger, B.; Arnold, C.R.; Maier, A.B.; Westendorp, R.G.; Grubeck-Loebenstein, B. The effect of chronological age on the inflammatory response of human fibroblasts. *Exp. Gerontol.* **2012**, *47*, 749–753. [CrossRef] [PubMed]
33. Cavinato, M.; Jansen-Durr, P. Molecular mechanisms of UVB-induced senescence of dermal fibroblasts and its relevance for photoaging of the human skin. *Exp. Gerontol.* **2017**, *94*, 78–82. [CrossRef] [PubMed]
34. Kenny, F.N.; Drymoussi, Z.; Delaine-Smith, R.; Kao, A.P.; Laly, A.C.; Knight, M.M.; Philpott, M.P.; Connelly, J.T. Tissue stiffening promotes keratinocyte proliferation through activation of epidermal growth factor signaling. *J. Cell Sci.* **2018**, *131*, jcs.215780. [CrossRef]
35. Ghosh, A.K.; Yuan, W.; Mori, Y.; Varga, J. Smad-dependent stimulation of type I collagen gene expression in human skin fibroblasts by TGF-beta involves functional cooperation with p300/CBP transcriptional coactivators. *Oncogene* **2000**, *19*, 3546–3555. [CrossRef]
36. Wang, X.; Qian, Y.; Jin, R.; Wo, Y.; Chen, J.; Wang, C.; Wang, D. Effects of TRAP-1-like protein (TLP) gene on collagen synthesis induced by TGF-beta/Smad signaling in human dermal fibroblasts. *PLoS ONE* **2013**, *8*, e55899. [CrossRef]
37. Strnadova, K.; Sandera, V.; Dvorankova, B.; Kodet, O.; Duskova, M.; Smetana, K.; Lacina, L. Skin aging: The dermal perspective. *Clin. Derm.* **2019**, *37*, 326–335. [CrossRef]
38. Kabashima, K.; Honda, T.; Ginhoux, F.; Egawa, G. The immunological anatomy of the skin. *Nat. Rev. Immunol.* **2019**, *19*, 19–30. [CrossRef]
39. Ho, A.W.; Kupper, T.S. T cells and the skin: From protective immunity to inflammatory skin disorders. *Nat. Rev. Immunol.* **2019**, *19*, 490–502. [CrossRef]
40. Laidlaw, B.J.; Gray, E.E.; Zhang, Y.; Ramirez-Valle, F.; Cyster, J.G. Sphingosine-1-phosphate receptor 2 restrains egress of gammadelta T cells from the skin. *J. Exp. Med.* **2019**, *216*, 1487–1496. [CrossRef]
41. Duffy, D.; Perrin, H.; Abadie, V.; Benhabiles, N.; Boissonnas, A.; Liard, C.; Descours, B.; Reboulleau, D.; Bonduelle, O.; Verrier, B.; et al. Neutrophils transport antigen from the dermis to the bone marrow, initiating a source of memory CD8+ T cells. *Immunity* **2012**, *37*, 917–929. [CrossRef] [PubMed]
42. Dijkgraaf, F.E.; Matos, T.R.; Hoogenboezem, M.; Toebes, M.; Vredevoogd, D.W.; Mertz, M.; van den Broek, B.; Song, J.Y.; Teunissen, M.B.M.; Luiten, R.M.; et al. Tissue patrol by resident memory CD8(+) T cells in human skin. *Nat. Immunol.* **2019**, *20*, 756–764, Erratum in *Nat. Immunol.* **2020**, *21*, 696. [CrossRef] [PubMed]
43. Jee, M.H.; Mraz, V.; Geisler, C.; Bonefeld, C.M. gammadelta T cells and inflammatory skin diseases. *Immunol. Rev.* **2020**, *298*, 61–73. [CrossRef] [PubMed]
44. Choi, J.E.; Di Nardo, A. Skin neurogenic inflammation. *Semin. Immunopathol.* **2018**, *40*, 249–259. [CrossRef]
45. Lowy, D.B.; Makker, P.G.S.; Moalem-Taylor, G. Cutaneous Neuroimmune Interactions in Peripheral Neuropathic Pain States. *Front. Immunol.* **2021**, *12*, 660203. [CrossRef]
46. Sumpter, T.L.; Balmert, S.C.; Kaplan, D.H. Cutaneous immune responses mediated by dendritic cells and mast cells. *JCI Insight* **2019**, *4*, e123947. [CrossRef]
47. Kuroishi, T.; Bando, K.; Bakti, R.K.; Ouchi, G.; Tanaka, Y.; Sugawara, S. Migratory dendritic cells in skin-draining lymph nodes have nickel-binding capabilities. *Sci. Rep.* **2020**, *10*, 5050. [CrossRef]
48. Ibusuki, A.; Nishikawa, T.; Hiraki, T.; Okano, T.; Imai, K.; Kanegane, H.; Ohnishi, H.; Kato, Z.; Fujii, K.; Tanimoto, A.; et al. Prominent dermal Langerhans cells in an Omenn syndrome patient with a novel mutation in the IL2RG gene. *J. Derm.* **2019**, *46*, 1019–1023. [CrossRef]
49. Bastonini, E.; Bellei, B.; Filoni, A.; Kovacs, D.; Iacovelli, P.; Picardo, M. Involvement of non-melanocytic skin cells in vitiligo. *Exp. Derm.* **2019**, *28*, 667–673. [CrossRef]
50. Lowes, M.A.; Suarez-Farinas, M.; Krueger, J.G. Immunology of psoriasis. *Annu. Rev. Immunol.* **2014**, *32*, 227–255. [CrossRef]
51. Krishnan, V.; Mitragotri, S. Nanoparticles for topical drug delivery: Potential for skin cancer treatment. *Adv. Drug Deliv. Rev.* **2020**, *153*, 87–108. [CrossRef] [PubMed]

52. Shan, X.; Gong, X.; Li, J.; Wen, J.; Li, Y.; Zhang, Z. Current approaches of nanomedicines in the market and various stage of clinical translation. *Acta Pharm. Sin. B* **2022**, *12*, 3028–3048. [CrossRef] [PubMed]
53. Lee, H.; Song, C.; Baik, S.; Kim, D.; Hyeon, T.; Kim, D.H. Device-assisted transdermal drug delivery. *Adv. Drug Deliv. Rev.* **2018**, *127*, 35–45. [CrossRef] [PubMed]
54. Niu, L.; Chu, L.Y.; Burton, S.A.; Hansen, K.J.; Panyam, J. Intradermal delivery of vaccine nanoparticles using hollow microneedle array generates enhanced and balanced immune response. *J. Control. Release* **2019**, *294*, 268–278. [CrossRef] [PubMed]
55. Elmowafy, M. Skin penetration/permeation success determinants of nanocarriers: Pursuit of a perfect formulation. *Colloids Surf. B Biointerfaces* **2021**, *203*, 111748. [CrossRef] [PubMed]
56. Roberts, M.S.; Mohammed, Y.; Pastore, M.N.; Namjoshi, S.; Yousef, S.; Alinaghi, A.; Haridass, I.N.; Abd, E.; Leite-Silva, V.R.; Benson, H.; et al. Topical and cutaneous delivery using nanosystems. *J. Control. Release* **2017**, *247*, 86–105. [CrossRef] [PubMed]
57. Khabir, Z.; Guller, A.E.; Rozova, V.S.; Liang, L.; Lai, Y.J.; Goldys, E.M.; Hu, H.; Vickery, K.; Zvyagin, A.V. Tracing upconversion nanoparticle penetration in human skin. *Colloids Surf. B Biointerfaces* **2019**, *184*, 110480. [CrossRef]
58. Hung, C.F.; Chen, W.Y.; Hsu, C.Y.; Aljuffali, I.A.; Shih, H.C.; Fang, J.Y. Cutaneous penetration of soft nanoparticles via photodamaged skin: Lipid-based and polymer-based nanocarriers for drug delivery. *Eur. J. Pharm. Biopharm.* **2015**, *94*, 94–105. [CrossRef]
59. Hung, C.F.; Fang, C.L.; Al-Suwayeh, S.A.; Yang, S.Y.; Fang, J.Y. Evaluation of drug and sunscreen permeation via skin irradiated with UVA and UVB: Comparisons of normal skin and chronologically aged skin. *J. Derm. Sci.* **2012**, *68*, 135–148. [CrossRef]
60. Richards, G.M.; Oresajo, C.O.; Halder, R.M. Structure and function of ethnic skin and hair. *Derm. Clin.* **2003**, *21*, 595–600. [CrossRef]
61. Salimi, A.; Sharif Makhmal Zadeh, B.; Godazgari, S.; Rahdar, A. Development and Evaluation of Azelaic Acid-Loaded Microemulsion for Transfollicular Drug Delivery Through Guinea Pig Skin: A Mechanistic Study. *Adv. Pharm. Bull.* **2020**, *10*, 239–246. [CrossRef] [PubMed]
62. Jung, S.; Otberg, N.; Thiede, G.; Richter, H.; Sterry, W.; Panzner, S.; Lademann, J. Innovative liposomes as a transfollicular drug delivery system: Penetration into porcine hair follicles. *J. Investig. Derm.* **2006**, *126*, 1728–1732. [CrossRef] [PubMed]
63. Pena-Jimenez, D.; Fontenete, S.; Megias, D.; Fustero-Torre, C.; Grana-Castro, O.; Castellana, D.; Loewe, R.; Perez-Moreno, M. Lymphatic vessels interact dynamically with the hair follicle stem cell niche during skin regeneration in vivo. *EMBO J.* **2019**, *38*, e101688. [CrossRef] [PubMed]
64. Try, C.; Moulari, B.; Beduneau, A.; Fantini, O.; Pin, D.; Pellequer, Y.; Lamprecht, A. Size dependent skin penetration of nanoparticles in murine and porcine dermatitis models. *Eur. J. Pharm. Biopharm.* **2016**, *100*, 101–108. [CrossRef]
65. Pelikh, O.; Eckert, R.W.; Pinnapireddy, S.R.; Keck, C.M. Hair follicle targeting with curcumin nanocrystals: Influence of the formulation properties on the penetration efficacy. *J. Control. Release* **2021**, *329*, 598–613. [CrossRef]
66. Busch, L.; Keziban, Y.; Dahne, L.; Keck, C.M.; Meinke, M.C.; Lademann, J.; Patzelt, A. The impact of skin massage frequency on the intrafollicular transport of silica nanoparticles: Validation of the ratchet effect on an ex vivo porcine skin model. *Eur. J. Pharm. Biopharm.* **2021**, *158*, 266–272. [CrossRef]
67. Radtke, M.; Patzelt, A.; Knorr, F.; Lademann, J.; Netz, R.R. Ratchet effect for nanoparticle transport in hair follicles. *Eur. J. Pharm. Biopharm.* **2017**, *116*, 125–130. [CrossRef]
68. Patzelt, A.; Mak, W.C.; Jung, S.; Knorr, F.; Meinke, M.C.; Richter, H.; Ruhl, E.; Cheung, K.Y.; Tran, N.; Lademann, J. Do nanoparticles have a future in dermal drug delivery? *J. Control. Release* **2017**, *246*, 174–182. [CrossRef]
69. Lademann, J.; Richter, H.; Meinke, M.C.; Lange-Asschenfeldt, B.; Antoniou, C.; Mak, W.C.; Renneberg, R.; Sterry, W.; Patzelt, A. Drug delivery with topically applied nanoparticles: Science fiction or reality. *Skin Pharm. Physiol.* **2013**, *26*, 227–233. [CrossRef]
70. Kim, M.H.; Jeon, Y.E.; Kang, S.; Lee, J.Y.; Lee, K.W.; Kim, K.T.; Kim, D.D. Lipid Nanoparticles for Enhancing the Physicochemical Stability and Topical Skin Delivery of Orobol. *Pharmaceutics* **2020**, *12*, 845. [CrossRef]
71. Brown, M.B.; Martin, G.P.; Jones, S.A.; Akomeah, F.K. Dermal and Transdermal Drug Delivery Systems: Current and Future Prospects. *Drug Deliv.* **2006**, *13*, 175–187. [CrossRef] [PubMed]
72. Palmer, B.C.; DeLouise, L.A. Nanoparticle-Enabled Transdermal Drug Delivery Systems for Enhanced Dose Control and Tissue Targeting. *Molecules* **2016**, *21*, 1719. [CrossRef] [PubMed]
73. Wang, T.; Yin, L.; Ma, Z.; Zhang, Y. Chlorogenic Acid-Loaded Mesoporous Silica Nanoparticles Modified with Hexa-Histidine Peptides Reduce Skin Allergies by Capturing Nickel. *Molecules* **2022**, *27*, 1430. [CrossRef] [PubMed]
74. Kaur, J.; Anwer, M.K.; Sartaj, A.; Panda, B.P.; Ali, A.; Zafar, A.; Kumar, V.; Gilani, S.J.; Kala, C.; Taleuzzaman, M. ZnO Nanoparticles of Rubia cordifolia Extract Formulation Developed and Optimized with QbD Application, Considering Ex Vivo Skin Permeation, Antimicrobial and Antioxidant Properties. *Molecules* **2022**, *27*, 1450. [CrossRef] [PubMed]
75. Borges Rosa de Moura, F.; Antonio Ferreira, B.; Helena Muniz, E.; Benatti Justino, A.; Gabriela Silva, A.; de Azambuja Ribeiro, R.I.M.; Oliveira Dantas, N.; Lisboa Ribeiro, D.; de Assis Araujo, F.; Salmen Espindola, F.; et al. Antioxidant, anti-inflammatory, and wound healing effects of topical silver-doped zinc oxide and silver oxide nanocomposites. *Int. J. Pharm.* **2022**, *617*, 121620. [CrossRef]
76. Rao, Y.F.; Chen, W.; Liang, X.G.; Huang, Y.Z.; Miao, J.; Liu, L.; Lou, Y.; Zhang, X.G.; Wang, B.; Tang, R.K.; et al. Epirubicin-loaded superparamagnetic iron-oxide nanoparticles for transdermal delivery: Cancer therapy by circumventing the skin barrier. *Small* **2015**, *11*, 239–247. [CrossRef]

77. Pedram Rad, Z.; Mokhtari, J.; Abbasi, M. Fabrication and characterization of PCL/zein/gum arabic electrospun nanocomposite scaffold for skin tissue engineering. *Mater. Sci. Eng. C Mater. Biol. Appl.* **2018**, *93*, 356–366. [CrossRef]
78. Graff, P.; Honzke, S.; Joshi, A.A.; Yealland, G.; Fleige, E.; Unbehauen, M.; Schafer-Korting, M.; Hocke, A.; Haag, R.; Hedtrich, S. Preclinical Testing of Dendritic Core-Multishell Nanoparticles in Inflammatory Skin Equivalents. *Mol. Pharm.* **2022**, *19*, 1795–1802. [CrossRef]
79. Gehrcke, M.; de Bastos Brum, T.; da Rosa, L.S.; Ilha, B.D.; Soares, F.Z.M.; Cruz, L. Incorporation of nanocapsules into gellan gum films: A strategy to improve the stability and prolong the cutaneous release of silibinin. *Mater. Sci. Eng. C Mater. Biol. Appl.* **2021**, *119*, 111624. [CrossRef]
80. Gupta, T.; Kenjale, P.; Pokharkar, V. QbD-based optimization of raloxifene-loaded cubosomal formulation for transdemal delivery: Ex vivo permeability and in vivo pharmacokinetic studies. *Drug Deliv. Transl. Res.* **2022**, *12*, 2979–2992. [CrossRef]
81. Ghasemiyeh, P.; Azadi, A.; Daneshamouz, S.; Heidari, R.; Azarpira, N.; Mohammadi-Samani, S. Cyproterone acetate-loaded nanostructured lipid carriers: Effect of particle size on skin penetration and follicular targeting. *Pharm. Dev. Technol.* **2019**, *24*, 812–823. [CrossRef] [PubMed]
82. Tak, Y.K.; Pal, S.; Naoghare, P.K.; Rangasamy, S.; Song, J.M. Shape-Dependent Skin Penetration of Silver Nanoparticles: Does It Really Matter? *Sci. Rep.* **2015**, *5*, 16908. [CrossRef] [PubMed]
83. Jingge, M.; Chengtie, W. Bioactive inorganic particles-based biomaterials for skin tissue engineering. *Exploration* **2022**, *2*, 20210083. [CrossRef]
84. Muchova, J.; Hearnden, V.; Michlovska, L.; Vistejnova, L.; Zavadakova, A.; Smerkova, K.; Kociova, S.; Adam, V.; Kopel, P.; Vojtova, L. Mutual influence of selenium nanoparticles and FGF2-STAB((R)) on biocompatible properties of collagen/chitosan 3D scaffolds: In vitro and ex ovo evaluation. *J. Nanobiotechnol.* **2021**, *19*, 103. [CrossRef] [PubMed]
85. Chen, Y.; Feng, X. Gold nanoparticles for skin drug delivery. *Int. J. Pharm.* **2022**, *625*, 122122. [CrossRef]
86. Niu, J.; Chu, Y.; Huang, Y.F.; Chong, Y.S.; Jiang, Z.H.; Mao, Z.W.; Peng, L.H.; Gao, J.Q. Transdermal Gene Delivery by Functional Peptide-Conjugated Cationic Gold Nanoparticle Reverses the Progression and Metastasis of Cutaneous Melanoma. *ACS Appl. Mater. Interfaces* **2017**, *9*, 9388–9401. [CrossRef]
87. Ramadan, S.; Guo, L.; Li, Y.; Yan, B.; Lu, W. Hollow copper sulfide nanoparticle-mediated transdermal drug delivery. *Small* **2012**, *8*, 3143–3150. [CrossRef]
88. Sivasankarapillai, V.S.; Vishnu Kirthi, A.; Akksadha, M.; Indu, S.; Dhiviya Dharshini, U.; Pushpamalar, J.; Karthik, L. Recent advancements in the applications of carbon nanodots: Exploring the rising star of nanotechnology. *Nanoscale Adv.* **2020**, *2*, 1760–1773. [CrossRef]
89. Bankoti, K.; Rameshbabu, A.P.; Datta, S.; Roy, M.; Goswami, P.; Roy, S.; Das, A.K.; Ghosh, S.K.; Dhara, S. Carbon nanodot decorated acellular dermal matrix hydrogel augments chronic wound closure. *J. Mater. Chem. B* **2020**, *8*, 9277–9294. [CrossRef]
90. Zielinska, A.; Carreiro, F.; Oliveira, A.M.; Neves, A.; Pires, B.; Venkatesh, D.N.; Durazzo, A.; Lucarini, M.; Eder, P.; Silva, A.M.; et al. Polymeric Nanoparticles: Production, Characterization, Toxicology and Ecotoxicology. *Molecules* **2020**, *25*, 3731. [CrossRef]
91. Mittal, A.; Raber, A.S.; Schaefer, U.F.; Weissmann, S.; Ebensen, T.; Schulze, K.; Guzman, C.A.; Lehr, C.M.; Hansen, S. Non-invasive delivery of nanoparticles to hair follicles: A perspective for transcutaneous immunization. *Vaccine* **2013**, *31*, 3442–3451. [CrossRef] [PubMed]
92. Gao, F.; Li, W.; Deng, J.; Kan, J.; Guo, T.; Wang, B.; Hao, S. Recombinant Human Hair Keratin Nanoparticles Accelerate Dermal Wound Healing. *ACS Appl. Mater. Interfaces* **2019**, *11*, 18681–18690. [CrossRef] [PubMed]
93. Wang, M.; Wang, C.; Chen, M.; Xi, Y.; Cheng, W.; Mao, C.; Xu, T.; Zhang, X.; Lin, C.; Gao, W.; et al. Efficient Angiogenesis-Based Diabetic Wound Healing/Skin Reconstruction through Bioactive Antibacterial Adhesive Ultraviolet Shielding Nanodressing with Exosome Release. *ACS Nano* **2019**, *13*, 10279–10293. [CrossRef] [PubMed]
94. Permana, A.D.; Paredes, A.J.; Volpe-Zanutto, F.; Anjani, Q.K.; Utomo, E.; Donnelly, R.F. Dissolving microneedle-mediated dermal delivery of itraconazole nanocrystals for improved treatment of cutaneous candidiasis. *Eur. J. Pharm. Biopharm.* **2020**, *154*, 50–61. [CrossRef]
95. Jin, N.; Pyo, S.M.; Keck, C.M.; Muller, R.H. Azithromycin nanocrystals for dermal prevention of tick bite infections. *Pharmazie* **2019**, *74*, 277–285. [CrossRef]
96. Jeong, H.; Nam, S.; Song, J.; Park, S. Synthesis and physicochemical properties of pH-sensitive hydrogel based on carboxymethyl chitosan/2-hydroxyethyl acrylate for transdermal delivery of nobiletin. *J. Drug Deliv. Sci. Technol.* **2019**, *51*, 194–203. [CrossRef]
97. Junior, D.M.; Hausen, M.A.; Asami, J.; Higa, A.M.; Leite, F.L.; Mambrini, G.P.; Rossi, A.L.; Komatsu, D.; Duek, E.A.R. A New Dermal Substitute Containing Polyvinyl Alcohol with Silver Nanoparticles and Collagen with Hyaluronic Acid: In Vitro and In Vivo Approaches. *Antibiotics* **2021**, *10*, 742. [CrossRef]
98. Kanemaru, M.; Asai, J.; Jo, J.I.; Arita, T.; Kawai-Ohnishi, M.; Tsutsumi, M.; Wada, M.; Tabata, Y.; Katoh, N. Nanoparticle-mediated local delivery of pioglitazone attenuates bleomycin-induced skin fibrosis. *J. Derm. Sci.* **2019**, *93*, 41–49. [CrossRef]
99. Kim, H.; Lee, S.; Ki, C.S. Modular formation of hyaluronic acid/beta-glucan hybrid nanogels for topical dermal delivery targeting skin dendritic cells. *Carbohydr. Polym.* **2021**, *252*, 117132. [CrossRef]
100. Yan, Y.; Liang, H.; Liu, X.; Liu, L.; Chen, Y. Topical cationic hairy particles targeting cell free DNA in dermis enhance treatment of psoriasis. *Biomaterials* **2021**, *276*, 121027. [CrossRef]

101. Lorenzoni, R.; Contri, R.V.; Lima, C.K.F.; Barreto, F.; Araujo, B.V.; Pohlmann, A.R.; de Miranda, A.L.P.; Costa, T.D.; Guterres, S.S. Dermatopharmacokinetic and pharmacodynamic evaluation of a novel nanostructured formulation containing capsaicinoids for treating neuropathic pain. *Int. J. Pharm.* **2021**, *596*, 120294. [CrossRef] [PubMed]
102. Sanad, R.A.; Abdel-Bar, H.M. Chitosan-hyaluronic acid composite sponge scaffold enriched with Andrographolide-loaded lipid nanoparticles for enhanced wound healing. *Carbohydr. Polym.* **2017**, *173*, 441–450. [CrossRef] [PubMed]
103. Li, X.; Widjaya, A.S.; Liu, J.; Liu, X.; Long, Z.; Jiang, Y. Cell-penetrating corosolic acid liposome as a functional carrier for delivering chemotherapeutic drugs. *Acta Biomater.* **2020**, *106*, 301–313. [CrossRef] [PubMed]
104. Beaulac, C.; Sachetelli, S.; Lagace, J. In-vitro bactericidal efficacy of sub-MIC concentrations of liposome-encapsulated antibiotic against gram-negative and gram-positive bacteria. *J. Antimicrob. Chemother.* **1998**, *41*, 35–41. [CrossRef] [PubMed]
105. Khater, D.; Nsairat, H.; Odeh, F.; Saleh, M.; Jaber, A.; Alshaer, W.; Bawab, A.; Mubarak, M. Design, Preparation, and Characterization of Effective Dermal and Transdermal Lipid Nanoparticles: A Review. *Cosmetics* **2021**, *8*, 39. [CrossRef]
106. Lebron, J.A.; Lopez-Lopez, M.; Garcia-Calderon, C.B.; Rosado, V.I.; Balestra, F.R.; Huertas, P.; Rodik, R.V.; Kalchenko, V.I.; Bernal, E.; Moya, M.L.; et al. Multivalent Calixarene-Based Liposomes as Platforms for Gene and Drug Delivery. *Pharmaceutics* **2021**, *13*, 1250. [CrossRef]
107. Keck, C.M.; Specht, D.; Brussler, J. Influence of lipid matrix composition on biopharmaceutical properties of lipid nanoparticles. *J. Control. Release* **2021**, *338*, 149–163. [CrossRef]
108. Anantaworasakul, P.; Anuchapreeda, S.; Yotsawimonwat, S.; Naksuriya, O.; Lekawanvijit, S.; Tovanabutra, N.; Anantaworasakul, P.; Wattanasri, W.; Buranapreecha, N.; Ampasavate, C. Nanomaterial Lipid-Based Carrier for Non-Invasive Capsaicin Delivery; Manufacturing Scale-Up and Human Irritation Assessment. *Molecules* **2020**, *25*, 5575. [CrossRef]
109. Shahraeini, S.S.; Akbari, J.; Saeedi, M.; Morteza-Semnani, K.; Abootorabi, S.; Dehghanpoor, M.; Rostamkalaei, S.S.; Nokhodchi, A. Atorvastatin Solid Lipid Nanoparticles as a Promising Approach for Dermal Delivery and an Anti-inflammatory Agent. *AAPS PharmSciTech* **2020**, *21*, 263. [CrossRef]
110. Rostamkalaei, S.S.; Akbari, J.; Saeedi, M.; Morteza-Semnani, K.; Nokhodchi, A. Topical gel of Metformin solid lipid nanoparticles: A hopeful promise as a dermal delivery system. *Colloids Surf. B Biointerfaces* **2019**, *175*, 150–157. [CrossRef]
111. Essaghraoui, A.; Belfkira, A.; Hamdaoui, B.; Nunes, C.; Lima, S.A.C.; Reis, S. Improved Dermal Delivery of Cyclosporine A Loaded in Solid Lipid Nanoparticles. *Nanomaterials* **2019**, *9*, 1204. [CrossRef] [PubMed]
112. de Souza Guedes, L.; Martinez, R.M.; Bou-Chacra, N.A.; Velasco, M.V.R.; Rosado, C.; Baby, A.R. An Overview on Topical Administration of Carotenoids and Coenzyme Q10 Loaded in Lipid Nanoparticles. *Antioxidants* **2021**, *10*, 1034. [CrossRef] [PubMed]
113. Pham, C.; Van, M.; Thi, H.; Thanh, C.; Ngoc, B.; Van, B.; Thien, G.; Van, B.; Nguyen, C. Development of ibuprofen-loaded solid lipid nanoparticle-based hydrogels for enhanced in vitro dermal permeation and in vivo topical anti-inflammatory activity. *J. Drug Deliv. Sci. Technol.* **2020**, *57*, 101758. [CrossRef]
114. Amasya, G.; Ozturk, C.; Aksu, B.; Tarimci, N. QbD based formulation optimization of semi-solid lipid nanoparticles as nano-cosmeceuticals. *J. Drug Deliv. Sci. Technol.* **2021**, *66*, 102737. [CrossRef]
115. Boskabadi, M.; Saeedi, M.; Akbari, J.; Morteza-Semnani, K.; Hassan-Hashemi, S.; Babaei, A. Topical Gel of Vitamin A Solid Lipid Nanoparticles: A Hopeful Promise as a Dermal Delivery System. *Adv. Pharm. Bull.* **2021**, *11*, 663–674. [CrossRef]
116. Qiu, T.; Gao, S.; Liang, Z.; Wang, D.G.; Tabassum, H.; Zhong, R.; Zou, R. Pristine Hollow Metal-Organic Frameworks: Design, Synthesis and Application. *Angew. Chem. Int. Ed. Engl.* **2021**, *60*, 17314–17336. [CrossRef]
117. Morris, R.E.; Wheatley, P.S. Gas storage in nanoporous materials. *Angew. Chem. Int. Ed. Engl.* **2008**, *47*, 4966–4981. [CrossRef]
118. Dhurjad, P.; Dhalaram, C.S.; Ali, N.; Kumari, N.; Sonti, R. Metal-organic frameworks in chiral separation of pharmaceuticals. *Chirality* **2022**, *34*, 1419–1436. [CrossRef]
119. Li, H.Y.; Zhao, S.N.; Zang, S.Q.; Li, J. Functional metal-organic frameworks as effective sensors of gases and volatile compounds. *Chem. Soc. Rev.* **2020**, *49*, 6364–6401. [CrossRef]
120. Huang, Y.B.; Liang, J.; Wang, X.S.; Cao, R. Multifunctional metal-organic framework catalysts: Synergistic catalysis and tandem reactions. *Chem Soc. Rev.* **2017**, *46*, 126–157. [CrossRef]
121. Haider, J.; Shahzadi, A.; Akbar, M.U.; Hafeez, I.; Shahzadi, I.; Khalid, A.; Ashfaq, A.; Ahmad, S.O.A.; Dilpazir, S.; Imran, M.; et al. A review of synthesis, fabrication, and emerging biomedical applications of metal-organic frameworks. *Biomater. Adv.* **2022**, *140*, 213049. [CrossRef] [PubMed]
122. Ma, Y.; Qu, X.; Liu, C.; Xu, Q.; Tu, K. Metal-Organic Frameworks and Their Composites Towards Biomedical Applications. *Front. Mol. Biosci.* **2021**, *8*, 805228. [CrossRef] [PubMed]
123. Zhou, Y.; Yang, T.; Liang, K.; Chandrawati, R. Metal-organic frameworks for therapeutic gas delivery. *Adv. Drug Deliv. Rev.* **2021**, *171*, 199–214. [CrossRef] [PubMed]
124. Wang, Y.; Hu, Y.; He, Q.; Yan, J.; Xiong, H.; Wen, N.; Cai, S.; Peng, D.; Liu, Y.; Liu, Z. Metal-organic frameworks for virus detection. *Biosens. Bioelectron.* **2020**, *169*, 112604. [CrossRef]
125. Mao, H.; Yu, L.; Tu, M.; Wang, S.; Zhao, J.; Zhang, H.; Cao, Y. Recent Advances on the Metal-Organic Frameworks-Based Biosensing Methods for Cancer Biomarkers Detection. *Crit. Rev. Anal. Chem.* **2022**, 1–17. [CrossRef]
126. Muldoon, P.F.; Collet, G.; Eliseeva, S.V.; Luo, T.Y.; Petoud, S.; Rosi, N.L. Ship-in-a-Bottle Preparation of Long Wavelength Molecular Antennae in Lanthanide Metal-Organic Frameworks for Biological Imaging. *J. Am. Chem Soc.* **2020**, *142*, 8776–8781. [CrossRef]

127. Tamames-Tabar, C.; Imbuluzqueta, E.; Guillou, N.; Serre, C.B.S.R.M.; Elkaïm, E.C.P.H.; Blanco-Prieto, M.J. A Zn azelate MOF: Combining antibacterial effect. *CrystEngComm* **2015**, *17*, 456–462. [CrossRef]
128. Quaresma, S.; Andre, V.; Antunes, A.M.M.; Vilela, S.M.F.; Amariei, G.; Arenas-Vivo, A.; Rosal, R.; Horcajada, P.; Duarte, M.T. Novel Antibacterial Azelaic Acid BioMOFs. *Cryst. Growth Des.* **2020**, *20*, 370–382. [CrossRef]
129. Yang, J.; Wang, C.; Liu, X.; Yin, Y.; Ma, Y.-H.; Gao, Y.; Wang, Y.; Lu, Z.; Song, Y. Gallium–Carbenicillin Framework Coated Defect-Rich Hollow $TiO_2$ as a Photocatalyzed Oxidative Stress Amplifier against Complex Infections. *Adv. Funct. Mater.* **2020**, *30*, 2004861. [CrossRef]
130. Duan, F.; Feng, X.; Jin, Y.; Liu, D.; Yang, X.; Zhou, G.; Liu, D.; Li, Z.; Liang, X.J.; Zhang, J. Metal-carbenicillin framework-based nanoantibiotics with enhanced penetration and highly efficient inhibition of MRSA. *Biomaterials* **2017**, *144*, 155–165. [CrossRef]
131. Xiao, J.; Zhu, Y.; Huddleston, S.; Li, P.; Xiao, B.; Farha, O.K.; Ameer, G.A. Copper Metal-Organic Framework Nanoparticles Stabilized with Folic Acid Improve Wound Healing in Diabetes. *ACS Nano* **2018**, *12*, 1023–1032. [CrossRef]
132. Liu, Z.; Wang, F.; Ren, J.; Qu, X. A series of MOF/Ce-based nanozymes with dual enzyme-like activity disrupting biofilms and hindering recolonization of bacteria. *Biomaterials* **2019**, *208*, 21–31. [CrossRef]
133. Zhang, L.; Liu, Z.; Deng, Q.; Sang, Y.; Dong, K.; Ren, J.; Qu, X. Nature-Inspired Construction of MOF@COF Nanozyme with Active Sites in Tailored Microenvironment and Pseudopodia-Like Surface for Enhanced Bacterial Inhibition. *Angew. Chem. Int. Ed. Engl.* **2021**, *60*, 3469–3474. [CrossRef]
134. Ren, X.; Yang, C.; Zhang, L.; Li, S.; Shi, S.; Wang, R.; Zhang, X.; Yue, T.; Sun, J.; Wang, J. Copper metal-organic frameworks loaded on chitosan film for the efficient inhibition of bacteria and local infection therapy. *Nanoscale* **2019**, *11*, 11830–11838. [CrossRef]
135. Xiao, J.; Chen, S.; Yi, J.; Zhang, H.; Ameer, G.A. A Cooperative Copper Metal-Organic Framework-Hydrogel System Improves Wound Healing in Diabetes. *Adv. Funct. Mater.* **2017**, *27*, 1604872. [CrossRef]
136. Yao, X.; Zhu, G.; Zhu, P.; Ma, J.; Chen, W.; Liu, Z.; Kong, T. Omniphobic ZIF-8@Hydrogel Membrane by Microfluidic-Emulsion-Templating Method for Wound Healing. *Adv. Funct. Mater.* **2020**, *30*, 1909389. [CrossRef]
137. Chen, G.; Yu, Y.; Wu, X.; Wang, G.; Gu, G.; Wang, F.; Ren, J.; Zhang, H.; Zhao, Y. Microfluidic Electrospray Niacin Metal-Organic Frameworks Encapsulated Microcapsules for Wound Healing. *Research* **2019**, *2019*, 6175398. [CrossRef]
138. Han, D.; Li, Y.; Liu, X.; Li, B.; Han, Y.; Zheng, Y.; Yeung, K.W.K.; Li, C.; Cui, Z.; Liang, Y.; et al. Rapid bacteria trapping and killing of metal-organic frameworks strengthened photo-responsive hydrogel for rapid tissue repair of bacterial infected wounds. *Chem. Eng. J.* **2020**, *396*, 125194. [CrossRef]
139. Zhang, M.; Wang, G.; Wang, D.; Zheng, Y.; Li, Y.; Meng, W.; Zhang, X.; Du, F.; Lee, S. Ag@MOF-loaded chitosan nanoparticle and polyvinyl alcohol/sodium alginate/chitosan bilayer dressing for wound healing applications. *Int. J. Biol. Macromol.* **2021**, *175*, 481–494. [CrossRef]
140. Zhang, M.; Qiao, R.; Hu, J. Engineering Metal-Organic Frameworks (MOFs) for Controlled Delivery of Physiological Gaseous Transmitters. *Nanomaterials* **2020**, *10*, 1134. [CrossRef]
141. Malone-Povolny, M.J.; Maloney, S.E.; Schoenfisch, M.H. Nitric Oxide Therapy for Diabetic Wound Healing. *Adv. Healthc. Mater.* **2019**, *8*, e1801210. [CrossRef]
142. Pinto, R.V.; Wang, S.; Tavares, S.R.; Pires, J.; Antunes, F.; Vimont, A.; Clet, G.; Daturi, M.; Maurin, G.; Serre, C.; et al. Tuning Cellular Biological Functions Through the Controlled Release of NO from a Porous Ti-MOF. *Angew. Chem. Int. Ed. Engl.* **2020**, *59*, 5135–5143. [CrossRef]
143. Pinto, R.V.; Antunes, F.; Pires, J.; Graca, V.; Brandao, P.; Pinto, M.L. Vitamin B3 metal-organic frameworks as potential delivery vehicles for therapeutic nitric oxide. *Acta Biomater.* **2017**, *51*, 66–74. [CrossRef]
144. Marquez, A.G.; Hidalgo, T.; Lana, H.; Cunha, D.; Blanco-Prieto, M.J.; Alvarez-Lorenzo, C.; Boissiere, C.; Sanchez, C.; Serre, C.; Horcajada, P. Biocompatible polymer-metal-organic framework composite patches for cutaneous administration of cosmetic molecules. *J. Mater. Chem. B* **2016**, *4*, 7031–7040. [CrossRef]
145. Osorio-Toribio, G.; Velasquez-Hernandez, M.J.; Mileo, P.G.M.; Zarate, J.A.; Aguila-Rosas, J.; Leyva-Gomez, G.; Sanchez-Sanchez, R.; Magana, J.J.; Perez-Diaz, M.A.; Lazaro, I.A.; et al. Controlled Transdermal Release of Antioxidant Ferulate by a Porous Sc(III) MOF. *iScience* **2020**, *23*, 101156. [CrossRef]
146. Taherzade, S.D.; Rojas, S.; Soleimannejad, J.; Horcajada, P. Combined Cutaneous Therapy Using Biocompatible Metal-Organic Frameworks. *Nanomaterials* **2020**, *10*, 2296. [CrossRef]
147. Li, J.; Lv, F.; Li, J.; Li, Y.; Gao, J.; Luo, J.; Xue, F.; Ke, Q.; Xu, H. Cobalt-based metal–organic framework as a dual cooperative controllable release system for accelerating diabetic wound healing. *Nano Res.* **2020**, *13*, 2268–2279. [CrossRef]
148. McKinlay, A.C.; Allan, P.K.; Renouf, C.L.; Duncan, M.J.; Wheatley, P.S.; Warrender, S.J.; Dawson, D.; Ashbrook, S.E.; Gil, B.; Marszalek, B.; et al. Multirate delivery of multiple therapeutic agents from metal-organic frameworks. *APL Mater.* **2014**, *2*, 124108. [CrossRef]

*pharmaceutics*

*Article*

# Cataleptogenic Effect of Haloperidol Formulated in Water-Soluble Calixarene-Based Nanoparticles

**Nadezda E. Kashapova [1,*], Ruslan R. Kashapov [1,*], Albina Y. Ziganshina [1], Dmitry O. Nikitin [2], Irina I. Semina [2], Vadim V. Salnikov [3], Vitaliy V. Khutoryanskiy [4], Rouslan I. Moustafine [5] and Lucia Y. Zakharova [1]**

1 Arbuzov Institute of Organic and Physical Chemistry, FRC Kazan Scientific Center of RAS, 8 Arbuzov Str., 420088 Kazan, Russia
2 Department of Pharmacology, Kazan State Medical University, 49 Butlerov Str., 420012 Kazan, Russia
3 Kazan Institute of Biochemistry and Biophysics, FRC Kazan Scientific Center of RAS, 2/31 Lobachevsky Str., 420111 Kazan, Russia
4 School of Pharmacy, University of Reading, Whiteknights, Reading RG6 6DX, UK
5 Institute of Pharmacy, Kazan State Medical University, 16 Fatykh Amirkhan Str., 420126 Kazan, Russia
* Correspondence: kashapova.nadya@gmail.com (N.E.K.); kashapov@iopc.ru (R.R.K.)

**Abstract:** In this study, a water-soluble form of haloperidol was obtained by coaggregation with calix[4]resorcinol bearing viologen groups on the upper rim and decyl chains on the lower rim to form vesicular nanoparticles. The formation of nanoparticles is achieved by the spontaneous loading of haloperidol into the hydrophobic domains of aggregates based on this macrocycle. The mucoadhesive and thermosensitive properties of calix[4]resorcinol–haloperidol nanoparticles were established by UV-, fluorescence and CD spectroscopy data. Pharmacological studies have revealed low in vivo toxicity of pure calix[4]resorcinol ($LD_{50}$ is 540 $\pm$ 75 mg/kg for mice and 510 $\pm$ 63 mg/kg for rats) and the absence of its effect on the motor activity and psycho-emotional state of mice, which opens up a possibility for its use in the design of effective drug delivery systems. Haloperidol formulated with calix[4]resorcinol exhibits a cataleptogenic effect in rats both when administered intranasally and intraperitoneally. The effect of the intranasal administration of haloperidol with macrocycle in the first 120 min is comparable to the effect of commercial haloperidol, but the duration of catalepsy was shorter by 2.9 and 2.3 times ($p < 0.05$) at 180 and 240 min, respectively, than that of the control. There was a statistically significant reduction in the cataleptogenic activity at 10 and 30 min after the intraperitoneal injection of haloperidol with calix[4]resorcinol, then there was an increase in the activity by 1.8 times ($p < 0.05$) at 60 min, and after 120, 180 and 240 min the effect of this haloperidol formulation was at the level of the control sample.

**Keywords:** calixarene; haloperidol; mucoadhesion; self-assembly; TEM; nanoparticles; toxicity in vivo; open field; catalepsy

## 1. Introduction

Haloperidol is known as a psychotropic drug with antipsychotic, neuroleptic, and antiemetic activities. This drug has low water solubility and high permeability through biological tissues [1,2]. Due to the fact that the low water solubility of haloperidol limits its therapeutic potential, the effect of its action with various routes of administration is currently being widely studied. Nasal administration is considered as a promising approach to deliver drugs to the brain [3]. However, with intranasal administration of haloperidol, its bioavailability is limited since the drug must be in solution for its effective absorption. Dissolution becomes the rate-limiting step if it occurs more slowly than absorption. Varying the composition of the dosage form can change the rate of dissolution and thus control the overall absorption. Different approaches to overcome poor aqueous solubility of drugs, such as solid dispersion and liquisolid dispersion techniques [4,5], micellar solubilization [6,7], an inclusion of an active poorly water-soluble drug in various nanoparticles [8–10], cyclodextrins [11–14], and liposomes [15,16] are often used to increase a drug's solubility and, as a result, improve its bioavailability. In addition, there are several studies describing the inclusion of water-insoluble drugs into a calixarene cavity to form guest-host complexes [17–20], with a significant improvement of the in vitro dissolution profile and, in some cases, an increase in bioavailability [18,20] and a decrease of in vivo acute oral toxicity compared to the pure drug [20].

There are known examples of incorporating haloperidol into formulations based on lipids, surfactants and their mixtures [21], for the intranasal delivery of haloperidol, with improved pharmacokinetic profiles compared to the individual drug. In addition, the loading of haloperidol into nanoparticles based on anionic PEGylated Eudragit® L100-55 and cationic Eudragit® EPO polymers significantly increased the in vivo nose-to-brain delivery of haloperidol [22]. However, when haloperidol was loaded into hybrid nanoparticles based on the Eudragit L100-55 copolymer and the polymeric surfactant Brij98, its absorption was slowed down, which was expressed by a decrease in the pharmacological activity (cataleptogenic effect) compared to its free form [23]. Attempts to develop intranasal formulations are caused by problems with the oral delivery of haloperidol, when the drug enters systemic circulation after undergoing first-pass metabolism. In addition, haloperidol is 90% bound to plasma proteins, which leads to its low oral availability. Meanwhile, the intranasal administration of haloperidol can provide targeted delivery to the brain, bypassing the blood-brain barrier.

The nasal mucosa also acts as a barrier to drug penetration through the epithelial cells. The use of particles capable of adhering to mucous membranes as carriers may facilitate the retention of drugs on the surface providing more time for their absorption and increasing the effectiveness of their action. In our recent work, using porcine gastric mucin (PGM) as a model mucin, we have shown that viologen derivatives of calix[4]resorcinol interact with mucin strongly and, in combination with a drug (caffeine), the mixed systems exhibit mucoadhesive properties [24]. Due to their amphiphilic structure, the studied calixarenes are able to spontaneously self-assemble in aqueous solution with the formation of large aggregates, in which sparingly soluble drugs can be solubilized. In addition, $\pi$-electron-deficient 4,4′-bipyridinium units at the upper rim of the macrocyclic platform are able to selectively bind $\pi$-electron-rich molecules to form guest-host complexes [25], and also provide aqueous solubility, which is an important requirement for the development of efficient drug delivery carriers. Moreover, the search for new types of carriers of hydrophobic drugs, including haloperidol, remains an urgent task, since the previously studied formulations based on lipids, surfactants, their mixtures, and polymers are not without drawbacks, such as, for example, a laborious and multi-stage procedure for preparing nanoparticles using organic solvents and temperature, which does not meet the criteria of green chemistry. The formation of a complex between an amphiphilic calixarene and a hydrophobic drug can not only increase the aqueous solubility of the latter, but leads to the spontaneous formation of nanosized particles, which can make such macrocycles more preferable for formulating lipophilic biologically active substances. It should be noted that, to the best of our knowledge, there are no studies on the incorporation of haloperidol into calixarene molecules in the literature. The aim of this work was to prepare nanoparticles based on calix[4]resorcinol bearing viologen groups on the upper rim and decyl chains on the lower rim (**VC10**) and haloperidol (**Hal**) (Figure 1), to study the in vivo toxicity of **VC10** and its neurotropic properties, and to evaluate the cataleptogenic effect of the **VC10–Hal** formulation in comparison with a commercial formulation of **Hal**.

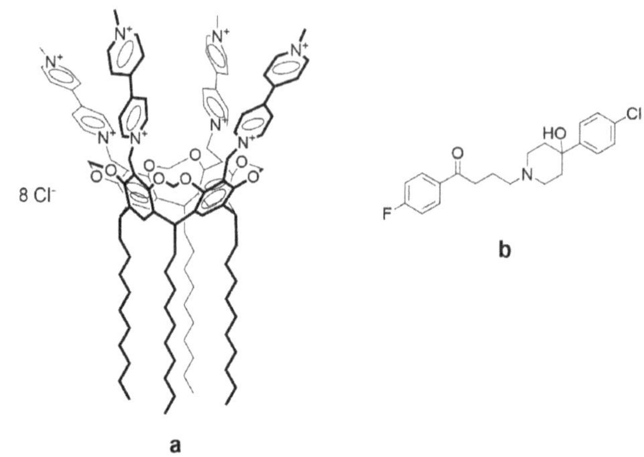

Figure 1. Molecular structures of calix[4]resorcinol **VC10** (**a**) and **Hal** (**b**).

## 2. Materials and Methods

### 2.1. Chemicals and Reagents

Calix[4]resorcinol **VC10** was synthesized by the reaction of tetra-(bromomethyl)calix[4] resorcinol with monomethylviologen using the procedure described in the literature [26]. Haloperidol, **Hal** (Alfa Aesar), $D_2O$ (99.9 atom% D, Carl Roth GmbH), mucin from porcine stomach, and PGM (Type III, bound sialic acid 0.5–1.5%, partially purified powder, Sigma-Aldrich (St. Louis, MO, USA)) were purchased and used without further purification. Deionized, ultrapure water with a resistivity of 18.2 MΩ was generated using a Direct Q-5 UV water purification system from Millipore SAS (Molsheim, France) and was used throughout this work.

### 2.2. Methods

#### 2.2.1. UV-Vis Spectroscopy

The UV-Vis absorption spectra were recorded using a Specord 250 Plus spectrophotometer (Analytik Jena AG, Jena, Germany) equipped with a temperature controller accessory (Peltier). Measurements were carried out using a 1-mm quartz cuvette at 25 °C, over a wavelength range of 220–500 nm. The turbidity (absorption, A) of the samples in turbidimetric titration was measured at $\lambda$ = 500 nm in a 1-cm quartz cuvette.

#### 2.2.2. NMR Spectroscopy

The $^1$H NMR spectra were recorded using a Bruker AVANCE(III)-600 spectrometer (Rheinstetten, Germany) operating at 600.1 MHz, which was equipped with a 5 mm broadband inverse probe head with z-gradient accessories to produce a field gradient up to 50 G·cm$^{-1}$. The samples were prepared in $D_2O$. The spectra were recorded at 303.0 ± 0.2 K. The chemical shifts are reported in the ppm scale and refer to the solvent (δ(HDO) 4.7 ppm).

#### 2.2.3. Dynamic Light Scattering

The hydrodynamic diameters of the **VC10–Hal** systems (molar ratio 1:1) at different concentrations (0.025 mM, 0.05 mM, 0.075 mM, 0.1 mM, 0.15 mM, 0.2 mM, 0.25 mM, 0.3 mM) were measured via the dynamic light scattering method using a Malvern Zetasizer Nano ZS particle size analyzer (Malvern Instruments Ltd., Worcestershire, UK). The light source was a 4 mW He-Ne laser with a wavelength of 632.8 nm. All measurements were carried out in disposable polystyrene cells in automatic mode at 25 °C, at a fixed scattering angle of 173°. The mean particle size ± standard deviation from three measurements was calculated using Malvern Zetasizer Software.

2.2.4. Transmission Electron Microscopy

The morphology of the **VC10–Hal** aggregates was examined using electron microscopy with a Hitachi HT7800 transmission electron microscope (Hitachi High-Tech Science Corporation, Tokyo, Japan). The sample for imaging was prepared in deionized water; 5 μL of the solution was applied straight onto a 3.05 mm diameter copper grid with a formvar film (01700-F, Ted Pella, Inc., Redding, CA, USA) and dried at room temperature. The grid with the dried sample was placed in the transmission electron microscope using a special holder, followed by imaging at an accelerating voltage of 80 kV in the TEM mode.

2.2.5. Fluorescence Spectroscopy

The fluorescence spectra were recorded by a Hitachi F-7100 Fluorescence Instrument (Hitachi High-Tech Science Corporation, Tokyo, Japan) with a xenon lamp as an excitation source and a temperature controller unit. Steady state fluorescence spectra were recorded using a 1 cm path length quartz cuvette (Hellma Analytics, Müllheim, Germany) in the range from 290 to 450 nm with an excitation light wavelength of 270 nm at temperatures of 298 K, 305 K, and 312 K. The slit widths of excitation and emission were set as 5 nm and 5 nm, respectively. The emission spectra of PGM at a constant concentration (0.05 mg/mL) were recorded in a titration series with a gradual increase in the concentration of **VC10** and **VC10–Hal** (molar ratio 1:1). The fluorescence intensity, at a wavelength of 330 nm, was used for the calculations given in Section 3.3.

2.2.6. Circular Dichroism Spectroscopy

Circular dichroism (CD) spectra were recorded on a JASCO J-1500 spectropolarimeter (JASCO Corporation, Tokyo, Japan). Measurements were carried out using a 1 mm path length quartz cuvette at room temperature (25 °C). CD spectra were recorded from 250 to 190 nm with a bandwidth of 1 nm, scanning speed of 100 nm/min, and data pitch of 1 nm. In all samples, the concentration of PGM was 1 mg/mL. CD spectra were the average of three scans in each of two independent measurements.

2.2.7. In Vivo Experiments

In vivo experiments were carried out using 62 male Wistar rats weighing 250–270 g and 54 white male mice weighing 18–22 g. Prior to the experiments, all animals were kept under standard vivarium conditions with a natural light regime and on a complete balanced diet in compliance with the International Recommendations of the European Convention for the Protection of Vertebrate Animals used in Experimental Research (1997), and the Rules of Laboratory Practice approved by the order of the Ministry of Health of the Russian Federation No. 199n, 1 April 2016. All in vivo experiments reported in this work were approved by the Ethical Committee of Kazan State Medical University (Protocol No. 8 of 30 October 2018).

Toxicity Assay

To determine the acute toxicity, a freshly prepared aqueous solution of **VC10** was administered intraperitoneally to male mice and male Wistar rats. Each study dose was applied to six animals. The dose that did not cause the death of any animal out of 6 (maximum tolerable dose) and the dose that caused the death of all 6 animals in the group (absolute lethal dose, $LD_{100}$) were determined. The intermediate doses were also determined, the introduction of which led to the death of some animals. The experimental data were processed according to the method described by Behrens; the average lethal dose ($LD_{50}$, the dose that causes the death of 50% of the animals) was determined graphically, and its error was determined using the Gaddam equation [27].

"Open Field" Test

The "Open Field" test is used to study the motor-exploratory activity of animals [28], the change in which reflects the effect of substances on the central nervous system (CNS).

The experiment on mice was carried out in a round chamber with opaque walls, with a diameter of 97 cm and a wall height of 42 cm (Open Science, Russia). The installation floor was divided into sectors for the convenience of visual registration. In addition, there were holes in the floor imitating minks (2 cm in diameter). The criterion for the transition from one sector to another was the location of the hind legs of the animal in the new sector. After testing each mouse, the deodorization of the installation surface using 3% hydrogen peroxide was carried out. After each group of mice, the installation was treated with a 70% ethanol solution. In these experiments, each animal was placed in the center of the field and within 3 min of testing the following parameters were recorded: (1) the number of crossed lines, which reflects the nonspecific level of excitation (motor activity); (2) the number of holes examined, which is an indicator of research activity [29]; (3) the number of entrances to the center, which reflects the psycho-emotional state.

Calix[4]resorcinol **VC10** was administered intraperitoneally to 8 mice at doses of 5 mg/kg of mice weight (1/100 of $LD_{50}$) and 10 mg/kg of mice weight (1/50 of $LD_{50}$), 30 min prior to testing. Control animals were injected with an equivalent volume of saline.

Behavioral changes were recorded using EthoVision XT video tracking software for automatic track analysis by Noldus (Netherlands). This provided a more accurate quantification of the behavioral differences in the animals.

Catalepsy Test

In order to assess the effect of the **VC10–Hal** formulation, the method of cataleptogenic effect of haloperidol in rats was used, which reflects the pharmacological properties of neuroleptics [30]. The severity of catalepsy was assessed by the duration of the "lecturer's posture" [31] using a special catalepsy device (Open Science, Russia), according to the protocol described in ref. [32]. Two series of experiments were carried out. In the first series, an aqueous solution of the binary **VC10–Hal** system was administered intranasally to 8 rats; in the second series it was administered intraperitoneally to 8 rats (the dose of haloperidol in all samples was 0.5 mg/kg of rat weight; the dose of **VC10** was 0.0028 mg/kg of rat's weight). A commercial haloperidol formulation (5 mg/mL of a sterile solution containing lactic acid (Gedeon-Richter, Budapest, Hungary)) was used as a control.

In the first series of experiments, the **VC10–Hal** formulation was instilled into the nostrils of rats for 5 min using a specially designed plastic cannula, and then each rat was placed in a special catalepsy device with a plastic bar at a height of 10 cm. Each rat was carefully placed on a plastic bar at 5, 10, 20, 30, 60, 120 and 180 min after the intranasal and intraperitoneal administration of the **VC10–Hal** formulation, or the commercial formulation of haloperidol as a control, and the ability to maintain the "lecturer's posture" (the duration on the bar) for 180 s was recorded. If the time spent on the bar reached 180 s, the rat was carefully removed. After each experiment, the rats were immediately returned to their cages. In the second series of experiments, intraperitoneal administration was carried out at the same dose and concentration as in the case of the intranasal administration.

Statistical Analysis

The obtained results were processed statistically according to the standard method using the two-sample Student's $t$-test, after checking the data for the normal distribution in the compared groups, as well as the equality of the general variances in the GraphPad Prism 8.0.1 program. The results of the behavioral tests are presented as the mean ± standard deviation. The critical level of significance was set at $p < 0.05$.

## 3. Results and Discussions

### 3.1. Coaggregation of Haloperidol and Viologen Decyl Calix[4]resorcinol

The choice of calix[4]resorcinol **VC10** as a solubilizer of haloperidol molecules was based on our previous studies, where it was shown that (1) the macrocycle has low cytotoxicity ($IC_{50}$ > 500) on the normal Chang liver cell line [33]; (2) has a low aggregation threshold of 0.3 mM in aqueous solutions and, due to its amphiphilic nature, is capable of solubilizing hydrophobic molecules into their aggregates [34]; (3) exhibits pronounced mucoadhesive properties both individually and in combination with drug molecules [24].

As mentioned above, **Hal** is practically insoluble in water. The UV-Vis absorption spectrum of **Hal** in ethanol shows that, at a concentration of 0.15 mM, it has limited absorption in the UV and visible region (Figure 2). With equimolar mixing of **VC10** with **Hal** after 15 min of sonication and 2 h of stirring at room temperature, the latter, visually, completely dissolves in aqueous solution due to solubilization by calix[4]resorcinol aggregates. The UV-Vis absorption spectrum of **VC10** in water shows a characteristic absorption peak at 260 nm (Figure 2). In the spectrum of the binary **VC10–Hal** system, there is an increase in the intensity of this peak and a slight hypsochromic shift by 3 nm. The maximum increase in absorbance is achieved after 24 h of mixing **VC10–Hal** at room temperature. The observed hyper- and hypsochromic effects in the UV-Vis absorption spectra indicate **Hal** binding in the hydrophobic domain of the **VC10** aggregates.

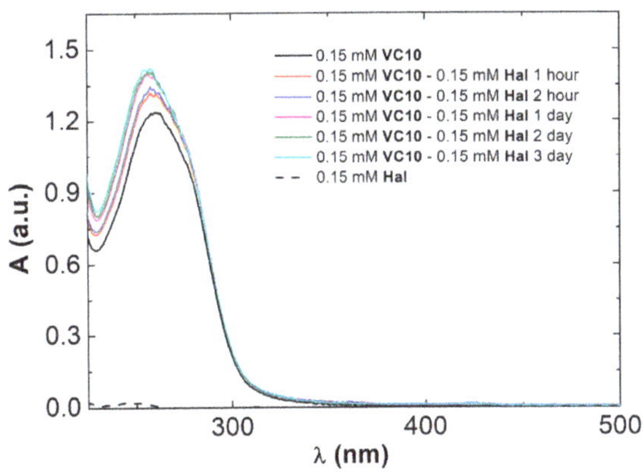


**Figure 2.** UV-Vis absorption spectra of 0.15 mM **VC10**, 0.15 mM **VC10**–0.15 mM **Hal** in $H_2O$, and 0.15 mM **Hal** in EtOH.

An equimolar mixture of **VC10–Hal** was studied by NMR spectroscopy. In the $^1$H-NMR spectrum of the binary **VC10–Hal** system, a new set of signals appears in the region of 6.85 and 7.71 ppm, as well as a broad peak in a strong field (2.39–2.90 ppm) in comparison with the spectrum of the pure **VC10** (Figure 3). In addition, an increase in the integral intensity is observed in the region of the H8 aromatic protons and H10 methylene protons of **VC10**, since in these regions there is an overlap with the signals of the aromatic (H8′) and aliphatic (H4′, H7′ H10′) protons of **Hal**, respectively. The appearance of the signals of hydrophobic **Hal** in $D_2O$ confirms its solubilization by amphiphilic **VC10** aggregates.

According to the DLS data, the **VC10–Hal** aggregates are formed at concentrations an order of magnitude lower than the critical aggregation concentration (CAC) of individual **VC10** equal to 0.3 mM [34]. The addition of **Hal** promotes aggregation of the amphiphilic **VC10**. It was shown that the equimolar addition of **Hal** to aqueous solutions of **VC10** with concentrations up to CAC leads to the formation of larger particles with an average diameter from ~127 to ~198 nm depending on the concentration of **VC10**, with a monomodal size distribution and a high-quality correlation function (Figures 4 and S1). This behavior is consistent with observations for conventional or polymeric surfactants, where the addition of apolar solutes promotes the aggregation of surfactant molecules, which otherwise tend to disperse in the aqueous phase [35].

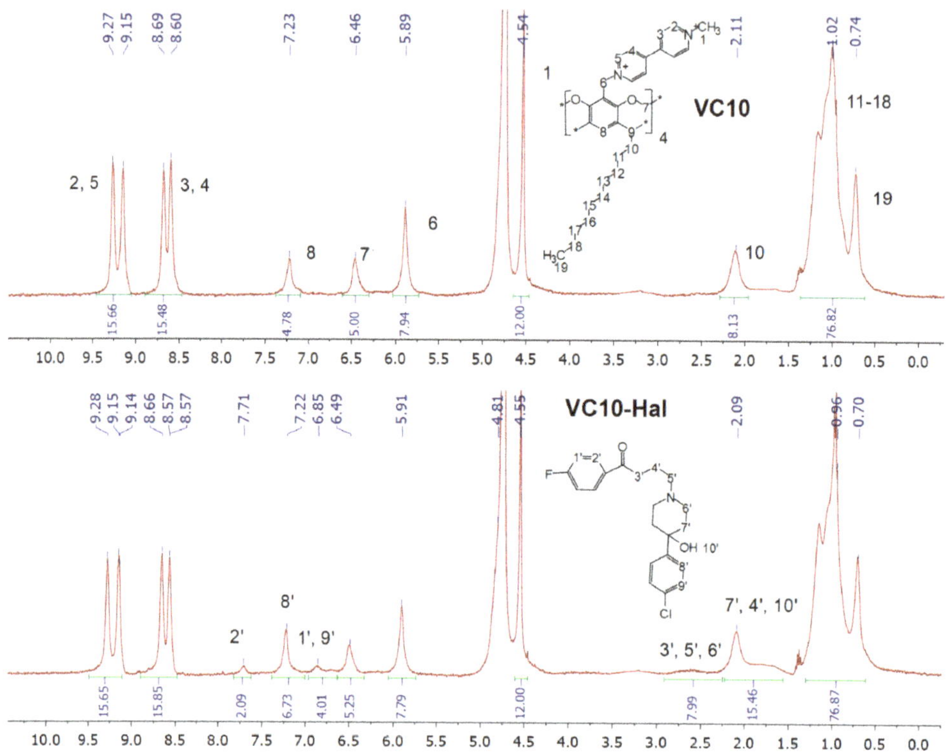


**Figure 3.** $^1$H-NMR spectra of 2 mM **VC10** and the binary 2 mM **VC10**–2 mM **Hal** system in $D_2O$.

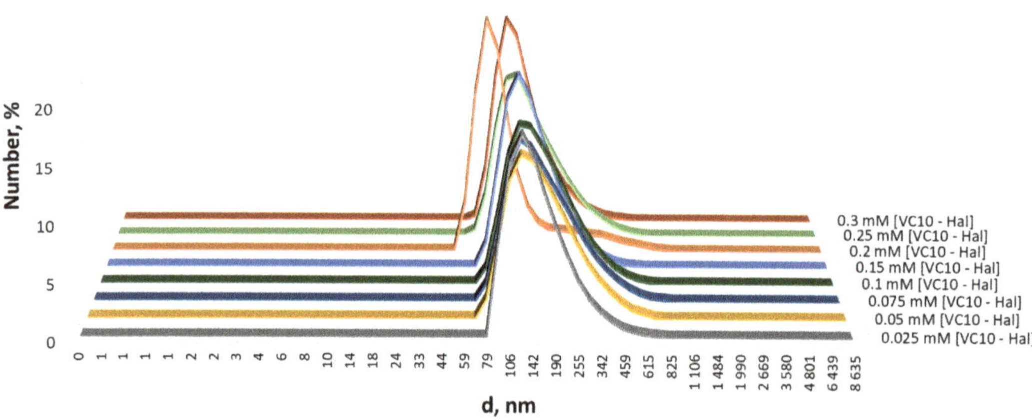


**Figure 4.** Particle size distribution by number in aqueous solutions of VC10–Hal (1:1) at different concentrations.

### *3.2. Morphology of Aggregates Based on Haloperidol and Viologen Decyl Calix[4]resorcinol*

The TEM images of the binary **VC10–Hal** system clearly show the presence of spherical vesicles, which are presented in Figure 5a as dark spherical particles; light spots do not have a clear spherical shape, it is a feature of sample drying during sample preparation. The aggregates based on **VC10–Hal** are uniformly distributed over the surface of the copper grid with the predominance of particles 100 nm in size (Figure 5b). It should be noted that micellar aggregates with a diameter of 10–50 nm were observed in the TEM image of pure **VC10** [33]. Binding of **Hal** by calix[4]resorcinol **VC10** leads to a significant change in the morphology of aggregates in aqueous solution with the transition of micelles to vesicles. Apparently, the solubilization of **Hal** molecules disrupts the high curvature of the surface of micellar aggregates, which leads to the formation of membrane structures. Morphological changes are typical during the solubilization of hydrophobic drugs by micellar systems. Thus, solubilization of 5-methyl salicylate within micelles of copolymers of polyoxyethylene and polyoxypropylene significantly enlarges and changes the shape of the micellar structures from spherical to ellipsoidal [36]. The localization of the drug in the hydrophobic micellar core promotes the formation of higher morphologies. In another work, hydrophobic perphenazine solubilized into taurocholate/lecithin aggregates caused a change in morphology from spherical particles to wormlike micelles [37]. Summarizing the results obtained by UV spectrophotometry, NMR spectroscopy, DLS and TEM, it can be concluded that haloperidol is located in the hydrophobic region within the bilayer formed by the non-polar alkyl tails of calix[4]resorcinol.

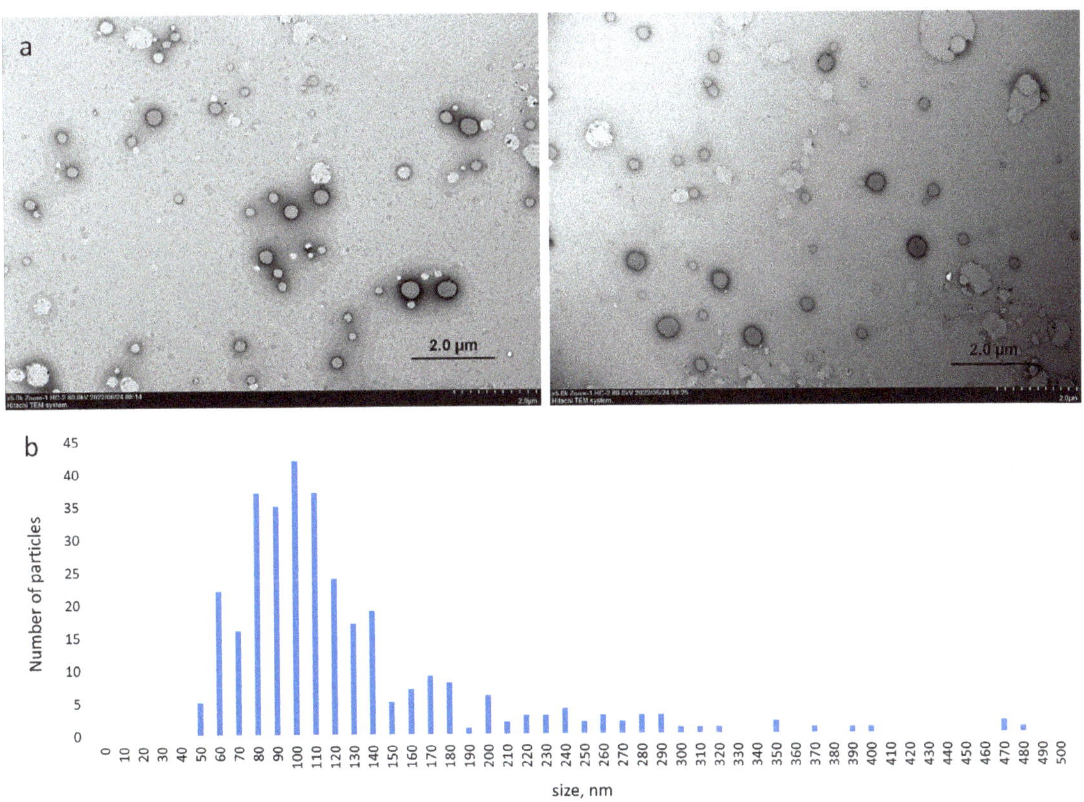


**Figure 5.** Transmission electron micrographs of **VC10–Hal** (**a**) and the histogram showing the average particle size obtained from the TEM images using ImageJ software (**b**).

### 3.3. *Mucoadhesive Properties of Calix[4]resorcinol–Haloperidol Nanoparticles*

To assess the mucoadhesive properties of calix[4]resorcinol–haloperidol nanoparticles, turbidimetric titration of PGM with a solution of binary **VC10-Hal** (1:1) system was carried out according to the procedure described in the literature [38]. The turbidity of solutions at various ratios was estimated from UV spectra at 500 nm, since at this wavelength there is no absorption in the UV spectra of **VC10** and **Hal**. The turbidimetric titration plot (Figure 6) shows that **VC10–Hal** aggregates have a good affinity for mucin due to the electrostatic interaction of positively charged viologen groups with negatively charged fragments in mucin. With an increase in the mass ratio of **VC10–Hal**, aggregation of mucin particles is observed with a maximum turbidity (absorption value A~1.4) at [**VC10–Hal**]/[mucin]~0.25, and with a further increase in the mass ratio, a decrease in turbidity and a disaggregation are observed. A similar profile was observed for the titration of mucin by individual **VC10** with a maximum absorption value of A~1.2 at 500 nm in our recent study [24]. A comparison of the turbidimetric titration curves of mucin by **VC10** and **VC10–Hal** shows that, despite the coaggregation of **VC10** and **Hal**, the ability of the macrocycle to effectively interact with mucin is maintained. Moreover, it should be noted that the maximum absorption on the turbidimetric curve for the **VC10–Hal** system is 0.2 units higher than that for the pure **VC10**, which indicates a more efficient interaction of **VC10** with mucin in the presence of **Hal**. Probably, the reason for the enhanced mucoadhesive effect is the vesicular form of the **VC10–Hal** aggregates, which has a lower surface curvature compared to the micellar structures of individual **VC10**.

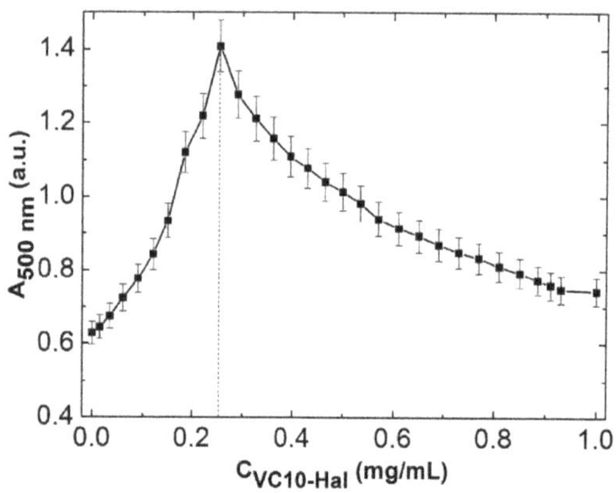


**Figure 6.** Turbidimetric titration of 1 mg/mL PGM with 1 mg/mL solution of **VC10–Hal** (1:1).

The binding of **VC10–Hal** aggregates to mucin was assessed from fluorescence quenching plots. It is known that mucin has intrinsic fluorescence due to fluorescent chromophores, namely amino acid residues, mainly tryptophan in the protein part of the molecule. In an aqueous solution, the excitation spectrum of tryptophan is in the wavelength range from 200 to 300 nm, and the fluorescence spectrum is recorded from 300 to 440 nm. The intensity of tryptophan fluorescence is highly dependent on the microenvironment, so the study of this fluorescence provides valuable information when binding proteins to various molecules. In our recent work, it was shown that the addition of **VC10** results in quenching of the mucin fluorescence intensity at 298 K [24]. In this work, we performed a series of fluorometric titrations of mucin with pure **VC10** and **VC10–Hal** at different temperatures (298 K, 304 K, 310 K) in order to determine the quenching mechanism. The concentration of mucin and calixarene was chosen so that the absorption value in their UV spectra did not exceed 0.1 unit. This minimizes the effect of the internal filter on the fluorescence spectra. With the gradual addition of **VC10** and **VC10–Hal** (at a ratio of 1:1) to PGM at a constant concentration (0.05 mg/mL) at different temperatures, the fluorescence of the latter is intensely quenched (Figures S2 and S3). These spectral changes clearly indicate the presence of specific interactions of **VC10** and **VC10–Hal** with PGM. The mechanism of the observed fluorescent quenching can be dynamic or static, or a combination of both of these processes. In general, the Stern–Volmer Equation (1) is used to reveal the quenching mechanism:

$$F_0/F = 1 + K_{SV}\cdot[Q], \quad (1)$$

where $F_0$ и F are the fluorescence intensities of PGM in the absence and in the presence of the quencher Q (**VC10–Hal** and **VC10**); $K_{SV}$ is the Stern–Volmer quenching constant; and Q is the concentration of the quencher (**VC10–Hal** and **VC10**).

Stern–Volmer plots for the fluorescence quenching of PGM by **VC10** and **VC10–Hal** at 298 K, 304 K and 310 K, are shown in Figure S4. The graphs have the *y*-intercept equal to one, and the slope equal to $K_{SV}$. In the case of one type of quenching, the graph in the Stern–Volmer coordinates is strictly linear, which is what we observe for our systems. The plots in Figure S4 showed a good linear relationship at every experimental temperature within the studied concentration range. From the obtained data (Table 1), it can be seen that the quenching constants $K_{SV}$ of PGM in the presence of the quencher (**VC10** and **VC10–Hal**) decrease with increasing temperature, which indicates static quenching [39]. When static quenching occurs, the fluorescent molecule forms a non-fluorescent complex with the quencher. As the quencher concentration increases, less unbound fluorophore remains in the solution and the fluorescence intensity decreases.

**Table 1.** Quenching constants of **PGM** in the presence of the quencher (**VC10** and **VC10–Hal**) at different temperatures.

| | $K_{SV}$ $10^3$ ($M^{-1}$) | | |
|---|---|---|---|
| | **298 K** | **304 K** | **310 K** |
| PGM–VC10 | 1762 ± 28 | 1635 ± 42 | 1516 ± 42 |
| PGM–[**VC10–Hal**] | 1702 ± 39 | 1563 ± 39 | 1405 ± 25 |

Further, to determine the binding constant ($K_a$), the number of binding sites (*n*), and the dissociation constants ($K_d$) for the PGM–**VC10** and PGM–[**VC10–Hal**] systems, the double logarithm regression curves as a function of quencher concentration were plotted based on Equation (2):

$$\log((F_0 - F)/F) = \log K_a + n\log(Q). \quad (2)$$

In the graph, *n* is equal to the tangent of the slope, and $K_a$ is the point of intersection with the y-axis. The dissociation constant ($K_d$) is the reciprocal of the association constant, $K_d = 1/K_a$. Table 2 summarizes the calculated data of *n*, $K_a$, $K_d$.

**Table 2.** Number of binding sites (*n*), binding constants ($K_a$), and dissociation constants ($K_d$), for the PGM–**VC10** and PGM–[**VC10–Hal**] systems at different temperatures.

| | PGM–VC10 | | | PGM–[VC10–Hal] | | |
|---|---|---|---|---|---|---|
| | *n* | $\log K_a$ | $K_d$ $10^{-8}$ (M) | *n* | $\log K_a$ | $K_d$ $10^{-8}$ (M) |
| 298 K | 1.21 ± 0.01 | 7.47 ± 0.06 | 3.40 | 1.30 ± 0.01 | 7.96 ± 0.04 | 1.10 |
| 304 K | 1.17 ± 0.03 | 7.18 ± 0.17 | 6.28 | 1.12 ± 0.02 | 6.87 ± 0.11 | 13.25 |
| 310 K | 1.13 ± 0.04 | 6.90 ± 0.29 | 11.06 | 1.05 ± 0.04 | 6.45 ± 0.22 | 32.71 |

It can be seen from Table 2 that the *n* value for both systems at different temperatures is close to 1, which indicates one binding site in the PGM–**VC10** and PGM–[**VC10–Hal**] systems. The probable site of PGM binding to the positively charged viologen calix[4]arene **VC10** is the sialic acid carboxyl groups in mucin. Considering that the binding constants ($\log K_a$) are in the range of 6.45–7.96, it can be assumed that **VC10** and **VC10–Hal** have a strong affinity for mucin at different temperatures. The strongest ability to bind with mucin is observed at 298 K ($\log K_a$ = 7.47 for PGM–**VC10** and $\log K_a$ = 7.96 for PGM–[**VC10–Hal**]). With increasing temperature, the values of the binding constants in both systems decrease, which additionally points to a static quenching mechanism. As the temperature rises, the intramolecular mobility increases, the stability of the formed complexes decreases, and, accordingly, the values of the static quenching constants decrease. It should be noted that for the PGM–[**VC10–Hal**] system, as the temperature rises to physiological, the binding constant decreases by 1.5 units, while the decrease occurs by 0.6 units in the PGM–**VC10** system. When comparing both systems, it can be concluded that the ternary system in the presence of a drug is more thermosensitive despite the greater stability of vesicular structures compared to micelles, which is an advantage in the development of a drug delivery system. A likely cause of thermosensitivity, in the case of using the binary system **VC10**–Hal, may be a destructive change in mucin morphology as a result of a stronger interaction in the PGM–[**VC10–Hal**] system compared to the PGM–**VC10** system. A possible explanation for this effect is the lower curvature of the vesicle surface, which ensures interaction with a larger surface of mucin compared to micellar particles. It should be additionally emphasized that, similar to micellar aggregates, the vesicles spontaneously formed in the binary system **VC10–Hal** are dynamic assemblies that can be subjected to structural rearrangements under different stimuli including temperature induced changes [40,41].

Using $K_a$ from Table 2, the Gibbs free energy variation ($\Delta G^o$) was calculated using Equation (3):

$$\Delta G^o = -RT \cdot \ln K_a, \tag{3}$$

where R is the gas constant (8.314 $Jmol^{-1}K^{-1}$), and T are the experimental temperatures (298 K, 304 K, 310 K). The calculated values of $\Delta G^\circ$ are summarized in Table 3. The negative sign for $\Delta G^o$ indicates that the binding of PGM with **VC10** and **VC10–Hal** is a spontaneous process.

**Table 3.** The Gibbs free energy variation ($\Delta G^o$) for the PGM–**VC10** and PGM–[**VC10–Hal**] systems at different temperatures.

| | **ΔG° (kJ·mol$^{-1}$)** | | |
|---|---|---|---|
| | **298 K** | **304 K** | **310 K** |
| PGM–**VC10** | −42.62 | −41.79 | −40.95 |
| PGM–[**VC10–Hal**] | −45.41 | −39.98 | −38.28 |

To determine the conformational stability of PGM upon its interaction with **VC10** and binary **VC10–Hal** system, circular dichroism (CD) spectra were recorded at a constant mucin concentration and a variable concentration of the studied systems (Figure 7). The CD spectrum of the individual PGM has a wide band in the far UV region, with a minimum at 206 nm and a negative ellipticity value, which indicates its secondary structure (random coil), and which is consistent with the literature data [42]. The signal is due to amino acid residues in the mucin having -NHCO- chromophores, which absorb in the 200–210 nm region. In the binary PGM–**VC10** and ternary PGM–[**VC10–Hal**] systems, the spectrum profile is typical for the pure PGM, which indicates that the random coil conformation of mucin is retained upon its interaction with the calix[4]arene **VC10** and **VC10–Hal** nanoparticles. With an increase in the proportion of the system (**VC10** and **VC10–Hal**) added to PGM, the value of negative ellipticity at the minimum decreases, and this minimum shifts to 209 nm, which is caused by a rather strong interaction in the binary and ternary systems, which was confirmed above by the UV and fluorescence spectroscopy data. The increase in the **VC10** concentration led to changes in the amplitude of the spectrum, indicating that the specific binding of the viologen groups of **VC10** to carboxylate groups in the glycoprotein increases the disorder of the secondary structure due to the inclusion of macrocycle molecules in the peptide backbone [43].

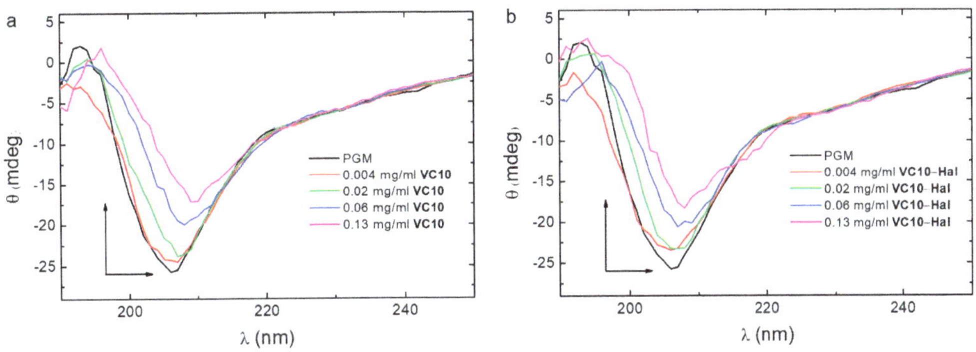


**Figure 7.** UV circular dichroism spectra of the PGM, PGM–**VC10** (**a**) and PGM–[**VC10–Hal**] (**b**) systems in aqueous solution. The concentration of PGM was constant (1 mg/mL) [**VC10–Hal**] = 1:1.

### *3.4. Toxicity Studies*

To identify the toxic and safe doses of **VC10** in order to use it as a carrier/delivery system, a study of acute toxicity and the effect of **VC10** on indicators in the "Open Field" in rodents (to assess the level of emotional and behavioral activity of animals) was carried out. The results of the study of acute toxicity of **VC10** when administered intraperitoneally allowed the calculation of the $LD_{50}$ values in mice and rats, which served as the basis for determining the working doses in further experiments. The $LD_{50}$ values of **VC10** were found to be 540 ± 75 mg/kg for mice and 510 ± 63 mg/kg for rats, which allows calix[4]resorcinol **VC10** to be classified as a toxicity category 4, i.e., as a compound with low toxicity [44].

The behavior in the "Open Field" indicates the functional state of the CNS of mice, which is the main marker of the toxic effects of any substances on the body. The "Open Field" test is used to study the behavior of rodents in new conditions and allows researchers to evaluate the dynamics of individual behavioral elements. This test creates a mild anxiety model. The calix[4]resorcinol **VC10** was administered intraperitoneally at doses of 1/100 and 1/50 of the $LD_{50}$ 30 min before the experiment. Mice from the control group received the appropriate volumes of saline. Table S1 shows that the average number of examined holes in the studied groups, taking into account the experimental error, is comparable to the control group, where the mice were not injected with the test compound. The maintenance of exploratory activity in the mice suggests that the cognitive functions of animals are not impaired by **VC10**. The number of crossed lines in all three groups was approximately the same (Table S2), which indicates the absence of an effect of **VC10** on the motor activity of mice. In the absence of any shelters, the animal feels more secure being near the wall. The number of entrances to the center did not change for the animals that received **VC10** in a dose of 1/50 of the $LD_{50}$, compared with the control group (Table S3). This means that calixarene does not have a depressing effect on the psycho-emotional status of mice. The primary pharmacological tests revealed the low toxicity of **VC10** and the absence of its effect upon behavioral characteristics at the studied doses, on the basis of which it can be concluded that **VC10**, when administered once, does not affect the CNS of laboratory mice. The obtained results gave us the basis to carry out further in vivo experiments on the study of the cataleptogenic effect of haloperidol in the formulation with **VC10**.

### *3.5. In Vivo Catalepsy Tests*

Catalepsy tests in rats were performed to estimate the efficacy of the **VC10–Hal** formulation compared to the commercial formulation of **Hal**. Cataleptogenic effect (catalepsy), i.e., the loss of the ability to make voluntary movements and the ability to maintain an artificially uncomfortable position for a long time, is one of the manifestations of extrapyramidal symptoms as a side effects of drugs with neuroleptic activity [45]. The study of the cataleptogenic action of **Hal** was carried out in two series of experiments, namely, with the intranasal and intraperitoneal administration of the studied formulations.

Intranasal administration for the treatment of diseases of the CNS is attractive because it allows the drug to be delivered directly to the brain, bypassing the blood-brain barrier. At the same time, neurotherapeutic drugs are delivered to the brain in significant concentrations with minimal exposure to systemic circulation [46]. The results of the cataleptogenic effect of **Hal** in the formulation with **VC10,** and the commercial formulation of **Hal** (as a control), with intranasal administration are shown in Figure 8. Analysis of intranasal administration showed the severity of the cataleptogenic effect of **Hal** in the formulation of **VC10–Hal** in the first 120 min of the study, which is comparable to the effect of commercial **Hal**. However, at 180 and 240 min, the catalepsy duration of the test sample was lower than in the control one.

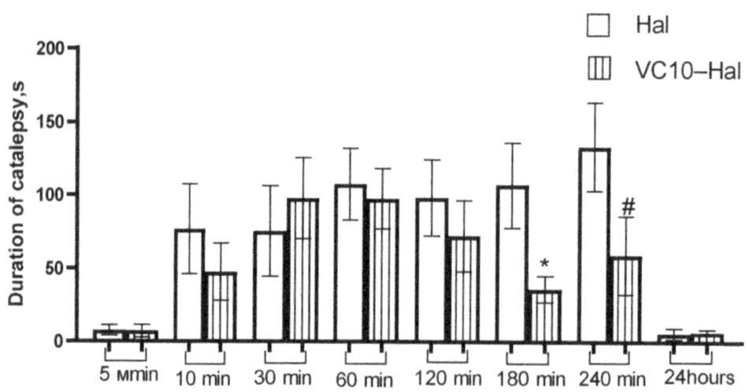


**Figure 8.** Duration of catalepsy after intranasal administration (s). * $p < 0.05$—Statistically significant difference compared to the haloperidol group. # $0.05 < p < 0.1$—Significance trend compared to haloperidol group.

As for the analysis of the intraperitoneal administration of the test sample in comparison with the commercial **Hal**, it should be noted that at 10 and 30 min there was a significant decrease in the intensity of the cataleptogenic effect of **Hal** in the formulation with **VC10**, and at 60 min, on the contrary, an increase in the effect (Figure 9). Further, at 120, 180 and 240 min, the effect of the formulated haloperidol was at the level of the control sample. The lower activity in the first 30 min may be due to the delayed release of **Hal** from the **VC10–Hal** formulation. The results of the cataleptogenic effect of **Hal** with intranasal and intraperitoneal administration of the studied samples showed that, depending on the route of administration, different results are observed over time, which, apparently, is due to the difference in pharmacokinetic parameters.

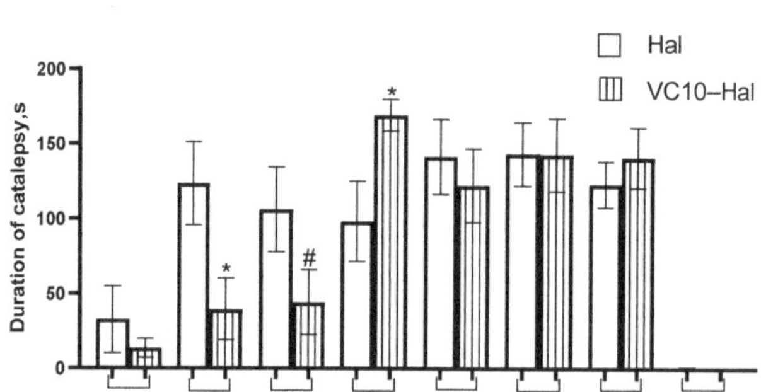


**Figure 9.** Duration of catalepsy after intraperitoneal administration (s). * $p < 0.05$—Statistically significant difference compared to the haloperidol group. # $0.05 < p < 0.1$—Significance trend compared to haloperidol group.

## 4. Conclusions

A water-soluble formulation of **Hal** was obtained by solubilizing it in the aggregates of calix[4]resorcinol **VC10** to form vesicles. **Hal** was found to be located in the hydrophobic region within the bilayer formed by the non-polar alkyl tails of calix[4]resorcinol. Effective mucoadhesive properties of **VC10–Hal** nanoparticles were shown by UV, fluorescence, and CD spectroscopy. A decrease in the binding constant in the PGM–[**VC10–Hal**] system with an increase in temperature to physiological level provides the thermosensitive properties of **VC10–Hal** nanoparticles. According to CD spectroscopy data, the spectrum profile of the PGM–[**VC10–Hal**] system corresponds to the spectrum of pure PGM, which indicates the conformational stability (random coil conformation) of mucin upon interaction with **VC10–Hal** nanoparticles.

In vivo experiments revealed the low toxicity of **VC10** ($LD_{50}$ is 540 ± 75 mg/kg for mice and 510 ± 63 mg/kg for rats), as well as the absence of its effect on motor activity and psycho-emotional status, which allows consideration of possibly using the binary **VC10–Hal** systems in further in vivo studies. The results of the experiments on the study of catalepsy in rats showed that with the various routes of drug administration (intranasal and intraperitoneal), **Hal** formulated with **VC10** exhibits a pronounced cataleptogenic effect comparable to commercial **Hal**. This work demonstrated the successful use of cationic calixarene as a carrier for a hydrophobic drug in vivo for the first time, which opens up a perspective for its application in the development of nanoscale systems for the delivery of poorly soluble drugs to the brain.

**Supplementary Materials:** The following supporting information can be downloaded at: https://www.mdpi.com/article/10.3390/pharmaceutics15030921/s1, Figure S1: Particle size distribution by number in aqueous solutions of **VC10–Hal**; Figure S2: Steady state fluorescence spectra of PGM at a constant concentration of 0.05 mg/mL in the presence of **VC10** at 298 K (a), 304 K (b), and 310 K (c); Figure S3: Steady state fluorescence spectra of PGM at a constant concentration of 0.05 mg/mL in the presence of **VC10-Hal** (1:1) at 298 K (a), 304 K (b), 310 K (c); Figure S4: Stern–Volmer plots for fluorescence quenching of PGM by **VC10** (a), and by **VC10-Hal** (b) at 298 K, 304 K, and 310 K. Table S1. Effect of viologen decyl calix[4]resorcinol **VC10** on the research activity of mice in the "Open field" test. (**VC10** in a dose of 1/100 of the $LD_{50}$ and 1/50 of the $LD_{50}$, intraperitoneally administration, n = 8); Table S2. Effect of viologen decyl calix[4]resorcinol **VC10** on the motor activity of mice in the "Open field" test. (**VC10** in a dose of 1/100 of the $LD_{50}$ and 1/50 of the $LD_{50}$, intraperitoneally administration, n = 8); Table S3. Effect of viologen decyl calix[4]resorcinol **VC10** on the the number of entrances to the center of mice in the "Open field" test. (**VC10** in a dose of 1/100 of the $LD_{50}$ and 1/50 of the $LD_{50}$, intraperitoneally administration, n = 8).

**Author Contributions:** Conceptualization, R.R.K., N.E.K. and V.V.K.; methodology, R.R.K., N.E.K. and V.V.K.; software, N.E.K.; validation, N.E.K. and D.O.N.; formal analysis, N.E.K. and A.Y.Z.; investigation, N.E.K. and D.O.N.; resources, A.Y.Z.; data curation, N.E.K., R.R.K., I.I.S. and R.I.M.; writing—original draft preparation, N.E.K.; writing—review and editing, R.R.K. and V.V.K.; visualization, V.V.S.; supervision, L.Y.Z. All authors have read and agreed to the published version of the manuscript.

**Funding:** This research was carried out with financial support from the government assignment for FRC Kazan Scientific Center of RAS.

**Institutional Review Board Statement:** Not applicable.

**Informed Consent Statement:** Not applicable.

**Data Availability Statement:** Data are contained within this article.

**Acknowledgments:** The authors thank the Assigned Spectral-Analytical Center, FRC Kazan Scientific Center of RAS; Laboratory of Microscopy of Kazan Institute of Biochemistry and Biophysics, FRC Kazan Scientific Center of RAS.

**Conflicts of Interest:** The authors declare no conflict of interest.

## References


1. Gozalbes, R.; Jacewicz, M.; Annand, R.; Tsaioun, K.; Pineda-Lucena, A. QSAR-based permeability model for drug-like compounds. *Bioorganic Med. Chem.* **2011**, *19*, 2615–2624. [CrossRef]
2. Šoltýsová, I.; Toropilová, D.; de Vringer, T. Lipid Based Formulations of Biopharmaceutics Classification System (BCS) Class II Drugs: Strategy, Formulations, Methods and Saturation. *Folia Vet.* **2016**, *60*, 63–69. [CrossRef]
3. Shan, X.; Williams, A.C.; Khutoryanskiy, V.V. Polymer structure and property effects on solid dispersions with haloperidol: Poly(N-vinyl pyrrolidone) and poly(2-oxazolines) studies. *Int. J. Pharm.* **2020**, *590*, 119884. [CrossRef] [PubMed]
4. Zhang, X.; Xing, H.; Zhao, Y.; Ma, Z. Pharmaceutical dispersion techniques for dissolution and bioavailability enhancement of poorly water-soluble drugs. *Pharmaceutics* **2018**, *10*, 74. [CrossRef] [PubMed]
5. Park, J.H.; Kim, D.S.; Mustapha, O.; Yousaf, A.M.; Kim, J.S.; Kim, D.W.; Yong, C.S.; Youn, Y.S.; Oh, K.T.; Lim, S.J.; et al. Comparison of a revaprazan-loaded solid dispersion, solid SNEDDS and inclusion compound: Physicochemical characterisation and pharmacokinetics. *Colloids Surf. B Biointerfaces* **2018**, *162*, 420–426. [CrossRef]
6. Zhang, Y.; Ren, T.; Gou, J.; Zhang, L.; Tao, X.; Tian, B.; Tian, P.; Yu, D.; Song, J.; Liu, X.; et al. Strategies for improving the payload of small molecular drugs in polymeric micelles. *J. Control. Release* **2017**, *261*, 352–366. [CrossRef]
7. Ibatullina, M.R.; Zhil'tsova, E.P.; Lukashenko, S.S.; Zakharova, L.Y. Supramolecular Systems of Metal Complexes of 1-Cetyl-4-aza-1-azoniabicyclo[2,2,2]octane Bromide for Increasing Griseofulvin Solubility. *Colloid. J.* **2020**, *82*, 8–15. [CrossRef]
8. Zhou, S.; Shang, Q.; Wang, N.; Li, Q.; Song, A.; Luan, Y. Rational design of a minimalist nanoplatform to maximize immunotherapeutic efficacy: Four birds with one stone. *J. Control Release* **2020**, *328*, 617–630. [CrossRef]
9. Zhang, M.; Qin, X.; Zhao, Z.; Du, Q.; Li, Q.; Jiang, Y.; Luan, Y. A self-amplifying nanodrug to manipulate the Janus-faced nature of ferroptosis for tumor therapy. *Nanoscale Horiz.* **2022**, *7*, 198–210. [CrossRef]
10. Wang, Y.; Zhang, C.; Xiao, M.; Ganesan, K.; Gao, F.; Liu, Q.; Ye, Z.; Sui, Y.; Zhang, F.; Wei, K.; et al. A tumor-targeted delivery of oral isoliquiritigenin through encapsulated zein phosphatidylcholine hybrid nanoparticles prevents triple-negative breast cancer. *J. Drug Deliv. Sci. Technol.* **2023**, *79*, 103922. [CrossRef]
11. Kicuntod, J.; Khuntawee, W.; Wolschann, P. Inclusion complexation of pinostrobin with various cyclodextrin derivatives. *J. Mol. Graph. Model.* **2016**, *63*, 91–98. [CrossRef] [PubMed]
12. Ezawa, T.; Inoue, Y.; Murata, I.; Takao, K.; Sugita, Y.; Kanamoto, I. Characterization of the Dissolution Behavior of Piperine/Cyclodextrins Inclusion Complexes. *AAPS PharmSciTech* **2018**, *19*, 923–933. [CrossRef] [PubMed]
13. Morina, D.; Sessevmez, M.; Sinani, G.; Mülazımoğlu, L.; Cevher, E. Oral tablet formulations containing cyclodextrin complexes of poorly water soluble cefdinir to enhance its bioavailability. *J. Drug Deliv. Sci. Technol.* **2020**, *57*, 101742. [CrossRef]
14. Sbârcea, L.; Tănase, I.-M.; Ledeți, A.; Cîrcioban, D.; Vlase, G.; Barvinschi, P.; Miclău, M.; Văruț, R.-M.; Trandafirescu, C.; Ledeți, I. Encapsulation of Risperidone by Methylated β-Cyclodextrins: Physicochemical and Molecular Modeling Studies. *Molecules* **2020**, *25*, 5694. [CrossRef]
15. Aloisio, C.; Antimisiaris, S.G.; Longhi, M.R. Liposomes containing cyclodextrins or meglumine to solubilize and improve the bioavailability of poorly soluble drugs. *J. Mol. Liq.* **2017**, *229*, 106–113. [CrossRef]
16. Qian, X.; Wang, G.; Li, J.; Zhang, X.; Zhang, M.; Yang, Q.; Zhang, Z.; Li, Y. Improving oral bioavailability of water-insoluble idebenone with bioadhesive liposomes. *J. Drug Deliv. Sci. Technol.* **2022**, *75*, 103640. [CrossRef]
17. Yang, W.; de Villiers, M.M. Aqueous solubilization of furosemide by supramolecular complexation with 4-sulphonic calix[n]arenes. *J. Pharm. Pharmacol.* **2004**, *56*, 703–708. [CrossRef]
18. Yang, W.; Otto, D.; Liebenberg, W.; de Villiers, M. Effect of para-Sulfonato-Calix[n]arenes on the Solubility, Chemical Stability, and Bioavailability of a Water Insoluble Drug Nifedipine. *Curr. Drug Discov. Technol.* **2008**, *5*, 129–139. [CrossRef]
19. Panchal, J.G.; Patel, R.V.; Menon, S.K. Preparation and physicochemical characterization of carbamazepine (CBMZ): Para-sulfonated calix[n]arene inclusion complexes. *J. Incl. Phenom. Macrocycl. Chem.* **2010**, *67*, 201–208. [CrossRef]
20. Patel, M.B.; Valand, N.N.; Modi, N.R.; Joshi, K.V.; Harikrishnan, U.; Kumar, S.P.; Jasrai, Y.T.; Menon, S.K. Effect of p-sulfonatocalix[4]resorcinarene (PSC[4]R) on the solubility and bioavailability of a poorly water soluble drug lamotrigine (LMN) and computational investigation. *RSC Adv.* **2013**, *3*, 15971–15981. [CrossRef]
21. Yasir, M.; Sara, U.V.S. Solid lipid nanoparticles for nose to brain delivery of haloperidol: In vitro drug release and pharmacokinetics evaluation. *Acta Pharm. Sin. B* **2014**, *4*, 454–463. [CrossRef] [PubMed]
22. Porfiryeva, N.N.; Semina, I.I.; Salakhov, I.A.; Moustafine, R.I.; Khutoryanskiy, V.V. Mucoadhesive and mucus-penetrating interpolyelectrolyte complexes for nose-to-brain drug delivery. *Nanomed. Nanotechnol. Biol. Med.* **2021**, *37*, 102432. [CrossRef] [PubMed]
23. Filippov, S.K.; Khusnutdinov, R.R.; Inham, W.; Liu, C.; Nikitin, D.O.; Semina, I.I.; Garvey, C.J.; Nasibullin, S.F.; Khutoryanskiy, V.V.; Zhang, H.; et al. Hybrid nanoparticles for haloperidol encapsulation: Quid est optimum? *Polymers* **2021**, *13*, 4189. [CrossRef]
24. Kashapov, R.R.; Kashapova, N.E.; Ziganshina, A.Y.; Syakaev, V.V.; Khutoryanskiy, V.V.; Zakharova, L.Y. Interaction of mucin with viologen and acetate derivatives of calix[4]resorcinols. *Colloids Surf. B Biointerfaces* **2021**, *208*, 112089. [CrossRef] [PubMed]
25. Wu, D.; Zhang, Z.; Yu, X.; Bai, B.; Qi, S. Hydrophilic Tetraphenylethene-Based Tetracationic Cyclophanes: NADPH Recognition and Cell Imaging with Fluorescent Switch. *Front. Chem.* **2021**, *9*, 1–8. [CrossRef] [PubMed]
26. Ziganshina, A.Y.; Kharlamov, S.V.; Korshin, D.E.; Mukhitova, R.K.; Kazakova, E.K.; Latypov, S.K.; Yanilkin, V.V.; Konovalov, A.I. Electrochemical behaviour of a molecular capsule based on methylviologen-resorcinarene and sulfonatomethylene-resorcinarene. *Tetrahedron Lett.* **2008**, *49*, 5312–5315. [CrossRef]

27. Mironov, A.N.; Bunyatyan, N.D.; Vasiliev, A.N.; Verstakova, O.L.; Zhuravleva, M.V.; Lepakhin, V.K.; Korobov, N.V.; Merkulov, V.A.; Orekhov, S.N.; Sakaeva, I.V.; et al. *Guidelines for Conducting Preclinical Studies of Drugs*; Grif and K: Tula, Russia, 2012; 944p, ISBN 9785812514663.
28. Sestakova, N.; Puzserova, A.; Kluknavsky, M.; Bernatova, I. Determination of motor activity and anxiety-related behaviour in rodents: Methodological aspects and role of nitric oxide. *Interdiscip. Toxicol.* **2013**, *6*, 126–135. [CrossRef]
29. Henry, B.L.; Minassian, A.; Young, J.W.; Paulus, M.P.; Geyer, M.A.; Perry, W. Cross-species assessments of motor and exploratory behavior related to bipolar disorder. *Neurosci. Biobehav. Rev.* **2010**, *34*, 1296–1306. [CrossRef]
30. Miyamoto, S.; Duncan, G.E.; Marx, C.E.; Lieberman, J.A. Treatments for schizophrenia: A critical review of pharmacology and mechanisms of action of antipsychotic drugs. *Mol. Psychiatry* **2005**, *10*, 79–104. [CrossRef]
31. Vogel, H.G. Psychotropic and Neurotropic Activity. In *Drug Discovery and Evaluation*; Springer: Berlin/Heidelberg, Germany, 2007; pp. 565–876, ISBN 978-3-540-71420-0.
32. Natfji, A.A.; Nikitin, D.O.; Semina, I.I.; Moustafine, R.I.; Khutoryanskiy, V.V.; Lin, H.; Stephens, G.J.; Watson, K.A.; Osborn, H.M.I.; Greco, F. Conjugation of haloperidol to PEG allows peripheral localisation of haloperidol and eliminates CNS extrapyramidal effects. *J. Control. Release* **2020**, *322*, 227–235. [CrossRef]
33. Kashapov, R.; Razuvayeva, Y.; Ziganshina, A.; Sapunova, A.; Lyubina, A.; Amerhanova, S.; Kulik, N.; Voloshina, A.; Nizameev, I.; Salnikov, V.; et al. Effect of preorganization and amphiphilicity of calix[4]arene platform on functional properties of viologen derivatives. *J. Mol. Liq.* **2022**, *345*, 117801. [CrossRef]
34. Kashapov, R.R.; Kharlamov, S.V.; Sultanova, E.D.; Mukhitova, R.K.; Kudryashova, Y.R.; Zakharova, L.Y.; Ziganshina, A.Y.; Konovalov, A.I. Controlling the size and morphology of supramolecular assemblies of viologen-resorcin[4]arene cavitands. *Chem.-A Eur. J.* **2014**, *20*, 14018–14025. [CrossRef] [PubMed]
35. Gadelle, F.; Koros, W.J.; Schechter, R.S. Solubilization of Aromatic Solutes in Block Copolymers. *Macromolecules* **1995**, *28*, 4883–4892. [CrossRef]
36. Shah, V.; Bharatiya, B.; Patel, V.; Mishra, M.K.; Shukla, A.D.; Shah, D.O. Interaction of salicylic acid analogues with Pluronic®micelles: Investigations on micellar growth and morphological transition. *J. Mol. Liq.* **2019**, *277*, 563–570. [CrossRef]
37. Hanio, S.; Schlauersbach, J.; Lenz, B.; Spiegel, F.; Böckmann, R.A.; Schweins, R.; Nischang, I.; Schubert, U.S.; Endres, S.; Pöppler, A.C.; et al. Drug-Induced Dynamics of Bile Colloids. *Langmuir* **2021**, *37*, 2543–2551. [CrossRef] [PubMed]
38. Albarkah, Y.A.; Green, R.J.; Khutoryanskiy, V.V. Probing the Mucoadhesive Interactions between Porcine Gastric Mucin and Some Water-Soluble Polymers. *Macromol. Biosci.* **2015**, *15*, 1546–1553. [CrossRef]
39. Fraiji, L.K.; Hayes, D.M.; Werner, T.C. Static and dynamic fluorescence quenching experiments for the physical chemistry laboratory. *J. Chem. Educ.* **1992**, *69*, 424–428. [CrossRef]
40. Lone, M.S.; Afzal, S.; Chat, O.A.; Aswal, V.K.; Dar, A.A. Temperature- and Composition-Induced Multiarchitectural Transitions in the Catanionic System of a Conventional Surfactant and a Surface-Active Ionic Liquid. *ACS Omega* **2021**, *6*, 11974–11987. [CrossRef]
41. Yang, Y.; Liu, L.; Huang, X.; Tan, X.; Luo, T.; Li, W. Temperature-induced vesicle to micelle transition in cationic/cationic mixed surfactant systems. *Soft Matter* **2015**, *11*, 8848–8855. [CrossRef]
42. Nikogeorgos, N.; Efler, P.; Kayitmazer, A.B.; Lee, S. "Bio-glues" to enhance slipperiness of mucins: Improved lubricity and wear resistance of porcine gastric mucin (PGM) layers assisted by mucoadhesion with chitosan. *Soft Matter* **2015**, *11*, 489–498. [CrossRef]
43. Shrivastava, H.Y.; Nair, B.U. Structural modification and aggregation of mucin by chromium(III) complexes. *J. Biomol. Struct. Dyn.* **2003**, *20*, 575–587. [CrossRef] [PubMed]
44. Kandsi, F.; Lafdil, F.Z.; Elbouzidi, A.; Bouknana, S.; Miry, A.; Addi, M.; Conte, R.; Hano, C.; Gseyra, N. Evaluation of Acute and Subacute Toxicity and LC-MS/MS Compositional Alkaloid Determination of the Hydroethanolic Extract of Dysphania ambrosioides (L.) Mosyakin and Clemants Flowers. *Toxins* **2022**, *14*, 475. [CrossRef] [PubMed]
45. Hoffman, D.C.; Donovan, H. Catalepsy as a rodent model for detecting antipsychotic drugs with extrapyramidal side effect liability. *Psychopharmacology* **1995**, *120*, 128–133. [CrossRef]
46. Pandey, M.; Jain, N.; Kanoujia, J.; Hussain, Z.; Gorain, B. Advances and Challenges in Intranasal Delivery of Antipsychotic Agents Targeting the Central Nervous System. *Front. Pharmacol.* **2022**, *13*, 865590. [CrossRef] [PubMed]

pharmaceutics

MDPI

Article

# Assessment of Different Niosome Formulations for Optogenetic Applications: Morphological and Electrophysiological Effects

**José David Celdrán [1,†], Lawrence Humphreys [1,2,†], Desirée González [1], Cristina Soto-Sánchez [1,2], Gema Martínez-Navarrete [1,2], Iván Maldonado [2,3], Idoia Gallego [2,3], Ilia Villate-Beitia [2,3], Myriam Sainz-Ramos [2,3], Gustavo Puras [2,3], José Luis Pedraz [2,3] and Eduardo Fernández [1,2,*]**

1 Biomedical Neuroengineering, Institute of Bioengineering (IB), University Miguel Hernández (UMH), 03020 Elche, Spain; jose.celdran.lopez@gmail.com (J.D.C.); lawrencehumphreys@hotmail.com (L.H.); dgonzalez@umh.es (D.G.); csoto@umh.es (C.S.-S.); gema.martinezn@umh.es (G.M.-N.)

2 Networking Research Centre of Bioengineering, Biomaterials and Nanomedicine (CIBER-BBN), Carlos III Health Institute (ISCIII), 28029 Madrid, Spain; ivan.maldonado@ehu.eus (I.M.); idoia.gallego@ehu.eus (I.G.); aneilia.villate@ehu.eus (I.V.-B.); miriam.sainz@ehu.eus (M.S.-R.); gustavo.puras@ehu.eus (G.P.); joseluis.pedraz@ehu.eus (J.L.P.)

3 Bioaraba, NanoBioCel Group, School of Pharmacy, University of the Basque Country (UPV/EHU), 01006 Vitoria-Gasteiz, Spain

* Correspondence: e.fernandez@umh.es

† These authors contributed equally to this work.

**Abstract:** Gene therapy and optogenetics are becoming promising tools for treating several nervous system pathologies. Currently, most of these approaches use viral vectors to transport the genetic material inside the cells, but viruses present some potential risks, such as marked immunogenicity, insertional mutagenesis, and limited insert gene size. In this framework, non-viral nanoparticles, such as niosomes, are emerging as possible alternative tools to deliver genetic material, avoiding the aforementioned problems. To determine their suitability as vectors for optogenetic therapies in this work, we tested three different niosome formulations combined with three optogenetic plasmids in rat cortical neurons in vitro. All niosomes tested successfully expressed optogenetic channels, which were dependent on the ratio of niosome to plasmid, with higher concentrations yielding higher expression rates. However, we found changes in the dendritic morphology and electrophysiological properties of transfected cells, especially when we used higher concentrations of niosomes. Our results highlight the potential use of niosomes for optogenetic applications and suggest that special care must be taken to achieve an optimal balance of niosomes and nucleic acids to achieve the therapeutic effects envisioned by these technologies.

**Keywords:** niosomes; optogenetics; morphological effects; electrophysiological effects

## 1. Introduction

Gene therapy aims to treat diseases by introducing genetic material (DNA or RNA) into the cells of the patients, either by correcting, adding, or removing a genetic sequence. It was first proposed in the 1970s for treating monogenic disorders [1] and has since been at the forefront of cancer treatment [2]. Gene therapy has achieved considerable success, with over two dozen official drugs approved for clinical trials [3,4]. One key component for delivering the genetic material into cells is the delivery system, classically referred to as a vector, of which there are many, each with its advantages and disadvantages. Among the most promising vectors that have proven to be suitable for genetic delivery are viral vectors [5–7]. They exhibit stable long-term expression and high transgene levels. Nevertheless, these vectors have some drawbacks, such as immunoreactivity, toxin production, insertional mutagenesis, and limitations in the size of genes that can be carried by the viral vector [6–10]. In this sense, non-viral nanoparticle vectors have been proposed as an interesting alternative that can overcome some of the aforementioned issues. More specifically, they have low immunogenicity and low cytotoxicity, are easily manufactured, and do not have the same gene-size restrictions [11]. In particular, niosomes have proven to be a promising candidate to deliver genetic material through the cell membrane [12–14].

Niosomes are bilayer vesicles composed of three main components—cationic lipids, "helper" components, and non-ionic surfactants—and can bind to DNA (forming nioplexes), exhibit long-term stability and proper physicochemical properties, and have relatively low preparation costs [15–19]. Our group already has extensive experience using niosomes as vectors for genetic material in the retina [19–23] and the brain cortex [24–26], achieving encouraging results in both. This opens the possibility of developing a safer and non-toxic genetic therapy for the treatment of multiple diseases that affect neural tissues. Other research groups have used niosomes for gene therapy, as well as for the delivery of genetic material into mesenchymal stem cells [27] and even in retinal tissue [28], but most of them have put their efforts into treating cancer by gene-silencing therapy with miRNAs [29], siRNAs [30,31], and oligodeoxynucleotides [32]. Though niosomes have many advantages, there is no scientific evidence related to their use for optogenetic applications.

Here, to the best of our knowledge, we are the first to combine niosome-based genetic delivery with optogenetic plasmids into cortical tissue. Optogenetics is a method that uses targeted ectopic expression of light-activated proteins (opsins) to control cell-specific neural activity with millisecond precision [33], allowing for precise activation of neural circuits using specific promoters [34,35]. Optogenetics has thus emerged as a promising alternative for treating diseases, such as epilepsy [36] and Parkinson's [37] and even a current clinical trial in a blind patient [38]. Two improved optogenetic variants have emerged with distinct advantages for photostimulations: ChrimsonR [39] and CatCh [40]. ChrimsonR is a red-shifted channelrhopsin (activated at 590 nm) with fast-kinetics and high cellular trafficking, while CatCh is a blue-light-activated channelrhodopsin (activated at 470 nm) that introduces calcium into cells and possesses fast-kinetics. However, these optogenetic proteins have been delivered into neuronal cells using viral vectors or in utero electroporation [38–40], but not niosomes. Therefore, delivering these optogenetic tools into neuronal cells using niosomes as vectors (which do not have some of the disadvantages of the viral vectors) could be a promising approach to explore.

In this study, we delivered optogenetic plasmids that codify for ChrimsonR and CatCh, as well as the ubiquitously used GFP plasmid as a control [41], combined with three different niosome formulations into rat cortical neurons in vitro. These niosome formulations varied among them in the "helper" compound (nanodiamonds (ND12), sphingolipids (P10), and chloroquine (CQ)), whose capabilities of delivering reporting genetic material into cells of multiple tissues have been previously successfully tested [42–44]. Our main objective was to determine the suitability of this approach for the photosensitization of cortical neurons in optogenetic therapies.

In this work, we characterized the morphology, electrophysiology, and cell viability of different combinations of niosomes and optogenetic plasmids in rat cortical in vitro cultures.

## 2. Material and Methods

### 2.1. Elaboration of Niosomes and Nioplexes

All niosome formulations were elaborated by the oil-in-water emulsification technique [17]. In the case of ND12 niosomes, nanodiamonds (NDs) were purchased as ultrananocrystalline diamonds with grain sizes smaller than 10 nm (Sigma-Aldrich, Burlington, MA, USA). A volume of 250 µL of NDs (10 mg/mL in $H_2O$) was ultrasonicated for 30 min and mixed with 2 mL of 0.5% Tween® (Sigma-Aldrich, Madrid, Spain), and 1.75 mL of MilliQ® water as the aqueous phase. A total of 5 mg of 1,2-di-O-octadecenyl-3-trimethylammonium propane chloride salt (DOTMA; Avanti Polar Lipids, Inc., Alabaster, AL, USA) was accurately weighted to obtain 1/2 ND/DOTMA mass ratios. The DOTMA was diluted in 1 mL of dichlorometane (DCM; Panreac, Castellar del Vallès, Barcelona, Spain), which constituted the organic phase. This phase was added to the aqueous phase and immediately sonicated for 30 min at 50 W (Branson Sonifier 250, Danbury). DCM was evaporated for 2 h at room temperature under magnetic stirring, obtaining a cationic lipid concentration of 1.2 mg/mL.

P10 niosomes were obtained by combining DOTMA with 2-[2-[(2R,3R)-3,4-bis(2-hydroxyethoxy)oxolan-2-yl]-2-(2-hydroxyethoxy)ethoxy]ethyl dodecanoate (Polysorbate 20, Bio-Rad, Alcobendas, Madrid, Spain) non-ionic surfactant and mixing them with sphingolipids from animal origin found in the intestinal mucosa of mammals with high levels of sphingomyelin (Bioiberica laboratory, Sus scrofa, pig) as helper components. Briefly, 3.4 mg of cationic lipid was gently grounded with 100 µg of sphingolipids, and then 500 µL of DCM was added to this lipid mixture and emulsified with 2.5 mL of polysorbate 20 (0.5%, *w:w*). Components were sonicated for 30 s at 50 W. Next, the DCM organic solvent was evaporated and eliminated from the emulsion by using a magnetic stirrer for 2 h at room temperature inside an extraction hood. Upon DCM evaporation, a colloidal dispersion carrying the formulations was obtained with a final cationic lipid concentration of 1.5 mg/mL.

CQ niosomes were prepared by dissolving 5 mg of cationic lipid 2,3-di(tetradecyloxy)propan-1-amine, 12.5 mg of non-ionic tensioactive poloxamer 407 (Sigma-Aldrich, Burlington, MA, USA), and 12.5 mg of non-ionic tensioactive polysorbate 80 (Sigma-Aldrich, USA) in 1 mL of DCM. The water phase contained 2.5 mg of "helper" lipid chloroquine diphosphate salt (Sigma-Aldrich, Burlington, MA, USA) dissolved in 5 mL of distilled water. The organic phase and the water phase were emulsified by sonication for 30 s at 50 W. The organic solvent was removed from the emulsion by evaporation under magnetic agitation for 3 h at room temperature, obtaining a cationic lipid concentration of 1 mg/mL.

Nioplexes were obtained by incubating each type of niosome with each plasmid. Optogenetic plasmids pCAG-ChrimsonR-tdT and pAAV-Syn-ChrimsonR-tdT were obtained from the Edward Boyden (Addgene plasmid # 59169 and Addgene plasmid # 59171, respectively), optogenetic plasmid pCMV-CatCh-EYFP was a gift from Peter Hegemann, and pCAG-GFP was obtained from Connie Cepko (Addgene plasmid # 11150). Plasmids were expanded and purified using the Qiagen endotoxin-free plasmid purification Maxi-prep kit (Qiagen, Valencia, CA, USA), according to the manufacturer's instructions. The concentration of the purified plasmid was quantified in a NanoDrop™ 2000 Spectrophotometer (Thermofisher Scientific, Waltham, MA, USA). Then, an appropriate volume of each plasmid was mixed and incubated for 30 min at room temperature with the corresponding volume of each niosome suspension (1 mg/mL cationic lipid) to obtain the respective nioplexes at cationic lipid:DNA ratios (*w:w*) of 2:1, 5:1, 8:1, and 10:1.

### 2.2. Physicochemical Characterization of Niosomes and Nioplexes

The hydrodynamic diameter, which includes the particle size and dispersity (Đ), and the zeta potential of all niosomes and their corresponding nioplexes were determined by Dynamic Light Scattering (DLS) and by Laser Doppler Velocimetry (LDV), respectively, using a Zetasizer Nano ZS (Malvern Instrument, Malvern, Worcestershire, UK), and the morphology of niosomes was determined by transmission electron microscopy (TEM), all as previously described [22].

### 2.3. Animal Models

E16-E19 rat embryos (Sprague Dawley) were used for the extraction of primary neuronal cells for in vitro experiments. All experimental procedures were carried out in accordance with the RD 53/2013 Spanish and 2010/63/EU European Union regulations for the use of animals in scientific research. Procedures were approved and supervised by the Miguel Hernández University Standing Committee for Animal Use in the Laboratory with code UMH.CID.DPC.01.17.2019/VSC/PEA/0010.

### 2.4. Primary Neuronal Cell Extraction and Culture

Primary neuronal cells were extracted from the cortical tissue of rat embryos (Sprague Dawley) and maintained in DMEM (GIBCO®, Thermofisher Scientific, Waltham, MA, USA) with 10% fetal bovine serum (FBS; Biowest®, Nuaillé, Pays de la Loire, France) during extraction. Afterwards, we removed DMEM with 10% FBS and added FBS-free DMEM in order to perform chemical dissociation. Chemical dissociation was carried out by adding trypsin 0.05% and incubating the mixture at 37 °C. Once the cell density was quantified in a hemocytometer, cells were re-suspended according to the desired morphological analysis. For morphological analysis of cortical neurons transfected with nioplexes, cells were resuspended in Neurobasal™ (GIBCO®) medium supplemented with FBS, B27, GlutaMAX, and penicillin-streptomycin (GIBCO®) and seeded at $1.5 \times 10^5$ cells per well in 24-well plates on glass coverslips, while for morphological analysis of cortical neurons transfected with only plasmids or niosomes, cells were resuspended in BrainPhys™ Imaging Optimized Medium (BPI; STEMCELL®, Saint-Égrève, Grenoble, France) supplemented with FBS, B27, GlutaMAX, and penicillin-streptomycin (GIBCO®) and seeded at $5 \times 10^4$ cells per well in 24-well plates on glass coverslips. Cell cultures were maintained in an incubator at 37 °C and 5% $CO_2$. This BPI medium was used in order to maintain alive the smaller number of cells per well (compared to Neurobasal™ cultures) and to facilitate cell imaging without the presence of genetically expressed fluorescent reporters. For cell viability analysis, cells were re-suspended in Neurobasal™ medium supplemented with FBS, B27, GlutaMAX, and penicillin-streptomycin and seeded at $1.5 \times 10^4$ cells per well in 96-well plates.

### *2.5. In Vitro Transfection in Primary Neuronal Cell Culture*

Cells in Neurobasal™ medium were seeded and incubated in 24-well plates between 21–28 days in vitro (DIV) before transfecting. Nioplexes, composed of niosomes and 1.25 µg of plasmid per well at their respective cationic lipid:DNA ratio (*w:w*), were formed by electrostatic interactions during 30 min at room temperature in serum-free OptiMEM solution (GIBCO®). Cells were transfected with nioplexes between these ages and not in younger cells (7–11 DIV) since they developed electrophysiological activity, which allowed correlating morphological results with electrophysiological results, also avoiding the loss of fluorescent cells while waiting for younger cells to develop electrophysiological activity. Transfection was carried out by exposing cells to nioplexes for 4 h at 37 °C in the incubator, followed by removal of the transfection medium and replacement with fresh Neurobasal™ medium. Lipofectamine™ 2000 (Invitrogen, Carlsbad, CA, USA) at a 1:1 ratio was employed as a positive control. In 96-well plates, the seeding, incubation, and transfection protocol was similar, but this time we also treated cells between 7–11 DIV, and the concentration of plasmid in each well was 0.25 µg.

Cells in BPI medium were seeded and incubated in 24-well plates, both between 21–28 and 7–11 DIV before transfecting. In addition, 1.25 µg of plasmid and niosomes at their respective cationic lipid/DNA ratio were incubated separately for 30 min at room temperature in OptiMEM solution. Transfection was carried out by exposing cells to either plasmid or niosomes for 4 h at 37 °C in the incubator, followed by removal of the transfection medium and replacement with fresh BPI medium. Untreated cells incubated with OptiMEM for 4 h were used as a positive control.

### *2.6. Morphological Evaluation of Transfected Cultured Cortical Neurons*

Neurobasal™ medium was removed from cells 24 h after their exposure to nioplexes, and they were fixed by 4% paraformaldehyde (PFA; Sigma-Aldrich, Burlington, MA, USA) for 20 min and washed 2 times with phosphate buffer (PB; Sigma-Aldrich, Burlington, MA, USA) concentrated at 0.1 M, 10 min each time. After washing, PB 0.1 M with 0.5% Triton X-100 was added for 5 min, and the cell nuclei were stained with Hoechst 33342 (Sigma-Aldrich, Burlington, MA, USA) for 10 min. Coverslips were mounted in slides with Mowiol® 4–88 (Sigma-Aldrich, Spain). Fluorescence images were taken with laser-confocal microscopy (Leica TCS SPE Microsystems GmbH, Wetzlar, Germany).

BPI medium was removed from cells 24 h after their exposure to either plasmids or niosomes, and they were fixed as described above and blocked with 10% FBS for 1 h, and then incubated overnight at 4 °C with anti-rabbit MAP2 monoclonal antibody (1 mg/mL,

1:500 dilution, Millipore, Burlington, MA, USA). After washing 2 times with PB 0.1 M for 10 min each time, cells were incubated for 1 h with a secondary antibody, AlexaFluor® 488 donkey anti-rabbit (2 mg/mL, 1:1000 dilution, Invitrogen, Themofisher Scientific, Waltham, MA, USA). After 3 washes with PB of 5 min each wash, 0.5% Triton X-100 and Hoechst 33342 addition, as well as coverslip mounting and fluorescence image taking, were carried out as described above.

Morphological analysis of fluorescence images was performed by the Fiji plugin NeuronJ. The morphological parameters evaluated in rat cortical neurons were number of dendrites, branching points, total length of all dendrites, mean length of all dendrites, and longest dendrite.

### 2.7. Electrophysiological Recordings

Transfected coverslips were removed from wells using tweezers when the cells had 21–28 DIV and were kept in extracellular medium containing (in mM): 136 NaCl, 2.5 KCl, 10 HEPES, 10 Glucose, 2 $CaCl_2$, 1.3 MgCl (pH = 7.3).

Borosilicate glass capillaries (1B150F-4, World Precision Instruments, USA) of 3–5 MΩ, obtained by a P97 puller (Sutter Instrument Co., Novato, CA, USA) for patch clamp recordings, were filled with an intracellular medium containing (in mM): 130 $K^+$-gluconate, 10 NaCl, 1 EGTA, 0.133 $CaCl_2$, 2 $MgCl_2$, 10 HEPES, 3.5 MgATP, 1 NaGTP (pH = 7.3). Cells were targeted with a patch electrode under visual guidance using the reporter tag's fluorescence, and whole-cell recordings were obtained using the HEKA EPC 10 USB double patch clamp amplifier (Harvard Bioscience, Inc., Holliston, MA, USA). Photocurrents were recorded while voltage-clamping cells at a potential of −60 mV, and also in the current clamp configuration in order to monitor the membrane potential during light stimulations.

A monochromatic light source (pE-300 ultra, CoolLED, Andover, UK) was used to stimulate cells during electrophysiological recordings. In order to measure the photostimulation of targeted cells, we used two 5 ms light flashes at 20 W, with a 1 s interspace of 590 nm for ChrimsonR positive cells and 470 nm for CatCh positive cells.

### 2.8. Cell Viability

The cell viability of primary neuronal cell cultures of both 21–28 and 7–11 DIV after their exposure to either plasmids or niosomes were analyzed 24, 48, and 72 h post-transfection by the tetrazolium salt 3-[4,5-dimethylthiazol-2-yl]-2,5-diphenyl tetrazolium bromide (MTT; Sigma-Aldrich, Burlington, MA, USA) colorimetric assay, and the absorbance was read at 570 nm in a 2100-C microplate reader (Neuvar Inc., Palo Alto, CA, USA), according to the manufacturer's instructions. Untreated cells incubated with OptiMEM were used as positive controls, and data were normalized relative to these positive controls.

A similar procedure was performed with primary neuronal cell cultures 21–28 DIV, which were treated with nioplexes and analyzed 24 h post-transfection.

### 2.9. Statistical Analysis

Differences between two groups were evaluated using a Mann–Whitney U test in non-parametric conditions, whereas for multiple comparison, it was either performed using a one-way ANOVA or multiple $t$-tests. Data are expressed as mean ± SD. A $p$-value $< 0.05$ was considered statistically significant. Analyses were performed with the GraphPad Prism 8.0 statistical package.

## 3. Results

### 3.1. Nioplexes Transfection and Neuron Morphology

We tested niosome formulations for their capacity to transfect optogenetic plasmids, as well as the widely used reporter GFP plasmid. More specifically, cortical neurons were transfected with the niosomes ND12, P10, and CQ, which were complexed with different plasmids (pCAG-ChrimsonR-tdT, pAAV-Syn-ChrimsonR-tdT, pCMV-CatCh-EYFP, and pCAG-GFP) at different cationic lipid/genetic material ratios (2:1, 5:1, 8:1, and 10:1) after

21 and 28 days in vitro (DIV). We did not observe the expression for any plasmid or niosome combination at a ratio of 2:1 after 24 h. However, with higher ratios (5:1, 8:1, and 10:1), we observed cell expression after 24 h. pCAG-ChrimsonR-tdT and pCAG-GFP plasmids expression was observed using a ratio of 5:1 and higher, pAAV-Syn-ChrimsonR-tdT plasmid expression was observed using a ratio of 8:1 and higher proportions, and pCMV-CatCh-EYFP plasmid expression was only observed using a ratio of 10:1.

All niosomes were able to deliver the optogenetic plasmids and successfully transfect neurons. However, the morphology of nioplex transfected cells appeared somehow different in comparison to cells treated with the commercially available reagent Lipofectamine. To quantify and characterize the differences, we measured (1) the number of dendrites, (2) branching points, (3) total length of all dendrites, (4) mean length of all dendrites, and (5) longest dendrite. Our results showed that neurons treated with niosome formulations and CAG-ChrimsonR plasmid had a significant reduction of all parameters in comparison with neurons transfected with Lipofectamine (Figures 1A,B and S1A–C). Similar results were observed in neurons treated with the Syn-ChrimsonR plasmid (Supplementary Figure S2A–E). This trend was also observed in neurons treated with niosome GFP complexes (Figures 1C,D and S1D,F), except for the treatment with ND12 at 5:1, which showed no statistical significance in the mean length of all dendrites ($p$-value = 0.1653) (Supplementary Figure S1E).

As previously mentioned, CatCh niosome complexes were only expressed at a ratio of 10:1. In general, we observed a similar trend in terms of changes to morphology. However, for cells transfected with P10 at a ratio of 10:1, we observed no statistical difference when we measured for the longest dendrite compared to controls ($p$-value = 0.7180). Additionally, all niosomes complexed with the CatCh plasmid did not exhibit any differences in the mean length of all the dendrites (Supplementary Figure S2F–J). All $p$-values can be found in Supplementary Table S1.

### 3.2. Electrophysiological Properties of Transfected Neurons

Having observed some morphological changes in neurons treated with niosome complexes, we set out to test if this also translated into any electrophysiological changes. We performed patch clamp electrophysiology on cells transfected after 21–28 DIV with our niosome complexes. Neurons transfected with optogenetic nioplexes or with Lipofectamine were photostimulated with 2 pulses (5 ms duration and 1 sec inter-pulse). In general, Lipofectamine-treated cells (n = 7) showed robust inward currents and light-driven action potentials (Figure 2A). When we performed voltage clamp (VC) recordings on cells treated with P10/CAG-ChrimsonR complexes (Figure 2B), in general, we observed similar rise times when compared to Lipofectamine controls, except for P10 at 8:1 (pulse 1 $p$-value = 0.0255 *, pulse 2 $p$-value = 0.0024 *, n = 6), which was slower (Figure 2C). Peak amplitudes values for all ratios were significantly smaller in comparison to controls (pulse 1 P10 vs. lipo, 10:1 $p$-value = 0.01 *, 8:1 $p$-value = 0.0006 ***, 5:1 $p$-value = 0.0005 ***, pulse 2, 10:1 $p$-value = 0.0119 * n = 6, 8:1 $p$ = 0.0006 ***, n = 6, 5:1 $p$ = 0.0006 ***, n = 12) (Figure 2D). When we performed current clamp (CC) recordings, we observed significant longer rise times only at a ratio of 8:1, but not with 10:1 or 5:1 (pulse 1 P10 vs. lipo, 10:1 $p$-value $\geq$ 0.9999, 8:1 $p$-value = 0.0141 *, 5:1 $p$-value = 0.8234, pulse 2, 10:1 $p$-value $\geq$ 0.9999 n = 6, 8:1 $p$-value = 0.0083 ***, n = 6, 5:1 $p$-value = 0.5691 n = 7, lipo n = 7) (Figure 2E). Peak amplitudes were significantly smaller for all ratios (pulse 1 P10 vs. lipo, 10:1 $p$-value = 0.0013 **, 8:1 $p$-value = 0.0024 **, 5:1 $p$-value = 0.0017 **, pulse 2, 10.1 $p$-value = 0.0011 **, n = 6, 8:1 $p$-value = 0.002** n = 6, 5:1 $p$-value = 0.0016 **, n = 7) (Figure 2F). Overall, the rise times between Lipofectamine-treated cells and P10 were not significantly different, except for cells treated with a ratio of 8:1. However, considerable electrophysiological changes were observed in terms of the peak amplitude when cells were photostimulated. This general trend was observed with cells treated with ND12 and CQ (Supplementary Figure S3).

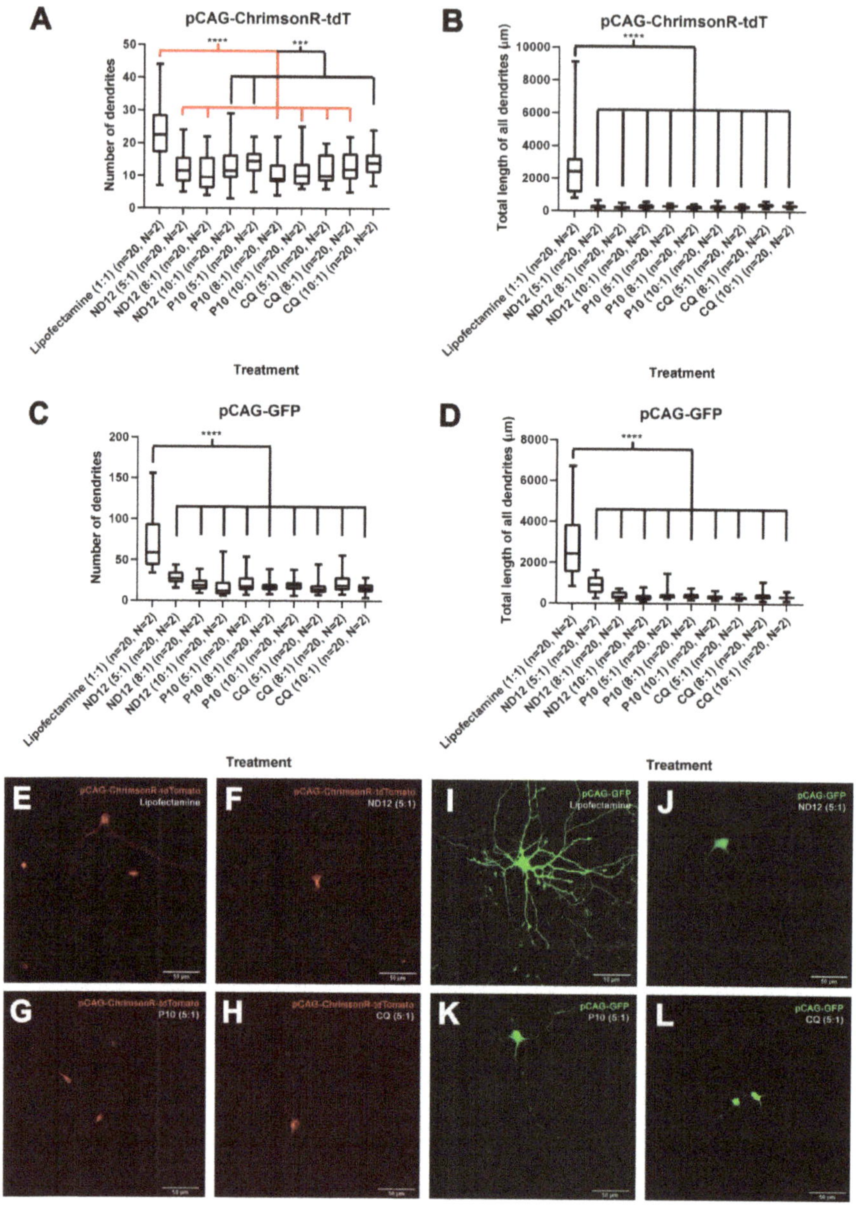

**Figure 1. Morphological changes induced by different niosome-based formulations.** The 21–28 DIV rat cortical neurons treated with nioplexes made of pCAG-ChrimsonR-tdTomato plus niosomes showed reduction in morphological parameters as number of dendrites (**A**) and total length of all dendrites (**B**) compared with the lipofectamine treatment, with the same outcome in pCAG-GFP (**C**,**D**) (Mann–Whitney test, *** $p < 0.001$, **** $p < 0.0001$, n = number of cells, N = number of cultures). (**E**–**H**) Morphological aspect of cortical neurons treated with pCAG-ChrimsonR-TdTomato plus lipofectamine (**E**), ND12(5:1) (**F**), P10(5:1) (**G**), and CQ(5:1) (**H**). (**I**–**L**) Morphological aspect cortical of neurons treated with pCAG-GFP plus lipofectamine (**I**), ND12(5:1) (**J**), P10(5:1) (**K**), and CQ(5:1) (scale bar = 50 μm) (**L**).

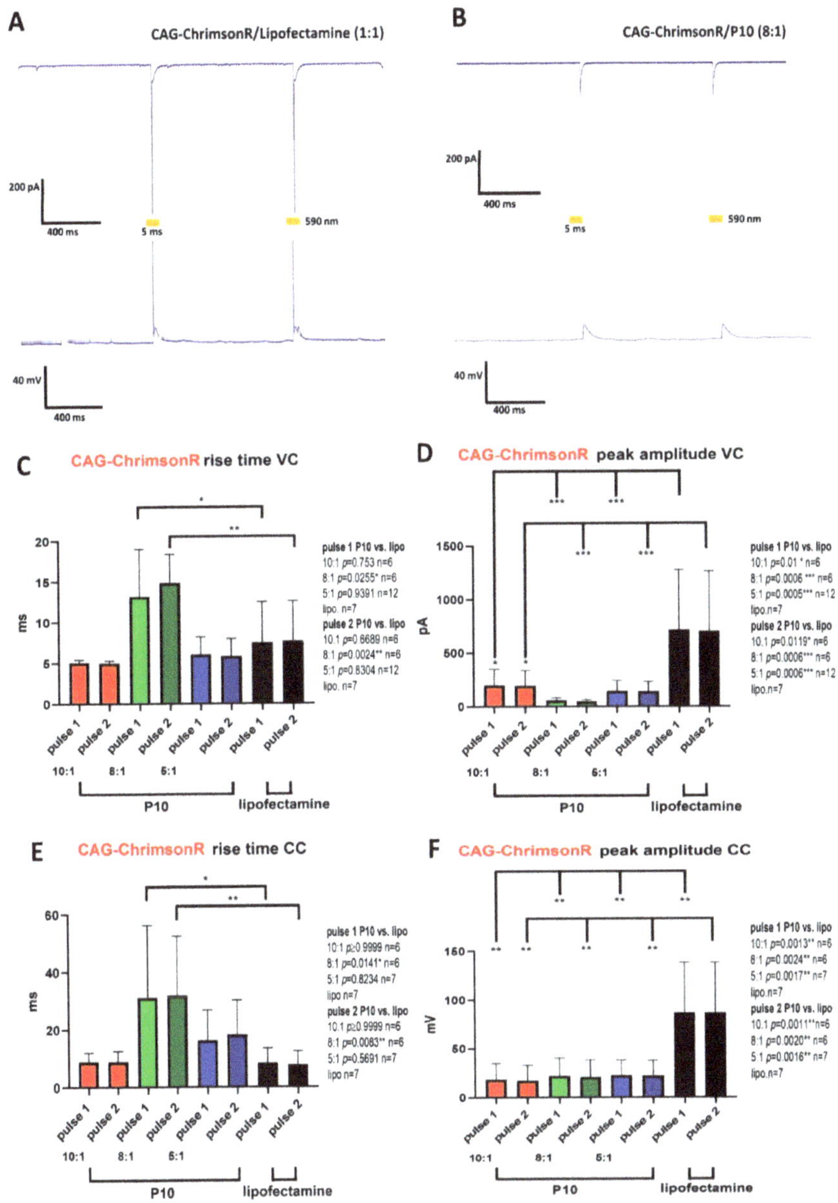

**Figure 2. Electrophysiological changes induced by different niosome-based formulations.** (**A**) Photostimulation of rat cortical neuron DIV 28 expressing CAG-ChrimsonR transfected with lipofectamine (1:1), showing AP firing. (**B**) Photostimulation of a rat cortical neuron DIV28 transfected with P10 (8:1) niosomes, showing depolarization, but no AP firing. Voltage clamp (VC, top) and current clamp (CC, bottom) recordings were performed while cells were photostimulated with 2 pulses of 5 ms (590 nm) with a 1-s interspace. (**C**–**F**) Comparison between lipofectamine and P10 niosomes at different ratios in rise time and peak amplitude electrophysiological parameters in each light pulse (ordinary one-way ANOVA, * $p < 0.05$, ** $p < 0.01$, *** $p < 0.001$). Graphs bars are expressed as mean ± SD.

Neurons transfected with Syn-ChrimsonR plasmid and niosomes ND12 and P10 generally present statistical significance in rise time compared to Lipofectamine (Supplementary Figure S4), except in the ND12 (10:1) treatment in both pulses ($p$-value = 0.3775 and 0.0505, respectively, in VC recordings) (Supplementary Figure S4A) and the P10 (10:1) treatment in pulse 1 ($p$-value = 0.2445 in VC) (Supplementary Figure S4F). CQ-Syn-ChrimsonR-treated cells showed no significant differences in rise times, except for the first pulse ($p$-value = 0.019 *) when using a ratio of 10:1 in CC recordings (Supplementary Figure S4L).

Peak amplitude values in both VC and CC modes showed statistical significance, except the ND12 (10:1) treatment in both pulses ($p$-value = 0.5061 and 0.6587, respectively) (Supplementary Figure S4D), P10 (8:1) treatment in both pulses ($p$-value = 0.5944 and 0.6644, respectively), P10 (10:1) treatment in both pulses ($p$-value = 0.3274 and 0.3756, respectively) (Supplementary Figure S4I), and CQ (10:1) treatment in pulses 1 and 2 ($p$-value = 0.4276 and 0.4907, respectively) (Supplementary Figure S4M).

Using the CatCh plasmid, there was no difference in any niosome treatment with any parameter (Supplementary Figure S5), except the peak amplitude in VC between Lipofectamine and the P10 (10:1) treatment in pulse 1 ($p$-value = 0.0349 *) (Supplementary Figure S5G).

Overall, niosome treatment results in variable changes to the rise time in light-driven responses either decreasing or increasing, depending on the niosome formulation. Peak amplitudes exhibited similar trends in that most treatments resulted in reduced peak amplitudes in both the VC and CC modes compared with Lipofectamine. Although cells depolarized upon illumination in almost all cases, they never reached a threshold to fire an action potential.

To establish whether there was a positive correlation between morphology and electrophysiology, we compared the total length of all dendrites and the peak amplitude for both the VC and CC modes. All niosomes complexed with CAG-ChrimsonR showed a strong positive correlation in both the VC and CC modes with pulses 1 and 2 (pulse 1, VC R squared = 0.9442, CC R squared = 0.9327, pulse 2, VC R squared = 0.9432, CC R squared = 0.9219) when compared to the Lipofectamine control (Figure 3A–D). Syn-ChrimsonR treatments showed a positive correlation and statistical significance between morphology and electrophysiology in the VC mode peak amplitude (Supplementary Figure S6A,B), but the CC mode peak amplitude showed no statistical significance and a weaker positive correlation (Supplementary Figure S6C,D). CatCh plasmid treatments showed no statistical significance and a weak positive correlation in the both VC and CC modes with both pulses (Supplementary Figure S6E–H).

The strong correlation we observe using the CAG-ChrimsonR nioplex confirms that the morphological changes have a direct influence on the electrophysiological behavior of these cells. This was observed to a lesser extent with Syn-ChrimsonR only in the VC mode, while cells treated with CatCh exhibited a weak correlation for both pulses in both recording modes.

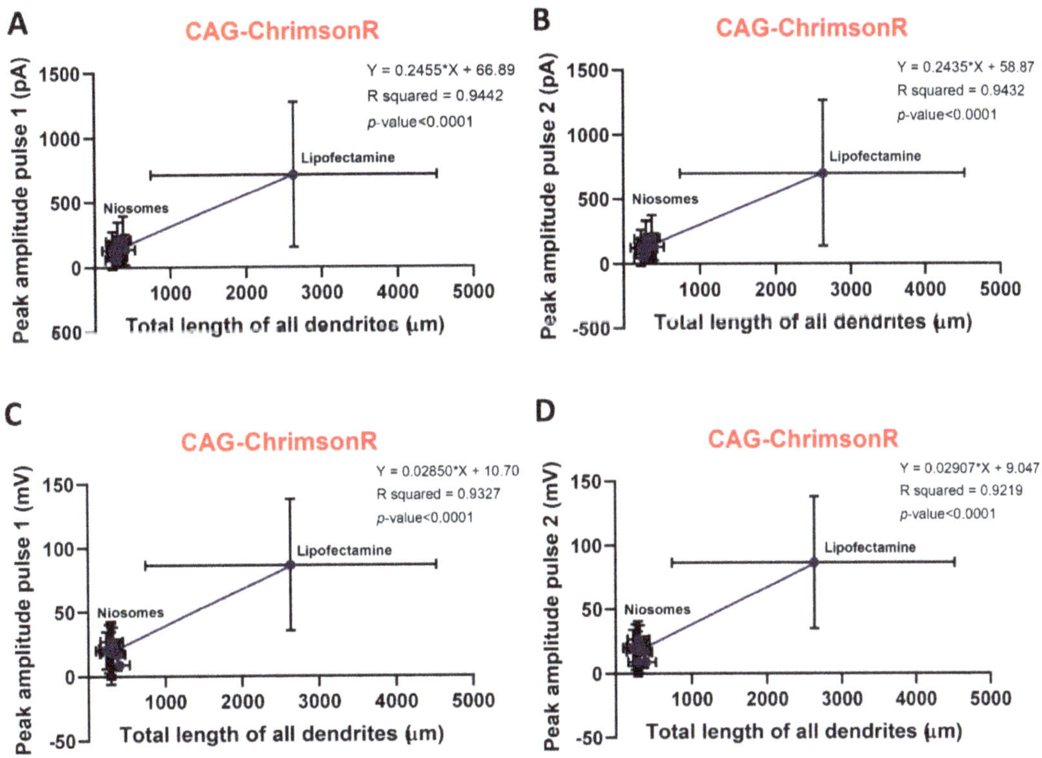


**Figure 3. Correlation of morphological and electrophysiological changes.** (**A–D**) Dispersion graphs correlating total length of all dendrites morphological parameters with peak amplitude electrophysiological parameters, existing positive correlation with VC recordings in pulses 1 (**A**) and 2 (**B**) and in CC recordings in pulses 1 (**C**) and 2 (**D**) (simple linear regression). Dots represent mean, horizontal graphs morphological (X-axis) SD, and vertical graphs electrophysiological (Y-axis) SD.

### *3.3. Morphological Characterization and Cell Viability Assesment of Niosomes, Nioplexes, and Naked Plasmids*

To discern whether the niosomes themselves were the negative factor affecting morphology, rather than a combination with the plasmids, we treated cortical neurons after 21–28 DIV with only the niosome formulations and characterized the morphology by marking cells with the anti-MAP2 antibody. We observed significant differences in the number of dendrites, as well as in the total length of all dendrites, for several niosomes treatments when compared to untreated cells (Figure 4A,B), except for the total length of all dendrites of neurons treated with CQ (5:1) ($p$-value = 0.1051). Furthermore, CQ (5:1)-treated cells had a similar appearance to untreated controls, and dendritic blebbing was absent (Figure 4C,D) which was observed in most other treatments (Figure 2E). On the other hand, in some of the treatments, no statistical differences were observed in certain morphological parameters, more specifically, in the mean length of all dendrites with treatments ND12 (8:1) ($p$-value = 0.0753), ND12 (10:1) ($p$-value = 0.0630), P10 (5:1) ($p$-value = 0.1431), P10 (8:1) ($p$-value = 0.0630), and CQ (10:1) ($p$-value = 0.1655) (Supplementary Figure S7B).

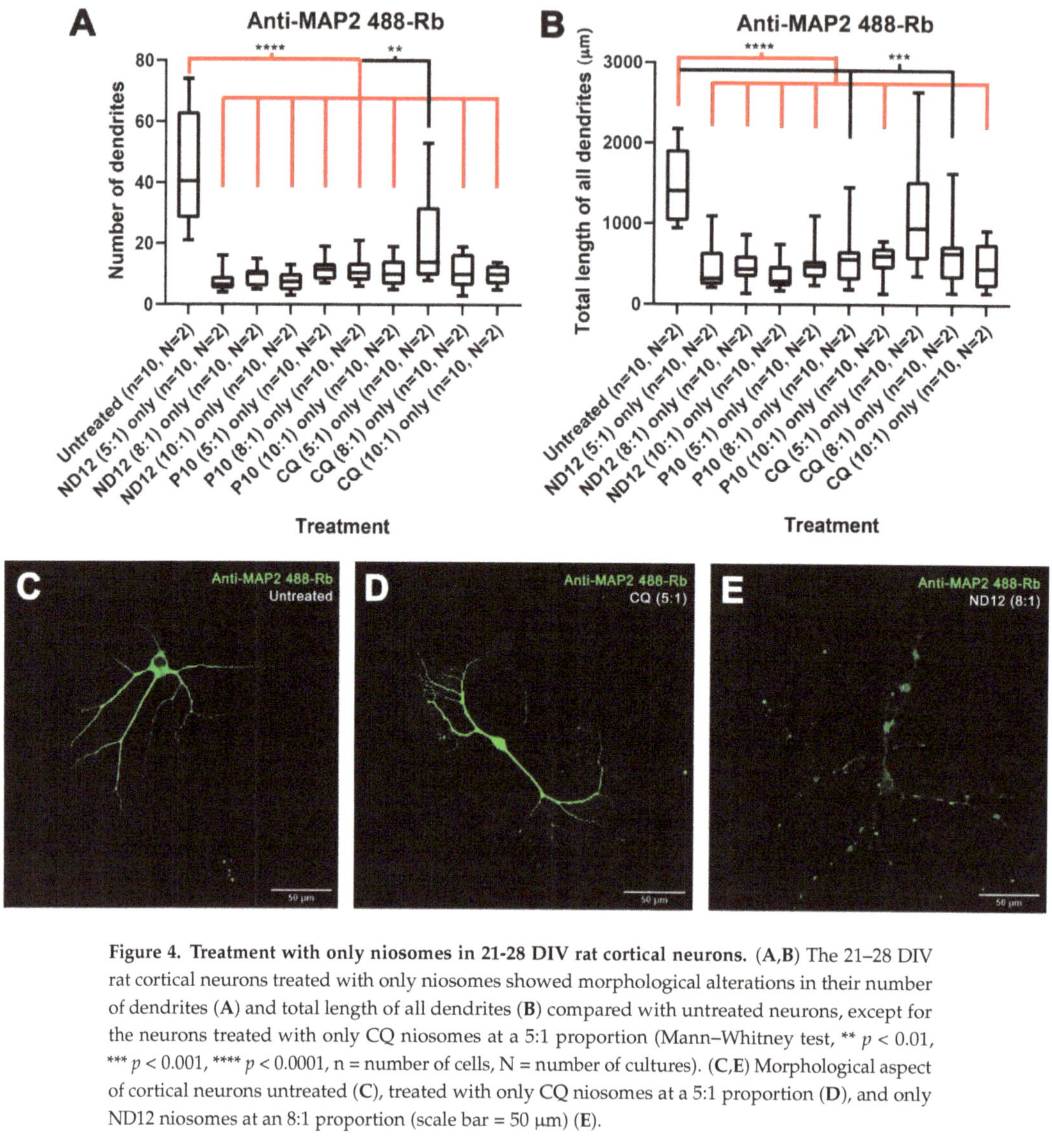


**Figure 4. Treatment with only niosomes in 21-28 DIV rat cortical neurons.** (**A**,**B**) The 21–28 DIV rat cortical neurons treated with only niosomes showed morphological alterations in their number of dendrites (**A**) and total length of all dendrites (**B**) compared with untreated neurons, except for the neurons treated with only CQ niosomes at a 5:1 proportion (Mann–Whitney test, ** $p < 0.01$, *** $p < 0.001$, **** $p < 0.0001$, n = number of cells, N = number of cultures). (**C**,**E**) Morphological aspect of cortical neurons untreated (**C**), treated with only CQ niosomes at a 5:1 proportion (**D**), and only ND12 niosomes at an 8:1 proportion (scale bar = 50 µm) (**E**).

To rule out the possibility that the plasmids themselves may have an adverse effect on neurons, we performed similar experiments by applying our naked plasmids, without niosome delivery systems, in 21–28 DIV cortical cultures. In general, no statistical differences were observed in the mean length of all dendrites and the longest dendrite in comparison to untreated controls (Supplementary Figure S8D,E). However, when using the CatCh and Syn-ChrimsonR plasmid, we did observe a reduction in the number of dendrites ($p$-value = 0.0136 * and 0.0014 **, respectively), branching points ($p$-value = 0.0081 ** and 0.0023 **, respectively), and total length of all dendrites ($p$-value = 0.0068 ** and 0.0039 **, respectively), and we also observed a reduction in the number of dendrites ($p$-value = 0.0498) and branching points ($p$-value = 0.0410) with the CAG-ChrimsonR plasmid, but not in the total length of all dendrites ($p$-value = 0.2799) (Supplementary Figure S8A–C). Experiments performed adding only Lipofectamine (1:1) showed no statistical difference in any morphological parameter compared with untreated neurons. All $p$-values can be found in Supplementary Table S2.

To investigate whether niosomes can affect the viability of neurons, we performed cell viability experiments. Neurons were seeded in a 96-well plate and divided into 3 groups: plasmid treated, niosome treated, and untreated controls. MTT was added to the wells 24, 48, and 72 h after the initial treatment. Values were normalized according to the absorbance values obtained in the untreated wells (Figure 5). The treatment with all nanoparticles at a 5:1 ratio did not show a statistically significant decrease in cell viability. On the other hand, wells treated with only nanoparticles at the 8:1 and 10:1 ratios showed a decrease in cell viability as early as 24 h, especially with the ND12 and CQ treatments ($p$-value < 0.0001 ****) and P10 to a lower extent (8:1 $p$-value = 0.03 *, 10:1 $p$-value = 0.038 *).

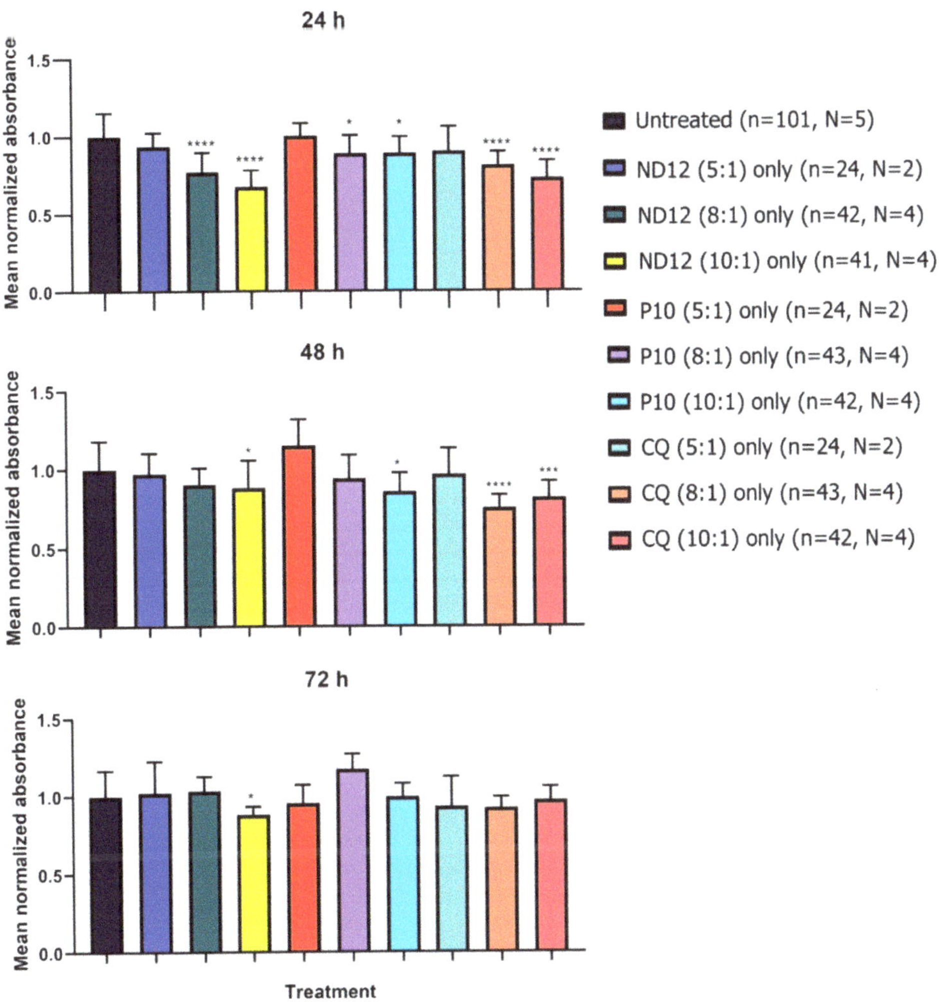


**Figure 5. Cell viability using different proportions of niosomes in 21–28 DIV cortical neurons.** MTT assays performed at 24, 48, and 72 h in 21–28 DIV rat cortical neurons showed reduced cell viability at niosome 8:1 and 10:1 proportions compared with lower proportions and untreated neurons (Multiple $t$-tests, * $p < 0.05$, *** $p < 0.001$, **** $p < 0.0001$, n = number of wells, N = number of cultures). Graph bars are expressed as mean ± SD.

After 48 h of treatment, we only observed a significant decrease in cell viability in ND12 and P10 at 10:1 (*p*-value = 0.0367 * and 0.0198 *, respectively), but not at 8:1. However, CQ treatment at 8:1 and 10:1 resulted in a significant decrease in cell viability (*p*-value = 0.0001 **** and 0.0011 **, respectively). After 72 h, only the ND12 treatment at a 10:1 ratio showed a significant decrease in cell viability (*p*-value = 0.0251 *). These results suggest that the majority of the deleterious effects produced by these niosomes occurs within the first 24 h once the cells have initially internalized them. All *p*-values can be found in Supplementary Table S3.

We then repeated these experiments with the niosomes complexed with the plasmids to assess any combinatorial effect on cell viability. Overall, we observed a more significant decrease in cell viability in comparison to the niosome treatment by itself. At ratios 8:1 and 10:1 with optogenetic plasmids, we observed significant decreases in cell viability for all nioplexes tested (Figure 6), except for P10 at 8:1 for all plasmids and P10 at 10:1 in the CatCh plasmid (*p*-value = 0.1531). GFP nioplexes also resulted in decreased viability for all ratios and niosome combinations, except for P10 8:1 (*p*-value = 0.1807), CQ 8:1 (*p*-value = 0.0663), and P10 10:1 (*p*-value = 0.7845) (Figure 6). When we only applied the plasmids or Lipofectamine, we observed no decrease in cell viability (Supplementary Figure S9). All *p*-values can be found in Supplementary Table S4.

To assess if these morphological changes could be age-dependent, we tested the niosomes on neurons cultured between 7 and 11 DIV. We observed robust statistical differences with all niosomes in the number of dendrites, total length of all dendrites (Figure 7), branching points, and longest dendrite (Supplementary Figure S7D,F) under all conditions. However, no statistical differences were found in any treatment in the mean length of all dendrites and some treatments for the longest dendrite (Supplementary Figure S7E). When we applied naked plasmids to younger cultures, no statistical differences were noted (Supplementary Figure S8F–J), except for the CAG-ChrimsonR plasmid in the total length of all dendrites (*p*-value = 0.0356 *) (Supplementary Figure S8H) and the naked GFP plasmid in the longest dendrite (*p*-value = 0.0199 *) (Supplementary Figure S8J) parameters. Additional experiments with only Lipofectamine (1:1) showed no statistical difference between untreated neurons in any morphological parameters, except in the branching points (*p*-value = 0.0122 *) and mean length of all dendrites (*p*-value = 0.0054 **) (Supplementary Figure S8G,I). All *p*-values can be found in Supplementary Table S5. Further comparisons of cell viability at different ages can be found in Figure 8 and Supplementary Figure S10. All *p*-values can be found in Supplementary Table S6. These results suggest that older neurons appear to be more resistant to niosome-induced alterations.

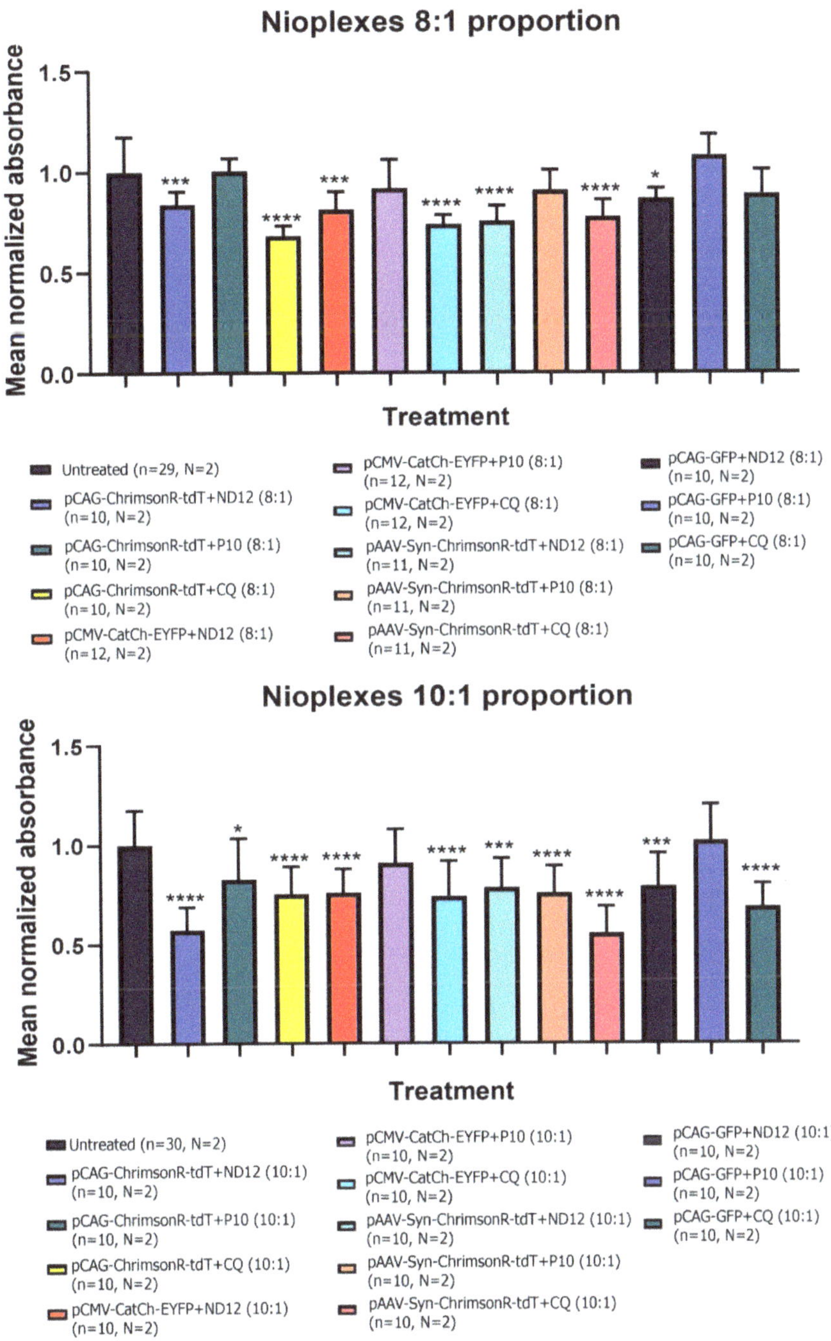


**Figure 6. Cell viability using different proportions of nioplexes.** MTT assays performed after 24 h of treatment in 21–28 DIV rat cortical neurons showed reduced cell viability with nioplexes both at 8:1 and 10:1 proportions compared with untreated neurons (Multiple *t*-tests, * $p < 0.05$, *** $p < 0.001$, **** $p < 0.0001$, n = number of wells, N = number of cultures). Graph bars are expressed as mean ± SD.

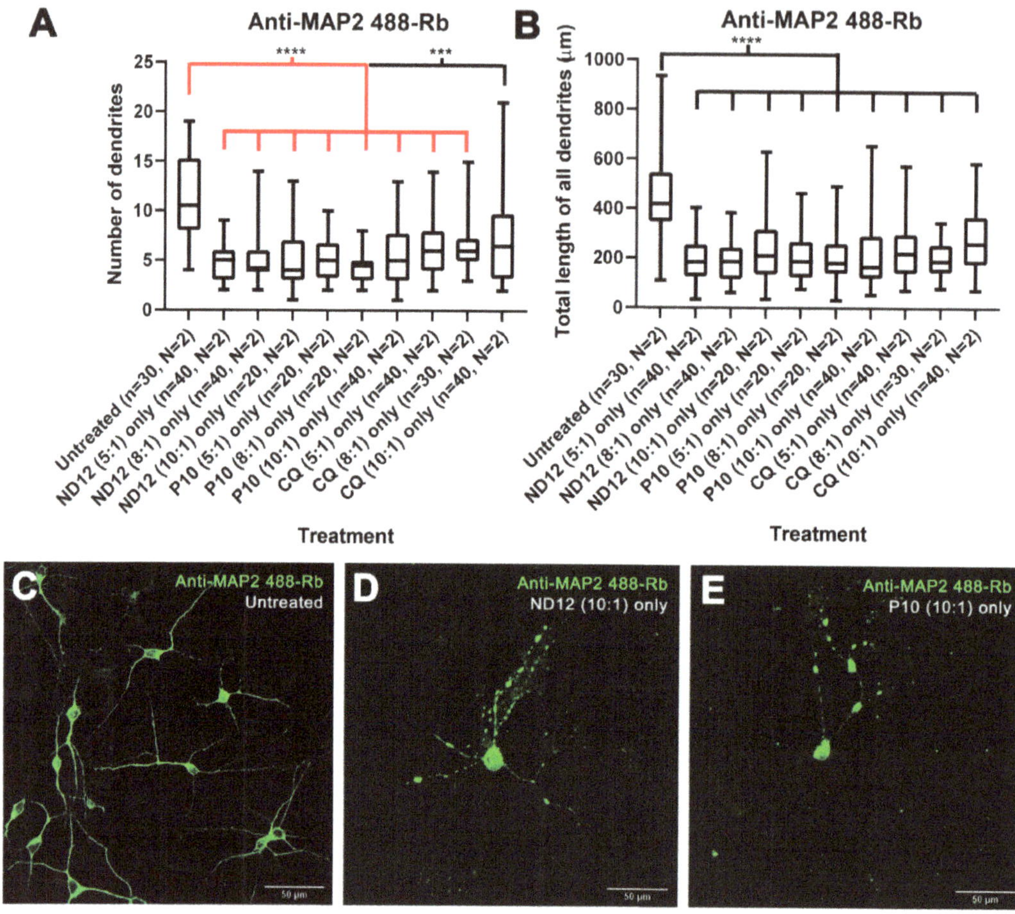


**Figure 7. Morphological changes induced by different niosome-based formulations in 7–11 DIV rat cortical neurons.** (**A**,**B**) The 7–11 DIV rat cortical neurons treated with only niosomes showed morphological alterations in their number of dendrites (**A**) and total length of all dendrites (**B**) compared with untreated neurons (Mann–Whitney test, *** $p < 0.001$, **** $p < 0.0001$, n = number of cells, N = number of cultures). (**C**–**E**) Morphological aspect of cortical neurons untreated (**C**), treated with only ND12 niosomes at a 10:1 proportion (**D**), and only P10 niosomes at a 10:1 proportion (scale bar = 50 μ) (**E**).

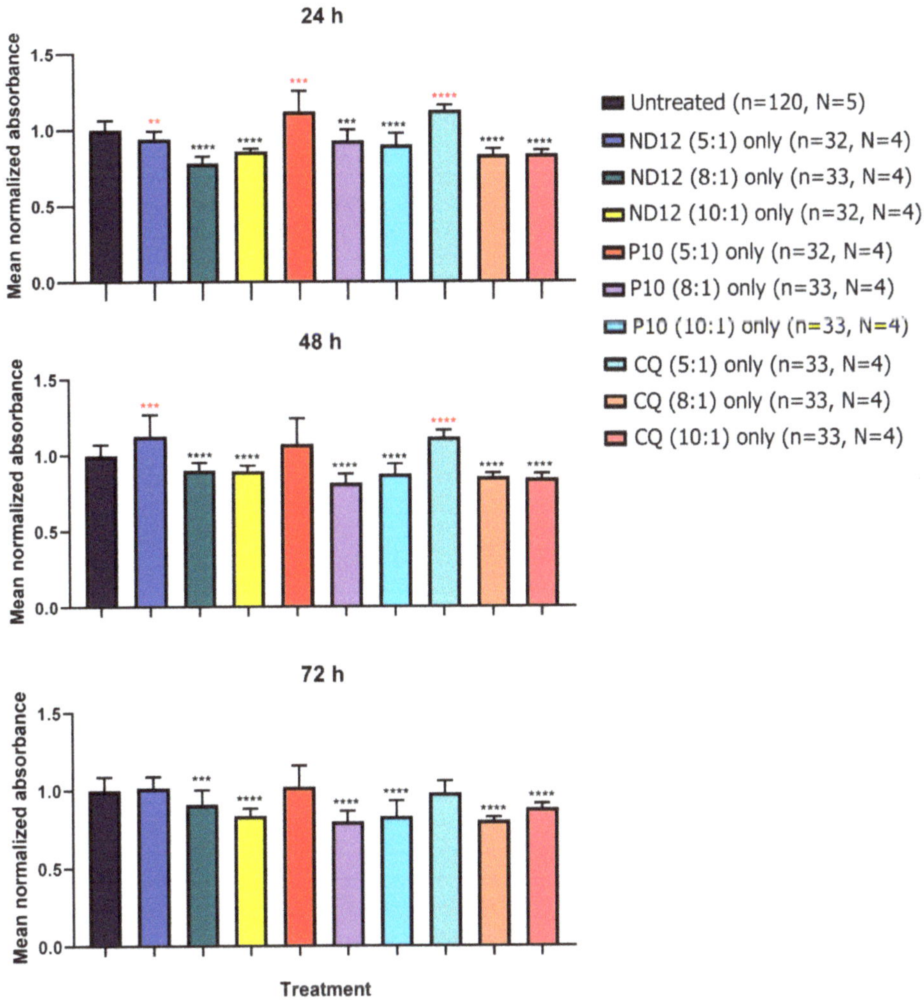


**Figure 8. Cell viability using different proportions of niosomes in 7–11 DIV cortical neurons.** MTT assays performed at 24, 48, and 72 h in 7–11 DIV rat cortical neurons showed reduced cell viability at niosome 8:1 and 10:1 proportions compared with lower proportions, naked plasmid treatments, and untreated neurons (Multiple *t*-tests, ** $p < 0.01$, *** $p < 0.001$, **** $p < 0.0001$, n = number of wells, N = number of cultures). Red *p*-values mean that there is a statistical difference with groups with higher mean values than the untreated groups, while black *p*-values mean that there is a statistical difference with groups with lower mean values than the untreated groups. Graph bars are expressed as mean ± SD.

## 4. Discussion

We have combined, for the first time, three different niosome formulations with three optogenetic plasmids and compared the transfections to a control GFP plasmid. Niosome ratios of 5:1, 8:1, and 10:1 demonstrated the capacity to transfect optogenetic material in rat cortical cells in vitro. However, a ratio of 2:1 proved to be insufficient with all plasmids tested. This is most likely due to the low concentration of niosomes and, in some cases, more negative zeta potential values hindering the electrostatic interaction between DNA and nanoparticles (Supplementary Table S7). Positively charged nioplexes are less likely to be formed that can easily interact with the negatively charged cell surface facilitating their uptake through endocytosis [22]. Although expression of the reporter confirmed the insertion of the optogenetic channels, we observed changes to the morphology of the neurons. These included a decrease in dendritic length and number, as well as arborization. This may be due to possible cytotoxic effects with the accumulation of high levels of cationic lipids and their headgroups (especially at the 8:1 and 10:1 proportions) [45]. When we used a ratio of 5:1, which has previously been reported to be optimal for transfection, here, once again, we observed a similar phenotype [22,42,44]. Some of the plasmids used required a minimal of an 8:1 ratio to observe expression (Syn-ChrimsonR). In some parameters, however, we did not observe any changes when compared to Lipofectamine-treated cells and niosomes, for example, with GFP and ND12 at a ratio of 5:1 in the mean length of all dendrites. This suggests that the size of the plasmid may also play some additional role, as the CAG-ChrimsonR plasmid is 7301 bp and the Syn-ChrimsonR plasmid is 6864 bp, while the GFP plasmid is 5551 bp.

Most of the literature on niosomes involves some form of stem cell or cancer cell line [27,29–32], which are generally more resistant to biological stresses in comparison to the more susceptible neurons, which may explain the effects we observed, especially at higher concentrations. However, previous studies on cell viability using niosomes on hepatocellular carcinoma, HepG2 cells, have shown that a 1.5 μM concentration results in 90% viability and 5 μM in less than 60% viability, corroborating the present results [46].

Interestingly, the CatCh plasmid would only express using a high ratio of 10:1; however, it showed no statistical difference in the mean length of all dendrites, even though the total number of dendrites and ramifications were reduced in comparison to Lipofectamine-treated cells. Considering that the CatCh plasmid is 7099 bp and, therefore, smaller than the CAG-ChrimsonR plasmid, the morphological alterations might be operating, at the molecular level, in a different way due to the size. One possible solution for solving problems related to plasmid size could be using lipid–polymer hybrid nanoparticles, which consist of nucleic acids polymers coated with a single lipid layer, allowing high nucleic acid condensation efficiency [47]. Others have reported improved efficiency of niosome drug delivery by magnetizing them and then modifying the surface by PEGylation to treat breast cancer cells with Carboplatin [48].

These morphological changes also translated into electrophysiological alterations. The nioplexes-treated neurons exhibit both reduced inward currents and depolarization, and generally were unable to fire when photostimulated, in contrast to Lipofectamine-treated neurons. During photostimulation, we did observe depolarization of the cells, but in almost all cases, these were sub-threshold and were unable to elicit any spikes. This suggests that the channels are transported to the cell membrane and are open during photoactivation; however, the reduction in the dendritic parameters is the most likely reason for the altered electrophysiological properties of the reduced photocurrents.

Peak amplitudes for all photocurrents were generally significantly reduced for all nioplexes when combined with CAG-ChrimsonR or Syn-ChrimsonR, while rise times depended on the plasmid and at which ratio. The CatCh plasmid, however, which was only expressed with all niosomes at a ratio of 10:1, exhibited in general slightly smaller peak amplitudes, but in most cases, they were not significantly different when compared to Lipofectamine. Rise times to peak amplitude were more varied and depended on the ratio and the nanoparticle being used. Neurons treated with the CatCh nioplexes had no differences in rise time compared with the CatCh with Lipofectamine.

We observed a strong correlation between the total length of all dendrites and peak amplitude between both pulses, suggesting that the morphological changes directly influence the cell's electrophysiological properties. CAG-ChrimsonR revealed a strong positive correlation between morphology and electrophysiology. The noxious effects that niosome uptake has on normal dendritic morphology development directly relates to the lower peak values recorded. However, this correlation was not always consistent, being weaker in the CC peak amplitude of Syn-ChrimsonR expressing neurons and, in general, in CatCh expressing neurons. The CatCh results are consistent with the lower differences in both the morphological and electrophysiological values observed after treatments. Therefore, the difficulty of nioplex-treated neurons to fire APs could be related to the amount of cationic lipid introduced in the membrane, compromising stability [49].

To discern whether niosomes or plasmids were damaging the cells, we tested just the niosomes and the naked plasmids and characterized the morphology of neurons in young and mature cultures. To our surprise, both the niosomes and the naked plasmids appeared to have a detrimental influence on some morphological properties of the cells. This suggests that there may be a combinatory effect. Interestingly, while naked plasmids did not generally affect the morphology of younger neurons, they did affect the mature cultures in some aspects, especially with the Syn-ChrimsonR and CatCh plasmids. As the purity of the plasmids was within an acceptable range of (A260/A280 = 1.8–2), we doubt this may have been due to contamination. This was intriguing, as bigger plasmids tend to degrade faster within cell medium [50]. Further, while adult neurons seem not to be affected by Lipofectamine alone, in younger neurons, it affects some morphological parameters (especially the mean length of all dendrites), suggesting that young neurons are more sensitive also to Lipofectamine.

The nanoparticles are predominantly taken up into the cell through the process of endocytosis and initially trapped within a membrane vesicle, which budded off from the cell membrane and eventually released into the cytosol. Once the plasmid has been released from the vesicle, the nanoparticles may continue to disrupt intracellular membranes, such as those of the mitochondria. Mitochondrial metabolism that has been disrupted can lead to the generation of reactive oxygen species (ROS), which can damage DNA and exhibit other toxic effects. Some suggestions have been made that lipids that act as mRNA carriers in vaccines could be responsible for possible cytotoxicity in a similar fashion [51].

Finally, the viability results revealed that high proportions (specially, 8:1 and 10:1) of only niosomes produced a decline in cell viability, which was not observed in either naked plasmids or niosomes at a ratio of 5:1. This decline was consistent in young neurons throughout all times tested, but not in adult neurons, in which the noxious effect of niosomes appears to diminish with time. This is probably due to younger cultures being more sensitive to environmental changes in comparison to mature cells [52]. The results of cell viability with nioplexes in adult neurons suggested that nioplexes caused, in some cases, higher cell damage than only niosomes, as a higher decrease in cell viability was observed. Therefore, it seemed as if a synergistic effect between the niosomes and the plasmid occurs. This, however, varied among niosomes, with P10 nioplexes exhibiting the lowest decreases in cell viability, suggesting that the composition of the helper compound may have a key role in the degree of harm produced.

Our results show for the first time that all the niosomes tested were able to transfect cortical neurons with optogenetic channels, suggesting that niosomes are good candidates to transfect optogenetic tools. However, our results also suggest that there is room for improvement. Thus, some transfected cells exhibit morphological and electrophysiological changes that affect them negatively, especially when using high niosome concentrations. Therefore, we should be aware of the importance of finding a correct balance between the concentration of niosomes and the ratio of niosomes to optogenetic plasmids. Engineering new formulations is a critical challenge for the development of advanced optogenetics applications based on these promising non-viral vectors.

**Supplementary Materials:** The following supporting information can be downloaded at: https://www.mdpi.com/article/10.3390/pharmaceutics15071860/s1, Figure S1: Additional morphological parameters in neurons treated with nioplexes made of pCAG-ChrimsonR-tdTomato and pCAG-GFP; Figure S2: Morphological parameters in neurons treated with nioplexes made of pAAV-Syn-ChrimsonR-tdTomato and pCMV-CatCh-EYFP; Table S1: *p*-values of 21–28 DIV neurons treated with nioplexes; Figure S3: Additional electrophysiological changes produced by nioplexes with CAG-ChrimsonR in rat cortical neurons; Figure S4: Electrophysiological changes produced by nioplexes with Syn-ChrimsonR in rat cortical neurons; Figure S5: Electrophysiological changes produced by nioplexes with CatCh in rat cortical neurons; Figure S6: Morphological and electrophysiological changes correlations in Syn-ChrimsonR and CatCh plasmids; Figure S7: Additional morphological parameters affected by niosomes themselves produce morphological changes in both 21–28 DIV and 7–11 DIV rat cortical neurons; Figure S8: Morphological parameters in neurons treated with naked plasmids and only lipofectamine in both 21–28 DIV and 7–11 DIV rat cortical neurons; Figure S9: Cell viability with naked plasmids and lipofectamine is not affected in 21–28 DIV cortical neurons; Figure S10: Cell viability with naked plasmids and lipofectamine is not affected in 7–11 DIV cortical neurons; Table S2: *p*-values of 21–28 DIV neurons treated with only niosomes or naked plasmids (morphological); Table S3: *p*-values of 21–28 DIV neurons treated with only niosomes or naked plasmids (MTT); Table S4: *p*-values of 21–28 DIV neurons treated with nioplexes (MTT); Table S5: *p*-values of 7–11 DIV neurons treated with only niosomes or naked plasmids (morphological); Table S6: *p*-values of 7–11 DIV neurons treated with only niosomes or naked plasmids MTT); Table S7: size, zeta potential, and polydispersity index of niosomes and nioplexes.

**Author Contributions:** J.D.C., L.H., C.S.-S., G.M.-N. and E.F. conceived the experiments; J.D.C. and L.H. performed the experiments and analyzed the results; D.G. performed the cell cultures; I.M., I.G., I.V.-B., M.S.-R., G.P. and J.L.P. conceived and elaborated the niosomes. All authors have read and agreed to the published version of the manuscript.

**Funding:** This research was funded in part by grants RTI2018-098969-B-I00, PRE2019-087693, DTS19/00175, and PDC2022-133952-100 from the Spanish "Ministerio de Ciencia, Innovación y Universidades" and by the European Union's Horizon 2020 Research and Innovation Programme under Grant Agreement No. 899287 (NeuraViPeR).

**Institutional Review Board Statement:** Not applicable.

**Informed Consent Statement:** Not applicable.

**Data Availability Statement:** Data are contained within the article and the Supplementary Materials.

**Acknowledgments:** The authors wish to give thanks for the intellectual and technical assistance of the Drug Formulation Unit (U10) of the ICTS "NANBIOSIS" from CIBER in Bioengineering, Biomaterials and Nanomedicine (CIBER-BBN) at the University of Basque Country (UPV/EHU). This work was supported by the Basque Country Government (Consolidated Groups, IT1448-22).

**Conflicts of Interest:** The authors declare no conflict of interest.

## References

1. Friedmann, T.; Roblin, R. Gene therapy for human genetic disease? *Science* **1972**, *175*, 949–955. [CrossRef]
2. Merz, B. Gene therapy may have future role in cancer treatment. *JAMA* **1987**, *257*, 150–151. [CrossRef]
3. Shahryari, A.; Saghaeian Jazi, M.; Mohammadi, S.; Razavi Nikoo, H.; Nazari, Z.; Hosseini, E.S.; Burtscher, I.; Mowla, S.J.; Lickert, H. Development and Clinical Translation of Approved Gene Therapy Products for Genetic Disorders. *Front. Genet.* **2019**, *10*, 868. [CrossRef]
4. Ma, C.-C.; Wang, Z.-L.; Xu, T.; He, Z.-Y.; Wei, Y.-Q. The approved gene therapy drugs worldwide: From 1998 to 2019. *Biotechnol. Adv.* **2020**, *40*, 107502. [CrossRef]
5. Powell, S.K.; Rivera-Soto, R.; Gray, S.J. Viral expression cassette elements to enhance transgene target specificity and expression in gene therapy. *Discov. Med.* **2015**, *19*, 49–57.
6. Chen, Y.H.; Keiser, M.S.; Davidson, B.L. Viral Vectors for Gene Transfer. *Curr. Protoc. Mouse Biol.* **2018**, *8*, e58. [CrossRef]
7. Bulcha, J.T.; Wang, Y.; Ma, H.; Tai, P.W.L.; Gao, G. Viral vector platforms within the gene therapy landscape. *Signal Transduct. Target. Ther.* **2021**, *6*, 53. [CrossRef] [PubMed]
8. Almarza, D.; Bussadori, G.; Navarro, M.; Mavilio, F.; Larcher, F.; Murillas, R. Risk assessment in skin gene therapy: Viral–cellular fusion transcripts generated by proviral transcriptional read-through in keratinocytes transduced with self-inactivating lentiviral vectors. *Gene Ther.* **2011**, *18*, 674–681. [CrossRef] [PubMed]
9. Ibraheem, D.; Elaissari, A.; Fessi, H. Gene therapy and DNA delivery systems. *Int. J. Pharm.* **2014**, *459*, 70–83. [CrossRef] [PubMed]
10. Lundstrom, K. Viral Vectors in Gene Therapy. *Diseases* **2018**, *6*, 42. [CrossRef] [PubMed]
11. Foldvari, M.; Chen, D.W.; Nafissi, N.; Calderon, D.; Narsineni, L.; Rafiee, A. Non-viral gene therapy: Gains and challenges of non-invasive administration methods. *J. Control. Release* **2016**, *240*, 165–190. [CrossRef] [PubMed]
12. Choi, W.-J.; Kim, J.-K.; Choi, S.-H.; Park, J.-S.; Ahn, W.S.; Kim, C.-K. Low toxicity of cationic lipid-based emulsion for gene transfer. *Biomaterials* **2004**, *25*, 5893–5903. [CrossRef] [PubMed]

13. Rajera, R.; Nagpal, K.; Singh, S.K.; Mishra, D.N. Niosomes: A Controlled and Novel Drug Delivery System. *Biol. Pharm. Bull.* **2011**, *34*, 945–953. [CrossRef] [PubMed]
14. Ge, X.; Wei, M.; He, S.; Yuan, W.-E. Advances of Non-Ionic Surfactant Vesicles (Niosomes) and Their Application in Drug Delivery. *Pharmaceutics* **2019**, *11*, 55. [CrossRef]
15. Karmali, P.P.; Chaudhuri, A. Cationic liposomes as non-viral carriers of gene medicines: Resolved issues, open questions, and future promises. *Med. Res. Rev.* **2007**, *27*, 696–722. [CrossRef]
16. Dabkowska, A.P.; Barlow, D.J.; Campbell, R.A.; Hughes, A.V.; Quinn, P.J.; Lawrence, M.J. Effect of Helper Lipids on the Interaction of DNA with Cationic Lipid Monolayers Studied by Specular Neutron Reflection. *Biomacromolecules* **2012**, *13*, 2391–2401. [CrossRef]
17. Ojeda, E.; Puras, G.; Agirre, M.; Zarate, J.; Grijalvo, S.; Eritja, R.; DiGiacomo, L.; Caracciolo, G.; Pedraz, J.-L. The role of helper lipids in the intracellular disposition and transfection efficiency of niosome formulations for gene delivery to retinal pigment epithelial cells. *Int. J. Pharm.* **2016**, *503*, 115–126. [CrossRef]
18. Taymouri, S.; Varshosaz, J. Effect of different types of surfactants on the physical properties and stability of carvedilol nano-niosomes. *Adv. Biomed. Res.* **2016**, *5*, 48. [CrossRef]
19. Villate-Beitia, I.; Gallego, I.; Martínez-Navarrete, G.; Zárate, J.; López-Méndez, T.; Soto-Sánchez, C.; Santos-Vizcaíno, E.; Puras, G.; Fernández, E.; Pedraz, J.L. Polysorbate 20 non-ionic surfactant enhances retinal gene delivery efficiency of cationic niosomes after intravitreal and subretinal administration. *Int. J. Pharm.* **2018**, *550*, 388–397. [CrossRef]
20. Mashal, M.; Attia, N.; Puras, G.; Martínez-Navarrete, G.; Fernández, E.; Pedraz, J.L. Retinal gene delivery enhancement by lycopene incorporation into cationic niosomes based on DOTMA and polysorbate 60. *J. Control. Release* **2017**, *254*, 55–64. [CrossRef]
21. Ojeda, E.; Puras, G.; Agirre, M.; Zarate, J.; Grijalvo, S.; Eritja, R.; Martinez-Navarrete, G.; Soto-Sánchez, C.; Diaz-Tahoces, A.; Aviles-Trigueros, M.; et al. The influence of the polar head-group of synthetic cationic lipids on the transfection efficiency mediated by niosomes in rat retina and brain. *Biomaterials* **2016**, *77*, 267–279. [CrossRef]
22. Puras, G.; Mashal, M.; Zárate, J.; Agirre, M.; Ojeda, E.; Grijalvo, S.; Eritja, R.; Diaz-Tahoces, A.; Navarrete, G.M.; Avilés-Trigueros, M.; et al. A novel cationic niosome formulation for gene delivery to the retina. *J. Control. Release* **2014**, *174*, 27–36. [CrossRef]
23. Gallego, I.; Villate-Beitia, I.; Navarrete, G.M.; Menéndez, M.; López-Méndez, T.; Soto-Sánchez, C.; Zarate, J.; Puras, G.; Fernández, E.; Pedraz, J.L. Non-viral vectors based on cationic niosomes and minicircle DNA technology enhance gene delivery efficiency for biomedical applications in retinal disorders. *Nanomed. Nanotechnol. Biol. Med.* **2019**, *17*, 308–318. [CrossRef] [PubMed]
24. Attia, N.; Mashal, M.; Grijalvo, S.; Eritja, R.; Zárate, J.; Puras, G.; Pedraz, J.L. Stem cell-based gene delivery mediated by cationic niosomes for bone regeneration. *Nanomed. Nanotechnol. Biol. Med.* **2018**, *14*, 521–531. [CrossRef] [PubMed]
25. Attia, N.; Mashal, M.; Soto-Sánchez, C.; Martínez-Navarrete, G.; Fernández, E.; Grijalvo, S.; Eritja, R.; Puras, G.; Pedraz, J.L. Gene transfer to rat cerebral cortex mediated by polysorbate 80 and poloxamer 188 nonionic surfactant vesicles. *Drug Des. Dev. Ther.* **2018**, *12*, 3937–3949. [CrossRef]
26. Mashal, M.; Attia, N.; Soto-Sánchez, C.; Navarrete, G.M.; Fernández, E.; Puras, G.; Pedraz, J.L. Non-viral vectors based on cationic niosomes as efficient gene delivery vehicles to central nervous system cells into the brain. *Int. J. Pharm.* **2018**, *552*, 48–55. [CrossRef]
27. Carballo-Pedrares, N.; Kattar, A.; Concheiro, A.; Alvarez-Lorenzo, C.; Rey-Rico, A. Niosomes-based gene delivery systems for effective transfection of human mesenchymal stem cells. *Mater. Sci. Eng. C Mater. Biol. Appl.* **2021**, *128*, 112307. [CrossRef]
28. Qin, Y.; Tian, Y.; Liu, Y.; Li, D.; Zhang, H.; Yang, Y.; Qi, J.; Wang, H.; Gan, L. Hyaluronic acid-modified cationic niosomes for ocular gene delivery: Improving transfection efficiency in retinal pigment epithelium. *J. Pharm. Pharmacol.* **2018**, *70*, 1139–1151. [CrossRef] [PubMed]
29. Ghaffari, M.; Kalantar, S.M.; Hemati, M.; Firoozabadi, A.D.; Asri, A.; Shams, A.; Ghalekohneh, S.J.; Haghiralsadat, F. Co-delivery of miRNA-15a and miRNA-16–1 using cationic PEGylated niosomes downregulates Bcl-2 and induces apoptosis in prostate cancer cells. *Biotechnol. Lett.* **2021**, *43*, 981–994. [CrossRef]
30. Maurer, V.; Altin, S.; Seleci, D.A.; Zarinwall, A.; Temel, B.; Vogt, P.; Strauß, S.; Stahl, F.; Scheper, T.; Bucan, V.; et al. In-Vitro Application of Magnetic Hybrid Niosomes: Targeted siRNA-Delivery for Enhanced Breast Cancer Therapy. *Pharmaceutics* **2021**, *13*, 394. [CrossRef]
31. Pengnam, S.; Plianwong, S.; Patrojanasophon, P.; Radchatawedchakoon, W.; Yingyongnarongkul, B.-E.; Opanasopit, P.; Charoensuksai, P. Synergistic Effect of Doxorubicin and siRNA-Mediated Silencing of Mcl-1 Using Cationic Niosomes against 3D MCF-7 Spheroids. *Pharmaceutics* **2021**, *13*, 550. [CrossRef]
32. Gharbavi, M.; Johari, B.; Rismani, E.; Mousazadeh, N.; Taromchi, A.H.; Sharafi, A. NANOG Decoy Oligodeoxynucleotide–Encapsulated Niosomes Nanocarriers: A Promising Approach to Suppress the Metastatic Properties of U87 Human Glioblastoma Multiforme Cells. *ACS Chem. Neurosci.* **2020**, *11*, 4499–4515. [CrossRef]
33. Boyden, E.S.; Zhang, F.; Bamberg, E.; Nagel, G.; Deisseroth, K. Millisecond-timescale, genetically targeted optical control of neural activity. *Nat. Neurosci.* **2005**, *8*, 1263–1268. [CrossRef] [PubMed]
34. Aravanis, A.M.; Wang, L.-P.; Zhang, F.; Meltzer, L.A.; Mogri, M.Z.; Schneider, M.B.; Deisseroth, K. An optical neural interface: In vivo control of rodent motor cortex with integrated fiberoptic and optogenetic technology. *J. Neural Eng.* **2007**, *4*, S143–S156. [CrossRef] [PubMed]

35. Yamanaka, A.; Tsunematsu, T. New approaches for the study of orexin function. *J. Neuroendocr.* **2010**, *22*, 818–824. [CrossRef] [PubMed]
36. Zhang, H.; Zhao, H.; Zeng, C.; Van Dort, C.; Faingold, C.L.; Taylor, N.; Solt, K.; Feng, H.-J. Optogenetic activation of 5-HT neurons in the dorsal raphe suppresses seizure-induced respiratory arrest and produces anticonvulsant effect in the DBA/1 mouse SUDEP model. *Neurobiol. Dis.* **2018**, *110*, 47–58. [CrossRef]
37. Valverde, S.; Vandecasteele, M.; Piette, C.; Derousseaux, W.; Gangarossa, G.; Arbelaiz, A.A.; Touboul, J.; Degos, B.; Venance, L. Deep brain stimulation-guided optogenetic rescue of parkinsonian symptoms. *Nat. Commun.* **2020**, *11*, 2388. [CrossRef]
38. Sahel, J.-A.; Boulanger-Scemama, E.; Pagot, C.; Arleo, A.; Galluppi, F.; Martel, J.N.; Degli Esposti, S.; Delaux, A.; de Saint Aubert, J.-B.; de Montleau, C.; et al. Partial recovery of visual function in a blind patient after optogenetic therapy. *Nat. Med.* **2021**, *27*, 1223–1229. [CrossRef]
39. Klapoetke, N.C.; Murata, Y.; Kim, S.S.; Pulver, S.R.; Birdsey-Benson, A.; Cho, Y.K.; Morimoto, T.K.; Chuong, A.S.; Carpenter, E.J.; Tian, Z.; et al. Independent optical excitation of distinct neural populations. *Nat. Methods* **2014**, *11*, 338–346. [CrossRef] [PubMed]
40. Kleinlogel, S.; Feldbauer, K.; Dempski, R.E.; Fotis, H.; Wood, P.G.; Bamann, C.; Bamberg, E. Ultra light-sensitive and fast neuronal activation with the Ca2+-permeable channelrhodopsin CatCh. *Nat. Neurosci.* **2011**, *14*, 513–518. [CrossRef]
41. Matsuda, T.; Cepko, C.L. Electroporation and RNA interference in the rodent retina in vivo and in vitro. *Proc. Natl. Acad. Sci. USA* **2003**, *101*, 16–22. [CrossRef]
42. AL Qtaish, N.; Gallego, I.; Paredes, A.J.; Villate-Beitia, I.; Soto-Sánchez, C.; Martínez-Navarrete, G.; Sainz-Ramos, M.; Lopez-Mendez, T.B.; Fernández, E.; Puras, G.; et al. Nanodiamond Integration into Niosomes as an Emerging and Efficient Gene Therapy Nanoplatform for Central Nervous System Diseases. *ACS Appl. Mater. Interfaces* **2022**, *14*, 13665–13677. [CrossRef]
43. AL Qtaish, N.; Gallego, I.; Beitia, I.V.; Sainz-Ramos, M.; Martínez-Navarrete, G.; Soto-Sánchez, C.; Fernández, E.; Gálvez-Martín, P.; Lopez-Mendez, T.B.; Puras, G.; et al. Sphingolipid extracts enhance gene delivery of cationic lipid vesicles into retina and brain. *Eur. J. Pharm. Biopharm.* **2021**, *169*, 103–112. [CrossRef] [PubMed]
44. Sainz-Ramos, M.; Villate-Beitia, I.; Gallego, I.; Qtaish, N.A.; Lopez-Mendez, T.B.; Eritja, R.; Grijalvo, S.; Puras, G.; Pedraz, J.L. Non-viral mediated gene therapy in human cystic fibrosis airway epithelial cells recovers chloride channel functionality. *Int. J. Pharm.* **2020**, *588*, 119757. [CrossRef] [PubMed]
45. Cui, S.; Wang, Y.; Gong, Y.; Lin, X.; Zhao, Y.; Zhi, D.; Zhou, Q.; Zhang, S. Correlation of the cytotoxic effects of cationic lipids with their headgroups. *Toxicol. Res.* **2018**, *7*, 473–479. [CrossRef]
46. Torkzadeh-Mahani, M.; Hajizadeh, M.R.; Maleki, H.; Barani, M.; Fahmidehkar, M.A.; Mahmoodi, M. In vitro cytotoxicity assay of D-limonene niosomes: An efficient nano-carrier for enhancing solubility of plant-extracted agents. *Res. Pharm. Sci.* **2019**, *14*, 448–458. [CrossRef]
47. Guevara, M.L.; Persano, S.; Persano, F. Lipid-Based Vectors for Therapeutic mRNA-Based Anti-Cancer Vaccines. *Curr. Pharm. Des.* **2019**, *25*, 1443–1454. [CrossRef] [PubMed]
48. Davarpanah, F.; Yazdi, A.K.; Barani, M.; Mirzaei, M.; Torkzadeh-Mahani, M. Magnetic delivery of antitumor carboplatin by using PEGylated-Niosomes. *DARU J. Pharm. Sci.* **2018**, *26*, 57–64. [CrossRef] [PubMed]
49. Meng, N.; Grimm, D. Membrane-destabilizing ionizable phospholipids: Novel components for organ-selective mRNA delivery and CRISPR–Cas gene editing. *Signal Transduct. Target. Ther.* **2021**, *6*, 206. [CrossRef]
50. Zhao, N.; Fogg, J.M.; Zechiedrich, L.; Zu, Y. Transfection of shRNA-encoding Minivector DNA of a few hundred base pairs to regulate gene expression in lymphoma cells. *Gene Ther.* **2010**, *18*, 220–224. [CrossRef]
51. Palmer, M. On the Use of the Pfizer and the Moderna COVID-19 mRNA Vaccines in Children and Adolescents. 2022. Available online: https://doctors4covidethics.org/wp-content/uploads/2022/05/pfizer-moderna-public.pdf (accessed on 15 January 2023).
52. Kole, A.J.; Annis, R.P.; Deshmukh, M. Mature neurons: Equipped for survival. *Cell Death Dis.* **2013**, *4*, e689. [CrossRef] [PubMed]

*pharmaceutics*

MDPI

*Review*

# Functionalized Polymeric Micelles for Targeted Cancer Therapy: Steps from Conceptualization to Clinical Trials

**Ana Serras, Célia Faustino * and Lídia Pinheiro**

Research Institute for Medicines (iMed.ULisboa), Faculdade de Farmácia, Universidade de Lisboa (ULisboa), Avenida Professor Gama PintoGama Pinto, 1649-003 Lisboa, Portugal; anafiserras@hotmail.com (A.S.); lpinheiro@ff.ulisboa.pt (L.P.)

* Correspondence: cfaustino@ff.ulisboa.pt

**Abstract:** Cancer is still ranked among the top three causes of death in the 30- to 69-year-old age group in most countries and carries considerable societal and macroeconomic costs that differ depending on the cancer type, geography, and patient gender. Despite advances in several pharmacological approaches, the lack of stability and specificity, dose-related toxicity, and limited bioavailability of chemotherapy (standard therapy) pose major obstacles in cancer treatment, with multidrug resistance being a driving factor in chemotherapy failure. The past three decades have been the stage for intense research activity on the topic of nanomedicine, which has resulted in many nanotherapeutics with reduced toxicity, increased bioavailability, and improved pharmacokinetics and therapeutic efficacy employing smart drug delivery systems (SDDSs). Polymeric micelles (PMs) have become an auspicious DDS for medicinal compounds, being used to encapsulate hydrophobic drugs that also exhibit substantial toxicity. Through preclinical animal testing, PMs improved pharmacokinetic profiles and increased efficacy, resulting in a higher safety profile for therapeutic drugs. This review focuses on PMs that are already in clinical trials, traveling the pathways from preclinical to clinical studies until introduction to the market.

**Keywords:** cancer; nanomedicine; polymeric micelles; amphiphilic polymers; targeted drug delivery; stimuli-responsive micelles; clinical trials

## 1. Introduction

Cancer corresponds to a heterogeneous group of malignant diseases in which cells divide abnormally without control, with the potential to invade other tissues [1–3]. Cancer ranks second among the main causes of death worldwide (particularly in industrialized countries), and its incidence is expected to increase. According to the World Health Organization (WHO), global cancer statistics (2022) pointed to 20 million new cases and 9.7 million deaths, with a 77% increase expected by 2050 [4]. Lung, breast, colorectal, prostate, and stomach cancers are the most frequent ones (Table 1) as stated by the Global Cancer Observatory (GLOBOCAN) of the International Agency for Research on Cancer (IARC).

Cancer is a multifactorial disease that can be triggered by genetic predispositions, environmental influences, and lifestyle choices. Some risks are already known, including immune system diseases, high-fat diets, tobacco use, excessive alcohol consumption, and viral infections [5]. The incidence is influenced by genetic conditions, age, ethnicity, and geography. The majority of neoplasms are sporadic, however, genetic inheritance is known to play a significant role [5].

### *1.1. The Tumor Microenvironment*

Cancer complexity stems from both inter- and intratumoral heterogeneity and dynamic cell plasticity, which determines cancer cell progression, spread, and treatment resistance [2].

A network of signal transduction pathways, particularly those that promote the epithelial-to-mesenchymal transition and metabolic remodeling, are involved in the transformational nature of cancer and influence the evolutionary trajectory of cancer cells [2,6].

**Table 1.** Global prevalence, incidence, and years lived with disability (YLDs) ascribed to cancer for males, females, and both genders in 2021 with percentage change (numbers in parentheses) between 2010 and 2021. Data from Global Burden of Disease Collaborative Network 2022 [7].

| Cancer Type | Prevalence Cases (Millions) | Incidence Cases (Millions) | YLDs Counts (Millions) |
|---|---|---|---|
| Breast | 20.6 (34.0%) | 2.12 (32.8%) | 1.48 (31.8%) |
| female | 20.3 (33.8%) | 2.08 (32.6%) | 1.45 (31.5%) |
| male | 0.320 (53.6%) | 0.0388 (46.7%) | 0.0293 (49.0%) |
| both | 20.6 (34.0%) | 2.12 (32.8%) | 1.48 (31.8%) |
| Colorectal | | | |
| female | 4.92 (35.1%) | 0.931 (31.4%) | 0.450 (32.6%) |
| male | 6.76 (44.2%) | 1.26 (39.4%) | 0.632 (41.4%) |
| both | 11.7 (40.2%) | 25.6 (35.9%) | 1.08 (37.6%) |
| Prostate | | | |
| male | 10.4 (33.5%) | 1.32 (31.2%) | 0.848 (30.4%) |
| Trachea, bronchus, and lung | | | |
| female | 1.15 (37.0%) | 0.779 (37.3%) | 0.188 (35.8) |
| male | 2.10 (24.0%) | 1.50 (21.2%) | 0.361 (21.4%) |
| both | 3.25 (28.3%) | 2.28 (26.2%) | 0.548 (26.0%) |
| Stomach | | | |
| female | 0.695 (9.8) | 0.397 (9.8%) | 0.101 (9.8%) |
| male | 1.70 (14.2%) | 0.833 (9.5%) | 0.224 (1.0%) |
| both | 2.39 (12.9%) | 1.23 (9.6%) | 0.326 (10.6%) |
| Liver | | | |
| female | 0.219 (21.4%) | 0.165 (28.2%) | 0.0391 (26.8%) |
| male | 0.521 (23.3%) | 0.364 (25.0%) | 0.0874 (25.1%) |
| both | 0.739 (22.7%) | 0.529 (26.0%) | 0.127 (25.6%) |
| Pancreatic | | | |
| female | 0.201 (36.7%) | 0.235 (38.5%) | 0.0475 (37.6%) |
| male | 0.238 (35.9%) | 0.274 (38.1%) | 0.0561 (36.8%) |
| both | 0.439 (36.3%) | 0.509 (38.3%) | 0.104 (37.2%) |

Despite tumor heterogeneity, the tumor microenvironment (TME) shares common features that contribute to cancer development [8,9]. Various cell types, including mesenchymal stromal cells (MSCs), tumor endothelial cells (TECs), pericytes, and infiltrating immune cells (lymphocytes, neutrophils, tumor-associated macrophages (TAMs), and mast cells) are found in the TME, which also includes cancer cells, cancer-associated fibroblasts (CAFs), and the extracellular matrix (ECM) [8,9].

Genetic alterations in tumor cells lead to hyperplasia, uncontrolled growth and proliferation, and resistance to apoptosis. Several proteins, enzymes, cell surface receptors, growth factors, inflammatory mediators (e.g., cytokines and chemokines), and antigens are overexpressed in tumor cells [10,11]. The increased expression of matrix metalloproteinases (MMPs), responsible for the degradation of ECM proteins, plays an important role in TME remodeling associated with cell proliferation, migration, angiogenesis, and metastasis. Additionally, cancer cells often overexpress integrins, which are cell-adhesion transmembrane receptors involved in angiogenesis, recruitment of inflammatory cells, and tumor invasiveness [10,11]. Rapid proliferation of cancer cells is also associated with an increased demand for folate and iron. Thus, folate receptors (FRs) and transferrin receptors (TfRs), which mediate cellular uptake of folate and iron, respectively, are often overexpressed in cancer cells [10,11].

Moreover, the high oxygen requirement of fast proliferating tumor cells and the compromised tumor vasculature lead to low oxygen supply, and the resulting hypoxia environment triggers a metabolic shift from mitochondrial oxidative phosphorylation (the main pathway for energy production in normal cells) towards aerobic glycolysis [8,9]. Known as the Warburg effect [12], aerobic glycolysis leads to preferential glucose uptake and conversion into lactic acid, resulting in the acidic extracellular pH characteristic of solid tumors. This metabolic shift is mediated by hypoxia-inducible factor-1 (HIF-1), a transcription factor upregulated in cancer cells that responds to hypoxia by activating genes involved in glycolysis, angiogenesis, and cell survival [8,9]. Tumor hypoxia enhances the production of reactive oxygen species (ROS) and oxidative stress and affects the redox status of the TME by upregulating antioxidant enzymes involved in the synthesis of glutathione (GSH), an important intracellular antioxidant that regulates the cellular redox state by scavenging reactive oxygen and nitrogen species [8,9]. Despite the redox potential difference between the intra- and extracellular milieu of normal cells, this differential is increased in cancer cells due to 2- to 4-fold higher GSH content in the cytosol and subcellular organelles, contributing to the reductive TME.

Additionally, hypoxia drives the release of vascular endothelial growth factor-A (VEGF-A) that binds the VEGF receptor 2 (VEGFR2) at the surface of neighboring endothelial cells, inducing angiogenesis [8,9]. The overexpression of VEGF-A at the TME enhances neo-angiogenesis, producing primitive vasculature networks characterized by dysfunctional blood vessels with irregular and leaky lumen, which contribute to increased interstitial fluid pressure. VEGF-induced primitive vasculatures are shared in various solid tumors, promoting tumor growth, invasion, and metastasis [9]. Furthermore, TECs are known to overexpress $\alpha_V\beta_3$, an integrin involved in the regulation of the sprouting ability of endothelial cells during angiogenesis [9].

The hallmarks of the TME are summarized in Figure 1.

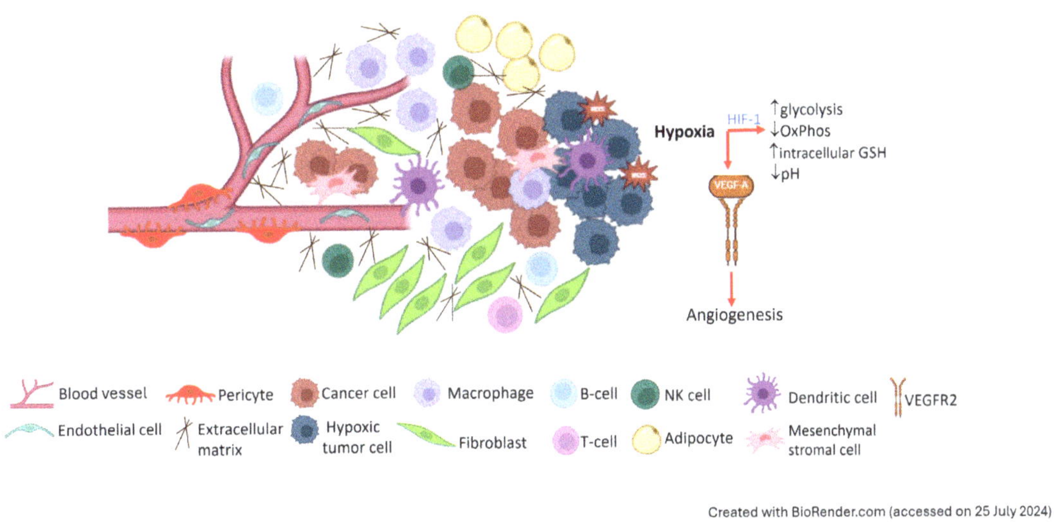


**Figure 1.** Characteristic features of the tumor microenvironment.

### 1.2. Cancer Chemotherapy

Chemotherapy is an effective treatment strategy for cancer, often combined with surgery and/or radiotherapy, depending on the tumor stage [13,14]. Despite the development of novel cancer treatment options, such as small-molecule targeted anticancer drugs (e.g., oncogene-targeted tyrosine kinase inhibitors, TKIs), immunotherapies (e.g., immune checkpoint inhibitors), and gene therapies (e.g., plasmid DNA, small interfering RNA, and microRNAs), conventional chemotherapy relying on cytotoxic drugs to kill and/or inhibit the growth and proliferation of cancer cells remains the first-line treatment for many cancers [1,13].

Traditional chemotherapeutic drugs are classified according to their primary mechanism of action (Table 2), which typically involves interaction with DNA and disruption of the cell cycle, although other secondary modes of action, such as the production of ROS and interference with mitochondrial pathways, also contribute to their cytotoxicity, ultimately leading to cell death in tumor tissues [13].

**Table 2.** Classification of conventional (cytotoxic) chemotherapeutic drugs based on their mode of action.

| Drug Class | Examples |
|---|---|
| Alkylating agents | Nitrogen mustards (bendamustine, chlorambucil, cyclophosphamide, ifosfamide, mechlorethamine, melphalan)<br>Nitrosoureas (carmustine, lomustine, streptozocin)<br>Platinum coordination complexes (cisplatin, carboplatin, oxaliplatin)<br>Triazenes (dacarbazine, procarbazine, temozolomide)<br>Alkyl sulfonate (busulfan)<br>Ethyleneimine (thiotepa) |
| Antimetabolites | Folate antagonists (methotrexate, pemetrexed, pralatrexate, raltitrexed)<br>Purine antagonists (fludarabine, 6-mercaptopurine, pentostatin, 6-thioguanine)<br>Pyrimidine antagonists (azacitidine, capecitabine, cytarabine, 5-fluorouracil, gemcitabine) |
| Antibiotics | Anthracyclines (daunorubicin, doxorubicin, epirubicin, idarubicin), mitoxantrone<br>Nonanthracyclines (bleomycin, dactinomycin, mitomycin) |
| Topoisomerase inhibitors | |
| • Topoisomerase I inhibitors | Camptothecin derivatives (irinotecan, topotecan) |
| • Topoisomerase II inhibitors<br>- catalytic inhibitors<br>- poisons | Epipodophylotoxins (etoposide, tenoposide)<br>Anthracyclines (daunorubicin, doxorubicin, epirubicin, idarubicin), mitoxantrone |
| Mitotic inhibitors | |
| • Microtubule-stabilizing agents | Taxanes (cabazitaxel, docetaxel, paclitaxel)<br>Epothilones (Ixabepilone) |
| • Microtubule-destabilizing agents | Vinca alkaloids (vinblastine, vincristine, vinorelbine) |

Chemotherapy is associated with toxic side effects due to the broad spectrum of activity and narrow therapeutic window of cytotoxic drugs, which do not distinguish between cancer cells and normal (healthy) cells. Most chemotherapeutic agents preferentially attack rapidly multiplying cells, such as cancer cells, but also bone marrow, gastrointestinal tract, and hair follicle cells [13]. Common adverse events (AEs) associated with cytotoxic anticancer drugs include myelosuppression, neutropenia, neurotoxicity, nephrotoxicity, hepatotoxicity, mucositis, nausea, vomiting, diarrhea, alopecia, cutaneous reactions, anemia, body weight loss, fatigue, and an increased risk of infections due to immunosuppression [1,13,15].

Moreover, most cytotoxic drugs in the clinic are highly hydrophobic (Figure 2), suffering from poor water solubility and low bioavailability, being administered as intravenous (IV) infusions (using body surface area dosing) at repeated, regular intervals (treatment cycles) to allow the recovery of normal tissues [13,15]. Nevertheless, neo-angiogenesis, dysfunctional tumor vasculature, increased interstitial fluid pressure, and efflux pumps, namely P-glycoprotein (P-gp), hinder intracellular therapeutic concentrations of cytotoxic drugs reaching the tumor site. The subtherapeutic drug availability in cancer cells can lead to the development of multidrug resistance (MDR), therefore a higher dose, often the maximum tolerated dose (MTD), is usually applied, causing systemic toxicity and potential severe AEs [13,15].

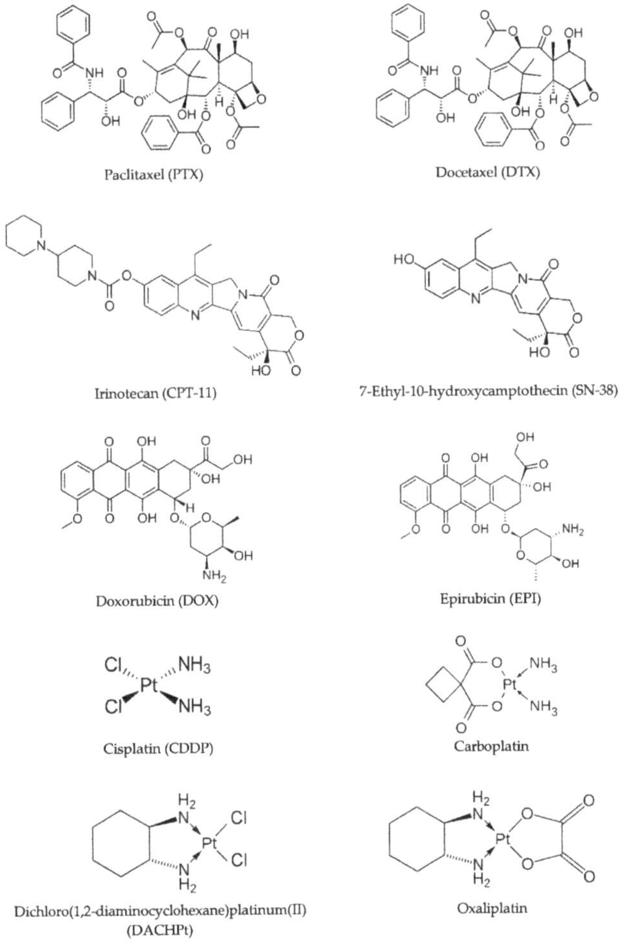


**Figure 2.** Some chemotherapeutic drugs under development as polymeric micellar formulations currently in different phases of clinical trials.

Combination chemotherapy involving the "cocktail" administration of multiple chemotherapy drugs simultaneously, preferentially with different mechanisms of action and non-overlapping toxicities, has shown considerable promise in overcoming MDR, preventing disease recurrence, and extending the survival of cancer patients when compared to monotherapy regimens [13,16]. Similarly, the combination of chemotherapy with phototherapy, gene therapy, and immunotherapy produces synergistic antitumoral effects and allows lower doses of the cytotoxic agent, reducing toxic side effects and enhancing the sensitivity of cancer cells toward the chemotherapeutic drug [16–18].

Improving the selectivity of anticancer drug delivery towards cancer cells while sparing normal (healthy) cells and tissues is a major challenge in cancer chemotherapy considering tumor heterogeneity and complexity. Therefore, targeting the TME or its (a)cellular components, which can reprogram tumor initiation, growth, invasion, metastasis, and therapy response, is a promising therapeutic strategy and nanomedicines are particularly suited to the task [19]. Several nanoformulations of hydrophobic cytotoxic drugs have been approved by the United States Food and Drug Administration (FDA) for cancer chemotherapy and are currently in the market, including Doxil®/Lipodox® (liposomal formulation of doxorubicin) and Abraxane® (nanoparticle albumin-bound paclitaxel), while many others are in clinical trials, including polymeric micelles [20]. The role of nanotechnology in the development of effective anticancer therapies for targeted and controlled drug delivery at the tumor site, thus improving drug efficacy and reducing systemic toxicity, is discussed in the next section.

## 2. The Role of Nanotechnology in Cancer Chemotherapy

The nanotechnological approach, involving drug encapsulation in polymer- or lipid-based nanoparticles (NPs), is a promising strategy for the delivery of hydrophobic chemotherapeutic agents. The nanocarriers solubilize the drug and protect it from chemical and enzymatic degradation, prolonging circulation in the bloodstream while simultaneously avoiding systemic toxicity [1]. Drugs can be physically encapsulated or chemically conjugated to the NP via labile bonds (prodrugs). In the former case, drug release rate is controlled by erosion of the biodegradable core material, diffusion across the polymeric matrix core, or polymer swelling followed by drug diffusion, while in the latter, drug release requires activation via bond cleavage by small molecules or enzymes [21,22].

Size is crucial for cellular uptake, drug release kinetics, biodistribution, and toxicity of NPs. NPs are usually internalized through endocytic pathways, becoming trapped in lysosomes and endosomes [1,23]. The cellular uptake of NPs with sizes in the range 20–100 nm involves caveolin-mediated endocytosis while larger NPs, within the submicron range (100–350 nm), are mainly internalized through clathrin-mediated endocytosis [23]. Therefore, targeting drug-loaded NPs to specific cellular organelles, such as endosomes and lysosomes, can circumvent recognition by drug efflux pumps, like P-gp, through internalization by endocytosis, thus overcoming MDR in cancer cells. Other mechanisms, like phagocytosis and micropinocytosis, may also contribute to NP internalization [23]. Besides size, cellular uptake is also influenced by surface charge of the NP. Cell membranes are negatively charged, which enhances cellular uptake of NPs with net positive surface charge (positive zeta potential) over negatively charged ones due to attractive electrostatic interactions, while selective uptake of anionic NPs by phagocytic cells has been reported [1,23,24].

NPs interact with serum proteins, which adsorb at the surface of the nanocarrier forming a protein corona that prevents NP agglomeration and reduces their toxicity, but also enhances their recognition and clearance by the mononuclear phagocytic system (MPS), which limits NP delivery and distribution [1,22,23,25]. Surface functionalization of NPs can reduce their cytotoxicity and promote cellular uptake by inhibiting protein corona formation in the presence of serum proteins. Hydrophilic surface coating minimizes protein adsorption and prolongs circulation in the bloodstream by escaping the MPS in the liver and spleen [1,22,23]. Poly(ethylene glycol) (PEG) is a hydrophilic, non-ionic synthetic polymer that is FDA-approved for clinical use and most often selected as hydrophilic coating due to its good biocompatibility and non-immunogenicity [1,23,26]. PEG is water-soluble and in aqueous environments forms a highly hydrated, dense brush-like shell that ensures NP solubility and stability, hindering NP aggregation as well as protein binding and opsonization, thus prolonging the NP circulation time upon systemic administration. Furthermore, PEG offers the additional advantage of being easily functionalized with appropriate ligands for targeted drug delivery, contributing to improving the efficacy and safety of anticancer drugs [26]. However, PEG is not biodegradable, and its excretion is dependent on the molecular weight (MW) of the polymer. Low-MW PEGs mainly undergo renal clearance by passive glomerular filtration while those with high MW are predominantly excreted into bile [27]. The MW threshold for kidney clearance of PEGs has been determined as 30 kDa, and PEGs with MWs in the range 2–15 kDa are often chosen to allow for complete renal excretion of the polymer [27].

Moreover, NPs can effectively target the drug to the local site(s) of action, i.e., tumor tissues, which can be achieved by passive or active targeting.

## 2.1. *Tumor-Targeting Mechanisms*

### 2.1.1. Passive Targeting

In passive targeting, NPs accumulate in tumor tissues due to the compromised leaky vasculature, which allows extravasation of nanosized particles (10–100 nm) that become trapped in the TME because of poor lymphatic drainage, a phenomenon known as the enhanced permeability and retention (EPR) effect [21,22,25]. After accumulating in tumors, NPs can act as intracellular Trojan horses, selectively delivering the chemotherapeutic drugs to their subcellular targets, thus overcoming drug resistance mechanisms. EPR based chemotherapeutics are known to alter the drug pharmacokinetics and biodistribution, minimizing the plasma concentration peak ($C_{max}$) and increasing the area under the concentration–time curve (AUC), both in plasma and in tumor, thus providing longer exposure to therapeutic levels of the drug at the target site that contribute to improving drug efficacy and safety [21,22].

### 2.1.2. Active Targeting

Active targeting makes use of the overexpression of certain cell surface receptors and antigens in cancer cells, aiming at increasing NP accumulation in tumor tissues and simultaneously enhancing selective uptake via receptor-mediated endocytosis [10,11,28]. Functionalization of the surface of NPs by conjugation with appropriate targeting ligands, such as folate, transferrin, monoclonal antibodies (mAbs), peptides, carbohydrates, and aptamers, is an efficient strategy for specific and selective drug delivery to cancer cells or intracellular components [10,11,22,28].

The targeting ligands can identify a variety of representative tumor biomarkers, such as FR, TfR, insulin receptor (IR), estrogen receptor $\alpha$ (ER$\alpha$), prostate-specific membrane antigen (PSMA), mucin-1 (MUC1), nucleolin, and human epidermal growth factor receptor 2 (HER2) [10,11,29–31]. TfR is overexpressed in cancer cells, and its endothelium expression is restricted to the endothelial cells forming the blood–brain barrier (BBB), which allows drug targeting to the central nervous system (CNS). Transferrin-targeted NPs can cross the BBB and enhance cellular uptake and brain accumulation of antiglioma drugs with poor BBB permeability [10,11,28]. NPs functionalized with carbohydrate moieties (e.g., galactose, lactose, glucose, or mannose) target the asialoglycoprotein receptor (ASGPR) overexpressed in hepatocellular carcinoma cells for selective drug delivery with high affinity [10,28]. Among the peptide ligands, arginine–glycine–aspartic acid (RGD), or other peptides containing this amino acid sequence, are often used for targeting $\alpha_v\beta_3$ integrin receptors overexpressed in cancer cells and angiogenic endothelial cells in the tumor vasculature [10,11,28].

Antibody-targeted NPs, prepared by attaching mAbs or antibody fragments to the hydrophilic surface of the NP (usually PEG), provide broad diversity of targets and specificity of interaction [10,28]. Aptamers are synthetic single-stranded RNA or DNA oligonucleotides designed to bind specific molecular targets. Aptamers are smaller and less immunogenic than mAbs, show better tissue penetration, and resist enzymatic degradation in vivo (unlike peptides), being easily synthesized and modified [10,28,31].

## 2.2. *Stimuli-Responsive Nanocarriers*

Controlled drug release at the target site is crucial to achieve therapeutic concentrations. Stimuli-responsive "smart" NPs are designed for effective on-site drug release by undergoing changes in chemical structure or physicochemical properties in response to specific environmental stimuli, either endogenous or exogenous, or a combination of two or more stimuli, to improve targetability and combinatorial drug delivery [21,22,28,32,33].

#### 2.2.1. Endogenous Stimuli

Endogenous stimuli include pH, redox status, hypoxia, and upregulated enzymes characteristic of the TME.

The acidic extracellular pH (6.5–6.9) in tumors due to the Warburg effect can be used to trigger drug release from pH-sensitive NPs, constructed by the introduction of ionizable chemical groups ("titratable" groups, such as amines or carboxylic acids) in the NP structure or by drug–NP conjugation through acid-labile linkers (e.g., ester, hydrazone), which are stable at physiological pH (7.4) but release their cargo in the acidic TME, induced by extensive protonation of the titratable group or hydrolysis of the linker, respectively [21,22,28,32–35]. The same strategy can be used for subcellular drug targeting to acidic organelles, namely endosomes (pH 6.5–6.9) and lysosomes (pH 4.0–5.0), ensuring effective intracellular drug concentrations [28,33].

By incorporating enzyme-labile linkages in the NP structure or in the conjugated drug, NPs can be engineered to release the encapsulated drug on demand, using enzymes overexpressed in the extracellular TME [21,22,24,32,36]. Proteinase substrates are commonly used for fabricating NPs with enzyme-responsive linkers [21,22,26,28,32,33]. For instance, NPs modified with short peptide substrates containing MMP-cleavable sequences release their cargo after exposure to MMP-2 overexpressed at the tumor site [26,28,33].

The difference in redox potential between the oxidative extracellular space and the reductive intracellular space, much richer in GSH, has been explored in the design of redox-responsive NPs. Redox-sensitive NPs containing disulfide bonds are stable in the bloodstream as well as in endocytic vesicles but release their cargo in the reductive TME upon reduction of the disulfide linker by cytosolic GSH, which is overexpressed in cancer cells [21,22,26,28,32,33]. ROS-responsive NPs able to respond to the altered oxidative microenvironment of tumor cells due to excessive ROS production have also been developed, mainly using thioether-based oxidation-sensitive polymers that exhibit variation in solubility in response to ROS overproduction and ROS-induced degradation [26,28,32,37–39].

#### 2.2.2. Exogenous Stimuli

Exogenous stimuli, such as temperature, magnetic field, light, ultrasound waves, and electrical fields, have also been used to trigger drug release from NPs accumulated at the target sites. Thermoresponsive NPs made from thermosensitive materials that exhibit a lower critical solution temperature (LCST), such as poly(*N*-isopropylacrylamide) (PNIPAM), release their cargo due to phase separation at temperatures above the LCST [21,22,28,32,33,40]. In drug targeting of thermoresponsive NPs to cancer cells, hyperthermia can be used as trigger. Magnetic NPs, such as iron oxide NPs, including $Fe_3O_4$ (magnetite), $\gamma$-$Fe_2O_3$ (maghemite), and $\alpha$-$Fe_2O_3$ (hematite) as well as superparamagnetic iron oxide nanoparticles (SPIONs), release their cargo when placed under an oscillating magnetic field. The latter do not retain magnetization upon its removal, which avoids NP aggregation in the absence of the magnetic field [28,32,33,41]. The rise in temperature (40–44 °C) by the electromagnetic waves (magnetic hyperthermia) can also be used to enhance drug efficacy [42].

Light-sensitive NPs are promising drug delivery systems (DDSs) for spatiotemporally controlled release of drugs at target sites upon stimulation with ultraviolet (UV), visible, or near-infrared (NIR) light, depending on the chromophore incorporated in the NP [21,22,32,43]. Photoactive agents are already used in phototherapy and optical imaging in clinical practice, including fluorescence imaging and fluorescence-guided surgery [44]. Ultrasound-responsive NPs release their payloads under the influence of ultrasound waves, which penetrate deeper into the body than light, and can induce drug release by both thermal (hyperthermia) and mechanical effects (cavitating bubbles) [28,32,33,45,46]. Non-thermal effects associated with oscillating or cavitating bubbles can disrupt the nanocarrier and contribute to micropore formation in target cell membranes, enhancing membrane permeability and passive diffusion with subsequent intracellular drug accumulation [28,32,33].

Drug release from electric-field-responsive NPs is triggered by an applied electric field, which is easy to generate and control [21,22]. This type of NP can be constructed using conductive polymers, such as poly(pyrrole) (PPy), and their properties depend on dopant selection and MW of the drug [47]. Biotin (an essential vitamin involved in cellular carbohydrate, amino acid, and lipid metabolism) is often the dopant of choice, and the biotin-doped polymer is reacted with streptavidin (with four biotin-binding sites) with subsequent incorporation of a biotinylated drug. Electrical stimulation leads to the reduction of the PPy backbone and triggers the release of the biotin and the attached payload [47].

Among the numerous nanoparticulate drug delivery systems available, including nanoliposomes, polymeric NPs, polymeric micelles, dendrimers, polymersomes, lipid NPs, and inorganic NPs, polymeric micelles have emerged as promising platforms for targeted and controlled delivery of anticancer agents, as discussed in the next section.

## 3. Structure and Preparation of Polymeric Micelles

Polymeric micelles (PMs) are spherical-shaped nanostructures with sizes typically ranging from 10 to 100 nm, formed by spontaneous self-assembly of amphiphilic block copolymers in an aqueous environment when the concentration reaches a critical value, known as the critical micelle concentration (CMC) [21,22]. PMs have a unique core–shell structure with the hydrophobic blocks forming an inner core surrounded by a shell of hydrophilic blocks creating a protecting layer (corona) at the micelle–water interface (Figure 3). The hydrophobic effect is the main driving force for the self-assembly process, which lowers the Gibbs energy of the system by removing the hydrophobic blocks from the aqueous milieu [21,22].

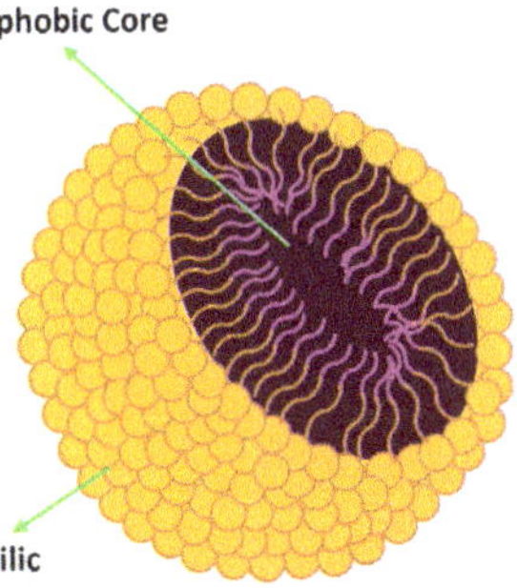


**Figure 3.** Schematic representation of a polymeric micelle.

The size and stability (CMC) of PMs depend on the hydrophilic–lipophilic balance (HLB) of the block copolymers and their MW [21,22]. The properties of the hydrophobic block strongly influence drug-loading capacity, stability, and drug release behavior while the properties of the hydrophilic block modulate the in vivo pharmacokinetic profile [1,21,22]. The failure of NPs in clinical trials is often due to poor pharmacokinetic profile. Pharmacokinetic parameters for some PMs that have completed or are still in clinical trials are presented in Table 3.

### 3.1. Polymers Used for the Manufacturing of Polymeric Micelles

Both natural and synthetic polymers can be used in the construction of PMs. Despite their good biocompatibility, biodegradability, and low immunogenicity, natural biopolymers like chitosan, alginate, and hyaluronan are susceptible to chemical and enzymatic degradation, have an associated risk of microbial contamination, may trigger allergic reactions in susceptible individuals, and display limited batch-to-batch reproducibility [21,22]. On the other hand, synthetic polymers have predictable and controllable physicochemical properties, which can be tailored by appropriate choice of monomer units, type of polymerization reaction, formation of copolymers, as well as easy functionalization [21,22].

Biocompatibility and biodegradability are key criteria for selection of hydrophobic core-forming blocks. Poly(esters), like poly(D,L-lactic acid) (PDLLA), poly(lactic-co-glycolic acid) (PLGA), and poly(ε-caprolactone) (PCL), and poly(amino acids), like poly(L-aspartic acid) (pAsp) and poly(L-glutamic acid) (pGlu), are usually employed since they undergo in vivo hydrolysis of their ester and amide bonds to yield the respective monomers, carboxylic acids and L-amino acids, which can be eliminated by natural metabolic pathways [21,22]. The poly(esters), namely FDA-approved PLGA and PDLLA, are usually selected due to their good safety profile, since their biodegradation generates glycolic and/or lactic acids, which are ultimately degraded to carbon dioxide and water via the Krebs cycle [21,22]. The side chains in the residues of poly(amino acids) allow functionalization to further enhance hydrophobicity and loading ability or for covalent coupling of the drug, leading to self-assembled block copolymer–drug conjugate micelles [21,22].

Non-biodegradable poly(ethers), like poly(propylene oxide) (PPO), can also be used, namely in poloxamers (Pluronics®), which are amphiphilic triblock copolymers composed of hydrophilic poly(ethylene oxide) (PEO) and hydrophobic PPO disposed in a PEO–PPO–PEO arrangement [21,22]. These non-ionic copolymers are often used due to their biocompatibility, intrinsic stealth effect, and commercial availability.

Among the available hydrophilic polymers, which include PEG, poly(vinyl alcohol) (PVA), poly(vinylpyrrolidone) (PVP), poly(ethylene imine) (PEI), poly(2-methyl-2-oxazoline) (PMeOx), poly(L-lysine) (PLL), and poly(2-hydroxyethyl methacrylate) (pHEMA), PEG is usually the polymer of choice due to its good biocompatibility, favorable safety profile, and ease of surface functionalization with appropriate ligands for targeted delivery to cancer cells or specific organelles [1,22,48,49].

The use of stimuli-responsive polymers leads to "smart" PMs, which usually release their cargo through micelle disassembly at the target site upon an endogenous or exogenous stimulus. Poly(aminoethyl acrylamide) (PAEA) and poly(2-(dimethylamino)ethyl methacrylate) (PDMAEMA) are pH-sensitive hydrophilic polymers while PNIPAM is also a thermosensitive polymer [21,22,24]. PNIPAM exhibits an LCST at 32 °C in aqueous media, corresponding to a reversible phase transition from an expanded coil state (hydrophilic) below the LCST to a collapsed globule state (hydrophobic) above the LCST through cooperative breaking of hydrogen bonding between the amide group of the polymer and water [21,22].

### 3.2. Crosslinked Polymeric Micelles

Although amphiphilic copolymers exhibit very low CMC ($10^{-6}$–$10^{-7}$ mol/L) when compared with low MW surfactants, extensive dilution after IV injection can lead to micelle dissociation and drug leakage with potential systemic toxicity. Thus, micelles can be crosslinked, either at the core or at the shell, to improve stability in the bloodstream and control drug delivery at the target site [29,50]. Despite shell-crosslinking imparting stabilization to PMs, it can also affect their hydrophilicity and stealth properties, therefore core-crosslinking is preferable for micelle stabilization [29,50]. Additionally, hydrophobic drugs physically encapsulated in the core-crosslinked polymeric micelles (CCPMs) can be attached to the crosslinkers of the core.

Covalent core-crosslinking of PMs is performed after micelle formation and usually requires side-chain- or end-group-functionalized block copolymers, employing radical polymerization or addition of a bifunctional agent as a crosslinker for PMs containing polymerizable groups (e.g., methacrylate) or reactive groups (e.g., carboxylic, amine), respectively, within the core [29,50]. Alternatively, core-crosslinking can be achieved under oxidative conditions through disulfide bridge formation if the PMs contain thiol groups, and the resulting crosslinked micelles are stable in the bloodstream, which contains very low levels of GSH (2–10 μmol/L compared with 0.5–10 mmol/L in the cytosol) [29,50]. These redox-responsive biodegradable micelles are cleaved and release their cargo in the reductive intracellular microenvironment of cancer cells overexpressing GSH.

**Table 3.** Pharmacokinetic parameters for polymeric micellar formulations of anticancer drugs in clinical trials in comparison with other nanoformulations and conventional chemotherapeutic drugs in the market, obtained upon intravenous administration.

| Formulation | Polymer | Drug | Drug-Loading Method | Size (nm) | Dose (mg/m$^2$) | n | $C_{max}$ (μg/mL) | $T_{max}$ (h) | AUC$_{0\to\infty}$ (μg·h/mL) | $t_{1/2z}$ (h) | Ref. |
|---|---|---|---|---|---|---|---|---|---|---|---|
| Genexol®-PM | mPEG$_{2k}$-PDLLA$_{1.75k}$ | PTX | Physical | 25 | 390 [a] | 2 | 6.567 ± 1.120 | | 27.490 ± 8.297 | 17.9 ± 1.0 (β) | [51] |
| | | | | | 300 [b] | 3 | 3.107 ± 1.476 | | 11.580 ± 4.277 | 11.4 ± 2.4 (β) | [51] |
| | | | | | 180 [a,b] | 3 | 4.6758 | | 7.4702 | 7.8 | [52] |
| Abraxane® | Albumin NP | PTX | Nab | 130 | 300 [a,b] | 5 | 13.520 | | 17.610 | 14.6 | [53] |
| Taxol® | Cremophor® EL (surfactant) | PTX | Free drug | | 250 [a] | 5 | 19.167 ± 5.324 | | 35.018 ± 12.758 | 0.33 ± 0.14 (α) 3.10 ± 1.08 (β) | [54] |
| | | | | | 175 [b] | 3 | 8.641 ± 0.985 | | 14.523 ± 1.936 | 0.30 ± 0.10 (α) 3.27 ± 0.95 (β) | [54] |
| PM-PTX | mPEG-PDLLA | PTX | Physical | 20 | 390 [a] | 3 | 4.044 ± 1.226 | | 19.381 ± 5.025 | 19.3 ± 3.29 | [55] |
| | | | | | 300 [b] | 6 | 3.736 ± 1.220 | | 13.751 ± 3.440 | 16.6 ± 6.55 | [55] |
| Nanoxel® | PVP-PNIPAM | PTX | Physical | 80–100 | 375 [a] | 6 | | | 32.758 | | [56] |
| | | | | | 300 [b] | 6 | | | 23.632 | | [56] |
| NK105 | PEG-p(Asp) | PTX | Physical | 85 | 180 [a] | 4 | 45.6278 ± 8.6430 | | 454.5 ± 119.1 | 11.3 ± 0.6 | [57] |
| | | | | | 150 [b] | 7 | 40.1699 ± 5.5334 | | 369.8 ± 35.2 | 10.6 ± 1.3 | [57] |
| | | | | | 100 [a] | 6 | 27.6 ± 5.3 | 0.80 ± 0.30 | 390 ± 64 | 12.3 ± 1.3 | [58] |
| | | | | | 80 [b] | 3 | 22.0 ± 3.3 | 0.80 ± 0.30 | 302 ± 104 | 12.7 ± 0.8 | [58] |
| CPC634 (CriPec® DTX) | mPEG$_{5k}$-pHPMA-Lac$_n$ | DTX | Conjugation | 65 | 100 | 3 | 44.1161 ± 8.6453 (T) 0.3219 ± 0.1206 (Rel) | 3.3 ± 2.3 (T) 1.8 ± 0.3 (Rel) | 1836.280 ± 385.084 (T) 8.4244 ± 0.5625 (Rel) | 35.0 ± 3.2 (T) 44.9 ± 9.9 (Rel) | [59] |
| | | | | | 60 [b] | 5 | 27.1444 ± 7.9993 (T) 0.2173 ± 0.0919 (Rel) | 1.5 ± 0.4 (T) 1.4 ± 0.4 (Rel) | 973.987 ± 246.491 (T) 4.0675 ± 2.9740 (Rel) | 31.6 ± 1.3 (T) 39.7 ± 9.4 (Rel) | [59] |
| | | | | | 75 | 26 | 44.4 (T) 0.262 (Rel) | | 1530 (T) 7.41 (Rel) | 38.03 (T) 59.05 (Rel) | [60] |
| Conventional DTX | Tween® 80 (surfactant) | DTX | Free drug | | 75 | 26 | 2.88 | | 5.74 | 100.09 | [60] |
| Taxotere® | Tween® 80 (surfactant) | DTX | Free drug | | 100 | 4 | 2.41 ± 0.35 | | 5.93 ± 0.53 | 18.5 ± 10.7 | [61] |
| NK012 | PEG$_{12k}$-p(Glu)$_{7k}$ | SN-38 | Conjugation | 20 | 28 | 9 | 19.1 ± 3.9 (PB) 0.114 ± 0.031 (Rel) 0.04 ± 0.01 (G) | 0.7 ± 0.3 (PB) 0.8 ± 0.3 (Rel) 6 ± 0 (G) | 294 ± 62 (PB) 2.12 ± 0.83 (Rel) 2.28 ± 0.57 (G) | 137 ± 19 (PB) 209 ± 25 (Rel) 205 ± 20 (G) | [62] |
| | | | | | 28 | 6 | 20.0 ± 4.6 (PB) 0.138 ± 0.024 (Rel) 0.0721 ± 0.0241 (G) | 0.75 ± 0.27 (PB) 0.56 ± 0.23 (Rel) 6.21 ± 0.51 (G) | 287 ± 60 (PB) 2.13 ± 0.28 (Rel) 4.95 ± 1.78 (G) | 153 ± 27 (PB) 282 ± 101 (Rel) 382 ± 179 (G) | [63] |
| CPT-11 | | CPT-11 | Free drug | | 250 | 5 | 7.58 ± 3.06 | | 27.86 ± 4.46 | 4.5 | [63] |
| SN-38 | | SN-38 | CPT-11 active metabolite | | 250 | 5 | 0.072 ± 0.018 | | 0.876 ± 0.301 | 13.9 | [63] |

**Table 3.** *Cont.*

| Formulation | Polymer | Drug | Drug-Loading Method | Size (nm) | Dose ($mg/m^2$) | n | $C_{max}$ (μg/mL) | $T_{max}$ (h) | $AUC_{0\to\infty}$ (μg·h/mL) | $t_{1/2z}$ (h) | Ref. |
|---|---|---|---|---|---|---|---|---|---|---|---|
| NK911 | $PEG_{5k}$-p$(Asp)_{4k}$ | DOX | Conjugation and physical | 40 | 67 [a] | 6 | | | 4.1741 ± 0.4712 | 0.13 ± 0.02 (α)<br>2.9 ± 0.5 (β)<br>73.6 ± 21.4 (γ) | [64] |
| | | | | | 50 [b] | 11 | | | 3.2627 ± 0.4252 | 0.12 ± 0.01 (α)<br>2.8 ± 0.3 (β)<br>64.2 ± 8.9 (γ) | [64] |
| Doxil® | HSPC:Chol: $mPEG_{2k}$-DSPE liposomes | DOX | Remote, via transmembrane ammonium sulfate gradient | <100 | 50 | 14 | | | 902 (T)<br>893 (LB) | 1.4 (α) (T)<br>45.9 (β) (T)<br>2.3 (α) (LB)<br>46.2 (β) (LB) | [65] |
| Adriamycin® | (DOX hydrochloride) | DOX | Free drug | | 50 | 4 | | | 3.5 | 0.06 (α)<br>10.4 (β) | [65] |
| SP1049C | Pluronics® | DOX | Physical | 22–27 | 70 [a,b] | 7 | | | 1.62–4.20 | 0.08–0.13 (α)<br>1.07–3.05 (β)<br>21.3–56.5 (γ) | [66] |
| NC-6300 | $PEG_{12k}$-p(Asp) | EPR | Conjugation | 40–80 | 185 [a] | 4 | 62.2 ± 10.0 (T)<br>0.357 ± 0.153 (Rel) | 2.125 ± 3.92 (T)<br>6.1 ± 11.9 (Rel) | 2835.3 ± 313.8 (T)<br>12.7 ± 7.1 (Rel) | 25.0 ± 1.11 (T)<br>32.1 ± 5.1 (Rel) | [67] |
| | | | | | 150 [b] | 4 | 49.4 ± 15.1 (T)<br>0.459 ± 0.354 (Rel) | 0.167 ± 0.00 (T)<br>14.1 ± 22.9 (Rel) | 2126.5 ± 573.0 (T)<br>17.1 ± 13.2 (Rel) | 23.6 ± 1.09 (T)<br>26.3 ± 6.9 (Rel) | [67] |
| NC-6004 | PEG-p(Glu) | CDDP | Metal complexation | 30 | 135 [a,b] | | 50.08 ± 9.84 (T) | | 2611.0 ± 520.7 (T) | 91.2 ± 19.5 (T) | [68] |
| | | | | | 120 [a] | 3 | 85.4 ± 10.8 (T)<br>84.6 ± 8.1 (mic)<br>0.131 (UF Pt) | 4.4 ± 2.5 (T)<br>3.1 ± 1.5 (mic)<br>26.4 (UF Pt) | 4377 ± 563 (T)<br>3857 ± 1171 (mic)<br>22.9 (UF Pt) | 158 ± 48 (T)<br>87 ± 37 (mic)<br>115 (UF Pt) | [69] |
| | | | | | 90 [b] | 6 | 60.8 ± 12.5 (T)<br>42.4 ± 20.3 (mic)<br>0.205 ± 0.114 (UF Pt) | 5.2 ± 2.2 (T)<br>4.8 ± 2.4 (mic)<br>20.5 ± 7.6 (UF Pt) | 2836 ± 554 (T)<br>1579 ± 939 (mic)<br>22.6 ± 10.0 (UF Pt) | 129 ± 40 (T)<br>39 ± 27 (mic)<br>123 ± 44 (UF Pt) | [69] |

[a] MTD; [b] RD. Abbreviations: Asp, aspartate; AUC, area under the plasma concentration–time curve; CDDP, cisplatin; Chol, cholesterol; $C_{max}$, maximum plasma concentration; CPT-11, irinotecan; DOX, doxorubicin; DSPE, distearoyl phosphatidylethanolamine; DTX, docetaxel; EPR, epirubicin; G, glucuronide; Glu, glutamate; HPMA, *N*-(2-hydroxypropyl)methacrylamide; HSPC, hydrogenated soy phosphatidylcholine; Lac, lactate; LB, liposome-bound; mic, micellar; MTD, maximum tolerated dose; Nab, nanoparticle albumin-bound; NP, nanoparticle; PB, polymer-bound; PDLLA, poly(D,L-lactic acid); PEG, poly(ethylene glycol); PNIPAM, poly(N-isopropylacrylamide); PTX, paclitaxel; PVP, poly(vinylpyrrolidone); RD, recommended dose; Rel, released; SN-38, 7-ethyl-10-hydroxycamptothecin; T, total; $t_{1/2z}$, terminal half-life; $T_{max}$, time to reach peak plasma concentration; UF Pt, ultrafiltrable platinum.

Non-covalent core-crosslinking has also been attempted, and functionalization of the hydrophobic copolymer with aromatic pendant groups (e.g., benzyl) increases micelle stability via crosslinked π–π-stacking interactions, simultaneously enhancing the loading of chemotherapeutic drugs containing aromatic rings, such as taxanes and anthracyclines (e.g., NK911 and NC-6300, Table 2) [50]. Moreover, since π–π stacking is a pH-sensitive force, these PMs constitute pH-responsive systems that release their payload in the acidic TME. For transition metal complexes, like the platinum-based chemotherapeutic agents, the drug itself can be used as a crosslinker, leading to core-crosslinked micelles through polymer–metal complexation and allowing for drug release upon ligand exchange at the target site (e.g., NC-6004 and NC-4016, Table 2) [50].

Core-crosslinking has been shown to improve in vivo stability, circulation time, and biodistribution of PMs, resulting in higher accumulation at the target site [29,50]. However, drug leakage may still occur, requiring drug attachment to the micellar core through covalent (and reversible) bonding to ensure drug retention during circulation and enable controlled and sustained release at the target site. The cocrosslinked prodrugs thus obtained show significantly improved biodistribution and pharmacokinetic profiles (e.g., CricPec® Docetaxel, Table 2) [50].

## 4. Polymeric Micelles for Cancer Chemotherapy

PMs have been extensively studied as smart DDSs for hydrophobic antitumor drugs for targeted cancer chemotherapy [21,22] (Figure 4). PMs loaded with two or more chemotherapeutic agents for targeted and controlled codelivery to cancer cells provide synergistic effects, hinder MDR, and avoid the side effects and multiple injections required in combination therapy regimens involving the free drugs [70–72]. Triolimus is a multidrug-loaded PM containing three complementary anticancer agents: paclitaxel, a microtubule stabilizer; rapamycin (sirolimus), the mammalian target of rapamycin (mTOR) inhibitor and potent immunosuppressor; and tanespimycin, a prototypical inhibitor of the 90 kDa heat shock protein (Hsp90) able to target compensatory pathways activated by mTOR inhibition [73]. The formulation exhibited potent synergistic cytotoxic activity in vitro against several human cancer cells lines [73] and in vivo in heterotopic and orthotopic tumor xenograft models [74]. Triolimus was granted orphan drug designation by the FDA for the treatment of angiosarcoma, in 2015 [75]. A similar formulation, obtained after replacement of paclitaxel by docetaxel, showed synergistic antitumor effects in a genetic mouse model of prostate cancer without inducing systemic toxicity [76].

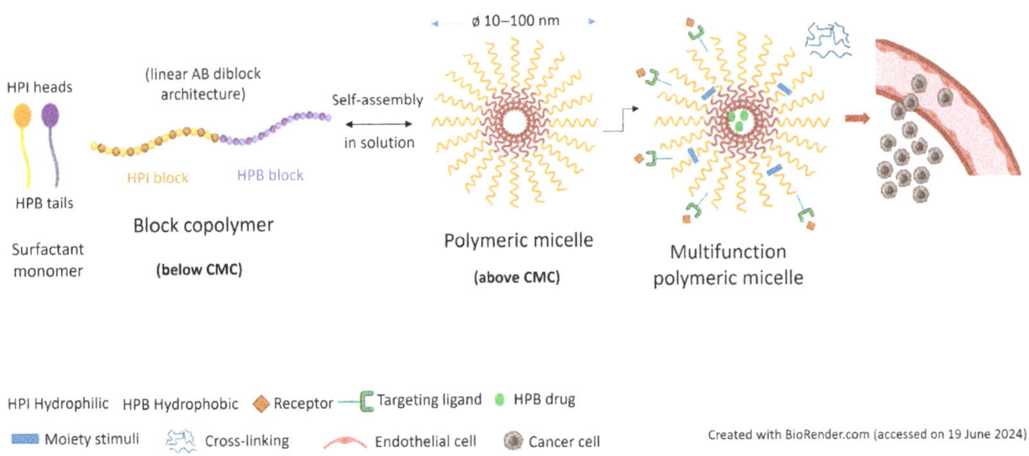


**Figure 4.** Multifunctional drug-loaded polymeric micelles for targeting cancer.

Moreover, multifunctional PMs loaded with both imaging and chemotherapeutic agents, which allow simultaneous diagnosis and treatment, provide a promising theranostic platform for personalized cancer therapy that maximizes drug specificity and efficacy [28,77]. Several polymeric micellar formulations for the delivery of antitumor drugs or imaging agents are under different stages of clinical development while others have already been approved in several countries and are currently in the clinic. Information regarding the various polymeric micellar formulations in clinical trials is summarized in Table 4 and will be discussed in the following sections.

### 4.1. Taxane Micellar Formulations

Taxanes are natural diterpenoids isolated from yew with potent cytotoxic activity, being among the most clinically used chemotherapeutic drugs despite their narrow therapeutic window [78]. Paclitaxel (PTX), isolated from the bark of the Pacific yew tree (*Taxus brevifolia*), is widely used in the treatment of breast, ovarian, esophageal, bladder, prostate, and cervical cancers, non-small cell lung carcinoma (NSCLC), head and neck cancer, and melanoma and also as second-line treatment for Kaposi's sarcoma [78]. PTX is a microtubule-stabilizing agent that binds to tubulin and inhibits microtubule disassembly, inducing mitotic arrest and cell apoptosis [78]. PTX is poorly water-soluble (0.3 μg/mL) [78,79], being conventionally formulated in a vehicle composed of a 50:50 (*v*/*v*) mixture of Cremophor® EL (polyethoxylated castor oil) and ethanol (Taxol®, Bristol-Myers Squibb Co., Princeton, NJ, USA), which is diluted in normal saline or 5% dextrose solution for IV administration [78,79]. However, the Taxol® formulation is commonly associated with several AEs, such as myelosuppression, neutropenia, anemia, nephrotoxicity, neurotoxicity (mainly peripheral neuropathy), and hypersensitivity reactions, the latter attributed to the high concentration of Cremophor® EL (CrEL) surfactant required to solubilize the drug [78,80]. Premedication with corticosteroids (e.g., dexamethasone) and antihistamines, both $H_1$ (e.g., diphenhydramine) and $H_2$ receptor antagonists (e.g., cimetidine or ranitidine), is thus required to avoid the severe hypersensitivity reactions due to systemic exposure to high CrEL amount [78]. Additionally, since CrEL can leach plasticizers like di(2-ethylhexyl)phthalate (DEPH) from polyvinyl chloride (PVC) materials, Taxol® administration requires PVC-free infusion systems (e.g., polyethylene-lined) with in-line filtration due to the risk of drug precipitation upon dilution [78,80]

Docetaxel (DTX) is a second-generation taxane obtained by semi-synthesis from 10-deacetyl baccatin III found in the needles of the European yew tree (*Taxus baccata*), being more potent than PTX at inhibiting microtubule depolymerization [81]. Like PTX, DTX is a microtubule-stabilizing agent approved in 2012 [82] and indicated as first-line chemotherapy for breast cancer, NSCLC, prostate cancer, head and neck squamous cell carcinoma (HNSCC), and stomach adenocarcinoma [83].

Due to poor water solubility (3 μg/mL) [81], DTX is solubilized using polysorbate 80 (Tween® 80) and ethanol as cosolvent in the conventional commercial formulation, Taxotere® (Sanofi-Aventis, Bridgewater, NJ, USA). The presence of the surfactant has been associated with AEs, including acute hypersensitivity and systemic immune reactions, hypotension, cutaneous reactions, fluid retention, and peripheral neuropathy [84]. Therefore, Taxotere® administration requires premedication with oral corticosteroids [84].

**Table 4.** Polymeric micellar formulations for intravenous delivery of anticancer drugs or imaging agents in clinical trials. Data from US clinical trial website (https://clinicaltrials.gov, accessed on 12 June 2024).

| Formulation | Drug (Combination Regimen) | Trial Identifier (Acronym) | Population (n) | Dose and Duration of Treatment | Phase | Start (Expected) Date–Completion (Estimated) Date (Status) |
|---|---|---|---|---|---|---|
| Polymeric micellar PTX | PTX (plus carboplatin and tislelizumab) | NCT06366945 | Clinical N-positive HNSCC (n = 85) | PM-PTX (300 mg/m$^2$), carboplatin (AUC 5), and tislelizumab (200 mg) every 3 weeks for 3 cycles | 2 | 04/2024–05/2029 (not yet rec.) |
| Polymeric micellar PTX | PTX (plus cisplatin and capecitabin) | NCT06301165 | Locoregionally advanced nasopharyngeal carcinoma (n = 162) | PM-PTX 200 mg/m$^2$ on day 1, cisplatin 75 mg/m$^2$ on day 1, and capecitabin 1000 mg/m$^2$ on days 1–14 *versus* gemcitabine 1000 mg/m$^2$ on days 1 and 8 and cisplatin 80 mg/m$^2$ on day 1, every 3 weeks, for 3 cycles, followed by concurrent chemoradiotherapy (cisplatin 100 mg/m$^2$, every 3 weeks, 3 cycles and IMRT) | 2 | 03/2024–12/2028 (recruiting) |
| PTX polymer micelles | PTX (plus cisplatin and cadonilimab) | NCT06356688 | Locally advanced esophageal squamous cell carcinoma (n = 30) | PM-PTX 230 mg/m$^2$ infusion over 3 h in cycle 1 then 260 mg/m$^2$ infusion over 3 h every 3 weeks in cycles 2–4, cisplatin 25 mg/m$^2$/day (IV drip) for 3 days, every 3 weeks, and cadonilimab 375 mg (IV drip) on day 3, every 3 weeks | 2 | 04/2024–06/2025 (not yet rec.) |
| Polymeric micellar PTX | PTX (plus cisplatin/carboplatin and sindilizumab) | NCT05782426 | Advanced non-squamous NSCLC (n = 28) | PM-PTX, platinum (cisplatin/carboplatin) in combination with sindilizumab injection for 4–6 cycles; maintenance with sindilizumab plus PTX-PM injection ($\leq$230 mg/m$^2$) | 2 | 03/2023–01/2026 (not yet rec.) |
| PTX polymeric micelles for injection | PTX | NCT06199895 | Taxane-resistant pancreatic adenocarcinoma, cholangiocarcinoma, lung cancer, gastric cancer, esophageal carcinoma, or breast cancer (n = 25) | PM-PTX 300 mg/m$^2$ infusion over 3 h once every 3 weeks (1 cycle treatment) | 2 | 11/2023–11/2025 (recruiting) |

**Table 4.** *Cont.*

| Formulation | Drug (Combination Regimen) | Trial Identifier (Acronym) | Population (n) | Dose and Duration of Treatment | Phase | Start (Expected) Date–Completion (Estimated) Date (Status) |
|---|---|---|---|---|---|---|
| PTX polymeric micelles for injection | PTX | NCT06143553 | HER2-negative MBC (n = 168) | PM-PTX 300 mg/m$^2$ infusion over 3 h, every 3 weeks (1 course treatment) versus albumin-bound PTX 260 mg/m$^2$ infusion over 30 min, every 3 weeks | 3 | 10/2023–07/2025 (recruiting) |
| DTX polymeric micelles for injection | DTX | NCT05254665 | Advanced solid tumors (n = 110) | Dose confirmation stage (evaluation of safety and tolerability of 3 dosing regimens) followed by expansion stage (evaluation of efficacy and safety of best dosing regimen) | 2 | 02/2022–03/2024 (unknown) |
| PTX micelles for injection | PTX | NCT04778839 | Chinese patients with advanced solid tumors (n = 98) | PM-PTX (175, 260, 320, or 390 mg/m$^2$ IV for 3 h) or conventional PTX injection (175 mg/m$^2$ IV for 3 h), every 3 weeks | 1 | 03/2021–03/2023 (recruiting) |
| PTX micelles for injection | PTX (plus cisplatin) | NCT02667743 | First-line therapy for advanced NSCLC (n = 454) | PM-PTX (230 or 300 mg/m$^2$ IV for 3 h) followed by cisplatin (70 mg/m$^2$ IV for 2 h), every 3 weeks versus conventional PTX injection (175 mg/m$^2$ IV for 3 h) followed by cisplatin (70 mg/m$^2$ IV, for 2 h), every 3 weeks | 3 | 05/2015–12/2021 (unknown) |
| Genexol®-PM | PTX | NCT03008512 | Hepatocellular carcinoma after failure of sorafenib (n = 5) | Genexol®-PM 100 mg/m$^2$ infusion for 1 h on days 1, 8, and 15 of a 28-day cycle, up to 8 cycles | 2 | 10/2016–02/2021 (terminated due to poor accrual) |
| Genexol®-PM | PTX (plus gemcitabine) | NCT02739633 | Recurrent/metastatic adenocarcinoma of the pancreas (n = 47) | Genexol®-PM (125 mg/m$^2$ IV over 60 min) and gemcitabine (1000 mg/m$^2$ IV) weekly, for 3 weeks, followed by 1 week of rest | 2 | 04/2016–12/2019 (unknown) |
| Genexol®-PM | PTX (plus carboplatin) | NCT02739529 | Gynecologic cancer (n = 18) | Genexol®-PM (100 or 120 mg/m$^2$) IV infusion once a week and carboplatin (AUC 5 or 6) IV infusion every 3 weeks | 1 | 04/2016–03/2018 (unknown) |

**Table 4.** *Cont.*

| Formulation | Drug (Combination Regimen) | Trial Identifier (Acronym) | Population (n) | Dose and Duration of Treatment | Phase | Start (Expected) Date–Completion (Estimated) Date (Status) |
|---|---|---|---|---|---|---|
| Genexol®-PM | PTX (plus carboplatin) | NCT05300828 | Ovarian cancer (n = 600) | Genexol®-PM (260 mg/m$^2$, IV infusion over 3 h) followed by carboplatin (AUC 5, IV over 3 h), every 3 weeks, as adjuvant treatment after cytoreductive surgery | Obs. | 10/2015–12/2022 (completed) |
| Genexol®-PM | PTX | NCT02064829 (TRIBECA) | Metastatic or locally recurrent breast cancer (n = 111) | Genexol®-PM or Nab-PTX, 260 mg/m$^2$ infusion over 30 min every 3 weeks (bioequivalence study) | N/A | 03/2014–07/2015 (completed) |
| Genexol®-PM | PTX (plus cisplatin) | NCT01689194 | Locally advanced HNSCC (n = 53) | N/A | 2 | 02/2013–08/2017 (completed) |
| Genexol®-PM | PTX (plus DOX) | NCT01784120 | Advanced breast cancer (n = 48) | N/A | 2 | 01/2011–12/2018 (unknown) |
| Genexol®-PM | PTX (plus gemcitabine) | NCT01770795 | Advanced NSCLC (n = 45) | N/A | 2 | 01/2011–10/2012 (completed) |
| Genexol®-PM | PTX (plus carboplatin) | NCT01276548 | Ovarian cancer (n = 102) | Genexol®-PM (260 mg/m$^2$, IV) or PTX (175 mg/m$^2$, IV) plus carboplatin (5 AUC, IV) | 2 | 10/2009–09/2012 (completed) |
| Genexol®-PM | PTX | NCT00912639 | Taxane-pretreated recurrent breast cancer (n = 90) | Genexol®-PM (300 mg/m$^2$ diluted in 500 mL of D5W or NS) infused for 3 h, every 3 weeks, for a minimum of 6 cycles | 4 | 05/2009–05/2011 (unknown) |
| Genexol®-PM | PTX | NCT00876486 | Recurrent or metastatic breast cancer (n = 213) | Genexol®-PM (260 mg/m$^2$) or Genexol (175 mg/m$^2$), IV infusion over 3 h, every 3 weeks | 3 | 12/2008–11/2013 (completed) |
| Genexol®-PM | PTX (plus cisplatin) | NCT01023347 | NSCLC (n = 276) | Genexol®-PM and cisplatin versus free PTX (Genexol®) and cisplatin | 2 | 06/2008–06/2012 (completed) |
| Genexol®-PM | PTX (plus gemcitabine) | NCT00882973 | Advanced pancreatic cancer (n = 18) | Genexol®-PM (220, 260, or 300 mg/m$^2$) ad gemcitabine (1250 mg/m$^2$) | 1 | 09/2008–11/2010 (completed) |

**Table 4.** *Cont.*

| Formulation | Drug (Combination Regimen) | Trial Identifier (Acronym) | Population (n) | Dose and Duration of Treatment | Phase | Start (Expected) Date–Completion (Estimated) Date (Status) |
|---|---|---|---|---|---|---|
| Genexol®-PM | PTX (plus carboplatin) | NCT00877253 | Advanced ovarian cancer (n = 18) | Genexol®-PM (220, 260, or 300 mg/m$^2$, IV infusion over 3 h) and carboplatin (AUC 5, IV infusion over 30–60 min), every 3 weeks | 1 | 05/2008–06/2009 (completed) |
| Genexol®-PM | PTX | NCT01426126 | Advanced urothelial cancer previously treated with gemcitabine and platinum (n = 37) | Genexol®-PM (240 mg/m$^2$ diluted in 500 mL of D5W) IV infusion for 3 h every 3 weeks | 2 | 12/2007–08/2011 (completed) |
| Genexol®-PM | PTX | NCT01169870 | Anthracycline-pretreated MBC (n = 0) | Genexol®-PM (300 mg/m$^2$ in 500 mL of D5W or NS, IV infusion over 1 h), every 3 weeks, up to 6 cycles versus PTX (175 mg/m$^2$ in 500 mL of D5W or NS, IV infusion over 3 h), every 3 weeks | 2 | 07/2007–10/2008 (withdrawn) |
| Genexol®-PM | PTX | NCT00111904 | Unresectable locally advanced or metastatic pancreatic cancer (n = 43) | Genexol®-PM IV infusion over 3 h, every 3 weeks | 2 | 05/2005–08/2007 (completed) |
| PTX-loaded polymeric micelle | PTX (plus carboplatin) | NCT00886717 | Advanced ovarian cancer (n = 74) | Determine MTD and RP2D (phase 1) and evaluate the efficacy of the regimen in terms of CA-125 response rate after 6 courses of therapy (phase 2) | 1/2 | 05/2008–n/a (unknown) |
| Nanoxel® | PTX (plus Herzuma®) | NCT03614364 | Metastatic salivary duct carcinoma (n = 41) | Nanoxel® 75 mg/m$^2$ plus D5W 100 mL MIV over 1 h and trastuzumab-pkrb (Herzuma®) 8 mg/kg loading dose plus NS 250 mL MIV over 90 min or 6 mg/kg maintenance dose plus NS 250 mL MIV over 30 min, since cycle 2, every 3 weeks | 2 | 09/2018–08/2023 (unknown) |
| Nanoxel® | PTX | NCT00915369 | Advanced breast cancer (n = 24) | Nanoxel® 220, 260, 310, or 375 mg/m$^2$, up to 6 cycles | 1 | 03/2009–04/2010 (unknown) |

**Table 4.** *Cont.*

| Formulation | Drug (Combination Regimen) | Trial Identifier (Acronym) | Population (n) | Dose and Duration of Treatment | Phase | Start (Expected) Date–Completion (Estimated) Date (Status) |
|---|---|---|---|---|---|---|
| Nanoxel® M | DTX, (plus DOX and cyclophosphamide | NCT05207514 | Breast cancer (n = 26) | DOX (60 mg/m$^2$, IV) and cyclophosphamide (600 mg/m$^2$) followed by Nanoxel® M (75 mg/m$^2$) or Taxotere® (75 mg/m$^2$), every 3 weeks, for 4 cycles, as neoadjuvant chemotherapy | 3 | 03/2022–05/2024 (terminated) |
| Nanoxel® M | DTX | NCT04066335 | NSCLC, breast, prostate, ovarian, head and neck, gastric, or esophageal cancers (n = 1498) | N/A | Obs. | 09/2019–08/2024 (recruiting) |
| Nanoxel® M | DTX (plus oxaliplatin) | NCT03585673 (DOSE) | Esophageal squamous cell carcinoma (n = 38) | Nanoxel® M (35 mg/m$^2$ IV over 1 h on days 1 and 8) and oxaliplatin (120 mg/m$^2$ IV over 2 h on day 1), every 3 weeks | 2 | 06/2018–03/2021 (unknown) |
| Nanoxel® M | DTX | NCT02982395 | BCG refractory non-muscle invasive bladder cancer (n = 36) | Nanoxel®M (75 mg in 100 mL NS, intravesical) or mitomycin (40 mg in 100 mL NS, intravesical) | 3 | 01/2017–08/2018 (terminated) |
| Nanoxel® M | DTX | NCT02639858 | Recurrent or metastatic HNSCC (n = 31) | Nanoxel® M (75 mg/m$^2$ IV infusion) | 2 | 10/2015–09/2020 (unknown) |
| NK-105 | PTX | NCT01644890 | Metastatic or recurrent breast cancer (n = 436) | NK-105 (65 mg/m$^2$) or free PTX (80 mg/m$^2$) on days 1, 8, and 15 of a 28-day cycle | 3 | 07/2012–01/2017 (completed) |
| [89Zr]-Df-CriPec® DTX | DTX | NCT03712423 (PICCOLO) | Immune-PET study in solid tumors (n = 7) | Low dose of [89Zr]-Df-CriPec® DTX (0.1–2 mg) on day 1 followed by maximally 3 [89Zr] PET scans; 2 weeks later, unlabeled CriPec® DTX (up to 60 mg/m$^2$, IV, every 3 weeks) followed by a low dose of [89Zr]-Df-CriPec® DTX and maximally 3 [89Zr] PET scans | 1 | 04/2018–05/2020 (completed) |

**Table 4.** *Cont.*

| Formulation | Drug (Combination Regimen) | Trial Identifier (Acronym) | Population (n) | Dose and Duration of Treatment | Phase | Start (Expected) Date–Completion (Estimated) Date (Status) |
|---|---|---|---|---|---|---|
| CriPec® DTX | DTX | NCT03742713 (CINOVA) | Platinum resistant ovarian cancer (n = 25) | CriPec® DTX (60 mg/m$^2$ IV) every 3 weeks | 2 | 10/2018–12/2020 (completed) |
| CriPec® DTX | DTX | NCT02442531 (NAPOLY) | Solid tumors (n = 33) | CriPec® DTX (dose escalation, start dose 15 mg/m$^2$ IV), every 6 weeks, up to 6 cycles | 1 | 08/2015–07/2018 (completed) |
| NK012 | SN-38 (plus 5-FU) | NCT01238939 | Solid tumors followed by dose expansion in patients with metastatic CRC (n = 35) | NK102 IV infusion over 30 min on day 1 and 5-FU IV continuous infusion (over 46 h) on days 1 and 15 of each 28-day cycle, for 6 cycles | 1 | 08/2010–03/2014 (completed) |
| NK012 | SN-38 (plus carboplatin) | NCT01238952 | Solid tumors with dose expansion in triple-negative breast cancer (n = 4) | NK012 and carboplatin IV infusion once every 28 days | 1 | 07/2010–03/2013 (completed) |
| NK012 | SN-38 | NCT00951054 | Advanced, metastatic triple-negative breast cancer (n = 61) | NK102 (28 mg/m$^2$ or 18 mg/m$^2$ depending on UGT1A1 polymorphism) IV infusion over 30 min, once every 28 days | 2 | 02/2009–02/2015 (completed) |
| NK012 | SN-38 | NCT00951613 | Relapsed small cell lung cancer (n = 72) | NK102 (28 mg/m$^2$ or 18 mg/m$^2$ depending on UGT1A1 polymorphism) IV infusion over 30 min, once every 28 days | 2 | 07/2009–01/2012 (completed) |
| NK012 | SN-38 | NCT00542958 | Refractory solid tumors (n = 39) | NK012 dose escalating (9.0, 12.0, 16.0, 21.0, and 28.0 mg/m$^2$) IV infusion over 30 min, every 3 weeks | 1 | 03/2007–12/2011 (completed) |
| NC-6300 | Epirubicin | NCT03168061 | Advanced solid tumors or advanced, metastatic, or unresectable soft tissue sarcoma (n = 150) | NC-6300 IV infusion at escalating doses every 3 weeks (phase 1) followed by NC-6300 at the RP2D (phase 2) | 1/2 | 06/2017–07/2020 (unknown) |

**Table 4.** *Cont.*

| Formulation | Drug (Combination Regimen) | Trial Identifier (Acronym) | Population (n) | Dose and Duration of Treatment | Phase | Start (Expected) Date–Completion (Estimated) Date (Status) |
|---|---|---|---|---|---|---|
| HA132 | Cisplatin | NCT05478785 | Advanced malignant solid tumors (n = 126) | HA132 IV, every 3 weeks | 1/2 | 08/2022–08/2025 (not yet recruit.) |
| NC-6004 | Cisplatin (plus pembrolizumab) | NCT03771820 | Recurrent or metastatic HNSCC that failed platinum or platinum-containing regimen (n = 136) | NC-6004 (90 mg/m$^2$ up to 135 mg/m$^2$ IV) followed by pembrolizumab (200 mg IV) infusion over 30 min, every 3 weeks | 2 | 07/2019–04/2022 (unknown) |
| NC-6004 | Cisplatin (plus 5-FU and cetuximab) | NCT03109158 | Recurrent/metastatic HNSCC (n = 1) | Cetuximab followed by NC-6004 (RP2D established in Phase 1 and 5-FU | 1/2 | 03/2017–03/2019 (completed) |
| NC-6004 | Cisplatin (plus 5-FU and cetuximab) | NCT02817113 | Recurrent and/or metastatic HNSCC (n = 4) | Cetuximab (400 mg/m$^2$ IV infusion over 2 h on day 1 then 250 mg/m$^2$ over 1 h, weekly) followed by NC-6004 (IV infusion over 1 h) on day 1, every 3 weeks, and 5-FU (1000 mg/m$^2$/day) on days 1–4 as continuous infusion, every 3 weeks | 1 | 06/2016–09/2018 (terminated, strategy changed) |
| NC-6004 | Cisplatin (plus gemcitabine) | NCT02240238 | Advanced solid tumors or NSCLC, biliary tract, and bladder cancers (n = 209) | NC-6004 at escalating doses (60, 75, 90, 105, 120, 135, 150, 165, or 180 mg/m$^2$) on day 1 followed by gemcitabine (1250 mg/m$^2$) IV infusion over 30 min on days 1 and 8 of each cycle | 1b/2 | 05/2015–05/2019 (completed) |
| NC-6004 | Cisplatin (plus gemcitabine) | NCT02043288 | Locally advanced or metastatic pancreatic cancer (n = 310) | NC-6004 90 mg/m$^2$ IV infusion over 60 min on day 1 and gemcitabine 1000 mg/m$^2$ IV infusion over 30 min on days 1 and 8, for 3-week cycle, or gemcitabine alone (1000 mg/m$^2$ IV infusion over 30 min on days 1, 8, and 15, for 4-week cycle) | 3 | 01/2014–12/2019 (completed) |

**Table 4.** *Cont.*

| Formulation | Drug (Combination Regimen) | Trial Identifier (Acronym) | Population (n) | Dose and Duration of Treatment | Phase | Start (Expected) Date–Completion (Estimated) Date (Status) |
|---|---|---|---|---|---|---|
| NC-6004 | Cisplatin (plus gemcitabine) | NCT00910741 | Locally advanced and metastatic pancreatic cancer (n = 40) | NC-6004 once every 3 weeks followed by gemcitabine on days 1 and 8 of the 3-week cycle | 1/2 | 05/2009–07/2013 (completed) |
| NC-4016 | DACHPt | NCT03168035 | Advanced solid tumors or lymphoma (n = 34) | NC-4016 dose escalating (15, 25, 30, 40, 60, and 80 mg/m$^2$ IV infusion over 2 h), once every 3 weeks | 1 | 11/2013–04/2017 (completed) |
| ONM-501 | cGAMP | NCT06022029 | Advanced solid tumors and lymphomas (n = 168) | ONM-501 intratumoral injection weekly, for 3 weeks, followed by a 3-week interval, w/o cemiplimab (Libtayo®) 350 mg IV infusion every 3 weeks | 1 | 10/2023–08/2026 (recruiting) |
| Pegsitacianine | ICG | NCT05048082 | Detection of lung malignancies in patients undergoing routine surgery (n = 24) | Pegsitacianine (1 mg/mL single dose, IV) infused 24–72 h prior to surgery | 2 | 04/2022–08/2022 (completed) |
| Pegsitacianine | ICG | NCT04950166 | Detection of peritoneal metastases in patients undergoing cytoreductive surgery (n = 50) | Pegsitacianine (1 mg/mL single dose, IV) infused 24–72 h prior to surgery | 2 | 11/2021–01/2023 (completed) |
| Pegsitacianine | ICG | NCT03735680 | Cancer detection in patients with solid tumors (n = 30) | Pegsitacianine single dose (1.0, 2.0, or 3.0 mg/kg) before surgery and fluorescence imaging at 3 ± 2 h, 6 ± 3 h, or 24 ± 8 h postdose | 2a | 08/2019–11/2021 (completed) |

Abbreviations: AUC, area under the plasma concentration–time curve; BCG, Bacillus Calmette–Guérin; CA-125, cancer antigen 125; cGAMP, cyclic guanosine monophosphate (GMP)-adenosine monophosphate (AMP); CRC, colorectal cancer; D5W, dextrose 5% in water; DACHPt, dichloro(1,2-diaminocyclohexane)platinum(II); DOX, doxorubicin; DTX, docetaxel; 5-FU, 5-fluorouracil; HNSCC, head and neck squamous cell carcinoma; ICG, indocyanine green; IMRT, intensity-modulated radiation therapy; IV, intravenous; MBC, metastatic breast cancer; MIV, multiple intravenous (infusions); MTD, maximum tolerated dose; N/A, not available; Nab, nanoparticle albumin-bound; NS, normal saline; NSCLC, non-small cell lung cancer; PET, positron emission tomography; PM, polymeric micelle; PTX, paclitaxel; RP2D, recommended phase 2 dose; SN-38, 7-ethyl-10-hydroxycamptothecin; UGT1A1, uridine diphosphate (UDP)-glucuronosyltransferase 1A1.

#### 4.1.1. Genexol®-PM

Genexol®-PM, developed by Samyang Biopharmaceuticals Corporation (Seoul, South Korea), is a polymeric micellar formulation of PTX made from a low-MW, non-toxic, and biodegradable amphiphilic diblock copolymer composed of monomethoxy PEG ($mPEG_{2k}$) and $PDLLA_{1.75k}$ at a 60:40 weight ratio that self-assembles to form 25 nm NPs [79,85,86]. Genexol®-PM is free of CrEL, like Abraxane®, and a nanoparticle albumin-bound (nab)-paclitaxel formulation (ABI-007, Abraxis BioScience, Los Angeles, CA, USA) [79], which allows higher dose administration compared to Taxol® without requiring premedication to prevent hypersensitivity reactions. Contrary to Abraxane®, Genexol®-PM does not contain human serum albumin, which is associated with a theoretical risk of viral transmission [75]). Moreover, Genexol®-PM, with a size around 25 nm, is able to penetrate tumor cells more easily and faster than nab-paclitaxel (Abraxane®), with a size around 130 nm, through the EPR effect.

Preclinical studies have shown that PTX biodistribution after administration of Genexol®-PM displayed 2- to 3-fold higher levels in several tissues, including liver, spleen, kidneys, lungs, heart, and tumor, as compared to Taxol®, with the highest PTX concentration found in the tumor [85]. The higher drug uptake and accumulation in tumor tissue are the result of polymeric micellar PTX targeting tumor cells through the EPR effect [85]. Despite showing comparable in vitro cytotoxicity against different human cancer cell lines, the in vivo antitumor efficacy of Genexol®-PM was significantly higher than that of Taxol® [85]. Genexol®-PM is also more effective than Taxol® as a radiosensitizer in chemoradiation therapy of NSCLC in the preclinical setting, preferentially accumulating in tumors and leading to lower PTX exposure of normal lung tissue than Taxol® [86]. Furthermore, Genexol®-PM exhibited a controlled and sustained drug release profile, with 40% PTX release after 16 h and 95% after 48 h, which can increase the synergistic effects of chemotherapy and radiation therapy [86].

Unlike Taxol®, Genexol®-PM exhibits a linear pharmacokinetic profile, as observed in patients with advanced malignancies [51] and solid tumors [52]. The plasma $AUC_{0\to\infty}$ and $C_{max}$ of Genexol®-PM in cancer patients revealed lower values than equivalent doses of Taxol® [51], since PTX entrapment in circulating CrEL micelles inhibits the partition of PTX from the vascular compartment to the tissues and results in non-linear pharmacokinetics and narrow distribution [80,85,87].

A phase 1 study (NCT03008512) of Genexol®-PM in patients with advanced malignancies [51] showed that the MTD was 390 $mg/m^2$, higher than that of Abraxane® (300 $mg/m^2$) [53], with neuropathy, myalgia, and neutropenia as the main dose-limiting toxicities (DLTs) [51]. Furthermore, acute hypersensitivity reactions were not observed, despite no premedication taken [51]. The recommended dose (RD) for phase 2 studies was established as 300 $mg/m^2$, higher than that of Taxol® (175 $mg/m^2$) in similar 3-week regimens [51]. At the phase 2 RD, Genexol®-PM was well tolerated and showed significant antitumor activity when administered as monotherapy for metastatic breast cancer [88], pancreatic cancer [89], and in combination with cisplatin for NSCLC [90], with an overall response rate (ORR) of 58.5%, 6.7%, and 37.7%, respectively. In the case of pancreatic cancer patients (NCT00111904), median overall survival (OS) and disease control rate (DCR) were improved when compared to gemcitabine monotherapy [89]. The most common AEs included neutropenia, fatigue, infection, dehydration, neuropathy, and abdominal pain [89]. A recent phase 1 study (NCT02739529) of weekly Genexol®-PM (100–120 $mg/m^2$) combined with carboplatin (5–6 AUC) every 3 weeks for gynecologic cancer (adult solid tumor) showed an acceptable safety profile and an ORR of 72.2% [91].

Several phase 2 studies have demonstrated the efficacy and safety of Genexol®-PM in patients with advanced malignancies, including metastatic breast cancer [88], NSCLC [90], pancreatic cancer (NCT00111904) [89], and ovarian cancer (NCT01276548) [92]. Genexol®-PM (230 $mg/m^2$) in combination with gemcitabine (1000 $mg/m^2$) as first-line treatment for patients with advanced NSCLC (NCT01770795) demonstrated significant antitumor efficacy, with an ORR of 46.5% [93]. This combination regimen had lower rates of myelotoxicity and emetogenicity in comparison with the platinum-based doublet regimen of Genexol®-PM in NSCLC patients [90]. Weekly Genexol®-PM (100 mg/m$^2$) combined with gemcitabine (1000 mg/m$^2$) for treatment of unresectable or metastatic biliary tract cancer revealed an ORR of 25.6% and a DCR of 71.8%, without severe side effects [94]. Genexol®-PM (230 mg/m$^2$) in combination with cisplatin (70 mg/m$^2$) was highly effective and tolerable as first-line palliative chemotherapy of unresectable thymic epithelial tumors [95]. The ORR was 62.5% with rates of 70% for thymic carcinoma and 46% for advanced thymoma [95]. On the other hand, in locally advanced HNSCC, induction therapy with Genexol®-PM (230 mg/m$^2$) and cisplatin (60 mg/m$^2$) (NCT01689194) exhibited modest tumor response compared with the most effective regimen of DTX, cisplatin, and 5-fluorouracil, although with a more favorable toxicity profile and promising 3-year progression-free survival (PFS) (54.3%) and OS (71.3%) rates [96].

Genexol®-PM (240–300 mg/m$^2$) as second-line chemotherapy in patients with advanced urothelial cancer after gemcitabine–cisplatin failure (NCT01426126) showed an ORR of 21% and a DCR of 65% [97]. These efficacy results were superior to second-line Taxol® after prior platinum-containing regimens and compared favorably with those of Abraxane® [97,98]. Moreover, Genexol®-PM monotherapy or in combination regimens allowed administration of higher PTX doses when compared with a conventional CrEL-based formulation (Genexol®), with lower incidence and severity of AEs, as observed in NSCLC [90,99], ovarian cancer [92,100], and urothelial cancer [97] patients. In a phase 3 study (NCT00876486) comparing the efficacy and safety of Genexol®-PM (260 mg/m$^2$) with Genexol® (175 mg/m$^2$) for recurrent or metastatic HER2-negative breast cancer, Genexol®-PM demonstrated superior clinical efficacy and a manageable safety profile, with an ORR of 39.1% compared with 24.3% for the conventional PTX formulation [101]. A recently completed prospective cohort study (NCT05300828) to evaluate the safety profile of Genexol®-PM (280 mg/m$^2$) plus carboplatin (AUC 5) as adjuvant therapy after cytoreductive surgery for newly diagnosed ovarian cancer patients showed that high-dose Genexol®-PM improved PFS compared to standard treatment (PTX 175 mg/m$^2$ plus carboplatin AUC 5) and was as effective as addition of bevacizumab (15 mg/kg) to standard therapy, particularly in patients with stages III–IV high-grade serous carcinoma of the ovary who underwent optimal debulking surgery [102].

Genexol®-PM was the first polymeric micellar product in the market [83], being introduced in South Korea in 2007 as first-line therapy for breast cancer [92] and NSCLC (in combination with cisplatin) [90], and more recently approved as first line therapy for ovarian cancer [92] in combination with other chemotherapeutic agents [83]. Genexol®-PM is also sold in India, Vietnam, the Philippines, and Indonesia, being commercialized as Paxus™ in some Asian countries [83] while in the US and several countries of the European Union it is licensed under the name Cynviloq™ [83].

Preliminary pharmacokinetic data from the TRIBECA study (NCT02064829), a phase 3 clinical trial aiming at establishing bioequivalence between Cynviloq™ and Abraxane®, at 260 mg/m$^2$, for patients with metastatic or locally recurrent breast cancer, supported potential for bioequivalence between the two formulations [75].

#### 4.1.2. Zisheng®

Zisheng® (PM-Pac or PM-PTX) is another nanoparticle polymeric micellar PTX formulation for injection, also made from mPEG-*b*-PDDLA, independently developed by Shanghai Yizhong Pharmaceutical Co., Ltd. (Shanghai, China), and the first approved PTX-loaded PM in China [3]. Similarly to Genexol®-PM, Zisheng® is CrEL-free and does not require premedication to prevent hypersensitivity reactions nor special non-PVC infusion systems or in-line filtration for administration, unlike a conventional CrEL-based formulation (Taxol®). The innovative PM-PTX dosage form showed improved efficacy and safety compared to a solvent-based (SB) PTX formulation (SB-PTX), both in vitro [103] and in vivo [103].

PM-PTX-induced apoptosis and cell viability inhibition in human NSCLC cell lines A549 and H226 in vitro was higher than that of SB-PTX [103]. In BALB/c nude mice, PM-PTX showed significantly enhanced tumor growth inhibition efficacy in the A549-derived xenograft tumor model when compared with SB-PTX at the same PTX dosage [103]. According to biodistribution studies, the ratios of PTX concentrations in major organ tissue to plasma concentrations were significantly higher in the PM-PTX group [55,103]. PM-PTX, with a size around 20 nm, passively targets tumor cells through the EPR effect and significantly reduces the retention time of PTX in the bloodstream, thus improving drug uptake and accumulation in tumor tissues [55,103]. Toxicity assessment and histopathological studies in healthy rats demonstrated that PM-PTX, at a 2–3-fold greater dosage than SB-PTX, significantly reduced the incidences of peripheral neuropathy, brain injury and liver damage, in terms of both short-term and long-term toxicity, but could induce potential male genital system toxicity (testicular and prostate atrophy) [103].

In a phase 1 study, patients with advanced solid malignancies (n = 18) received PM-PTX IV over 3 h, every 3 weeks, at escalating doses from 175 mg/m$^2$ (level 1) to 435 mg/m$^2$ (level 5), without acute hypersensitive reactions [55]. The ORR was 33.3% (including three patients with prior exposure to PTX chemotherapy), comparable with ORR for nab-PTX (Abraxane®) plus carboplatin (33%) [104] and for Genexol®-PM plus cisplatin (38%) [90] as first-line doublet regimens. All the patients treated with 435 mg/m$^2$ PM-PTX developed DLT grade 4 neutropenia as well as one patient treated with a 300 mg/m$^2$ dose (level 3). The incidence of neutropenia and peripheral sensory neuropathy became increasingly severe as the dose increased from 300 to 435 mg/m$^2$. Thus, the MTD of PM-PTX was determined as 390 mg/m$^2$ (level 4) while the recommended phase 2 dose was 300 mg/m$^2$ [55], similarly to Genexol®-PM [51]. The formulation exhibited a linear pharmacokinetic profile, with the peak concentration and AUC values of PTX increasing with dosage [55], and a relatively longer half-life compared to Genexol®-PM [51] (Table 3).

A phase 3 study (NCT02667743) comparing the efficacy and safety between PM-PTX (230–300 mg/m$^2$) plus cisplatin (70 mg/m$^2$) and conventional SB-PTX (175 mg/m$^2$) plus cisplatin (70 mg/m$^2$) as first-line therapy for advanced NSCLC showed an improved ORR for the PM-PTX formulation (50% versus 26% for SB-PTX), observed in both squamous (59% versus 37%) and non-squamous (44% versus 19%) histological types, with significantly lower incidence of serious AEs [105]. Furthermore, the study provided clinical evidence that PM-PTX administration prolonged PFS and also OS with a favorable safety profile in NSCLC patients without pleural metastasis when compared with conventional SB formulation (SB-PTX) [106].

A recent retrospective study evaluating the efficacy and safety of PM-PTX (360 mg/m$^2$) in combination with 5-fluorouracil (750 mg/m$^2$) and leucovorin (200 mg/m$^2$) as systemic chemotherapy for advanced gastric cancer demonstrated that the ORR was significantly higher than that of the conventional PTX (210 mg/m$^2$) group (31% versus 10%), with lower incidence of anemia, leukopenia, liver dysfunction, nausea, vomiting, diarrhea, and allergy [107].

Several clinical trials of PM-PTX are currently ongoing or planned, either as monotherapy or in combination regimens for the treatment of solid tumors, including a phase 3 study (NCT06143553) evaluating PM-PTX for HER2-negative metastatic breast cancer in comparison with nab-PTX (Table 4).

#### 4.1.3. Nanoxel®

Nanoxel® is another CrEL-free PTX polymeric micellar formulation developed in India by Dabur Pharma, Ltd., Ghaziabad, Uttar Pradesh, India (later integrated into Fresenius Kabi Oncology Ltd., Himachal Pradesh, India), marketed in the country since 2006 [108] for metastatic breast cancer chemotherapy and later approved for the treatment of ovarian cancer, NSCLC, and AIDS-related Kaposi's sarcoma [78]. The pH-sensitive PMs are composed of amphiphilic PVP-*b*-PNIPAM block copolymers [109]. The nanomicelles, with sizes in the range 80–100 nm, are stable at physiological pH (7.4) but in the acidic conditions of the TME, surface erosion of PNIPAM slowly releases PTX [109]. Due to their small sizes, the NPs passively target tumor cells by the EPR effect and selectively accumulate in the tumor, thus sparing normal tissue [110]. Contrary to Genexol®-PM and Abraxane®, which are lyophilized products that can be kept at room temperature, Nanoxel® is a liquid formulation that requires storage at 2–8 °C [78].

Transmission electron microscopy (TEM) studies revealed that Nanoxel® uptake in different human cancer cell lines, including NSCLC (A549), breast cancer (HBL-100), and ovarian cancer (PA-1) cells, is mediated by endocytosis, followed by intracellular drug release in the acidic endolysosomal compartment [110]. The intracellular drug uptake in Nanoxel® was comparable to Abraxane® and superior to a conventional CrEL-based PTX formulation (Intaxel®, Fresenius Kabi Oncology Ltd., Himachal Pradesh, India) in all the human cell lines tested, demonstrating the higher in vitro efficiency of the NP-based formulations for drug delivery to target cells [110].

A phase 1 dose escalation study evaluating a 3-weekly regimen of Nanoxel® (135–375 mg/m$^2$, administered as a 1 h infusion without premedication), for up to six cycles, in 23 patients with refractory or metastatic solid tumors showed that the formulation was well tolerated at a dose of 300 mg/m$^2$, higher than that of conventional PTX, with no incidence of hypersensitivity reactions, febrile neutropenia, or neuropathies above grade 1 [56]. The MTD was determined at 375 mg/m$^2$. Nanoxel® showed a linear pharmacokinetic profile and promising antitumoral activity in advanced breast cancer, with 50% of cases of heavily pretreated breast cancer showing objective responses [56].

A subsequent phase 2, open-label study showed an ORR of 40% each in patients with advanced or metastatic breast cancer (after failure of anthracycline chemotherapy) that received Nanoxel® (300 mg/m$^2$ or 220 mg/m$^2$) every 3 weeks for six cycles compared to 31% in patients treated with SB-PTX (Taxol®, 175 mg/m$^2$) [111]. Neutropenia incidence was lowest in the Nanoxel® 220 mg/m$^2$ arm (39.4% versus 50% in the Taxol® arm) but at the highest Naxoxel® dosage (300 mg/m$^2$), it was superior to Taxol® (56.3%) [111]. Grade 3 sensory neuropathy occurred in 12.5% of patients receiving 300 mg/m$^2$ Nanoxel® compared with 1.5% and 6.3% of patients on Nanoxel® 200 mg/m$^2$ and Taxol®, respectively. Hypersensitivity reactions were not observed with Nanoxel® despite the absence of premedication [111].

A retrospective study in a single hospital practice in India showed that in 84 cancer patients treated with Nanoxel® there were no infusion reactions for a total of 596 infusions while other AEs, like hematological and gastrointestinal side effects, were similar to conventional PTX [108]. Neutropenia was more frequent in the Nanoxel®-treated group (22.68% versus 9.8%) while nausea (2.58% versus 9.8%) and vomiting (9.79% versus 21.57%) were more common in the conventional PTX group. The same study compared the OS between Nanoxel® (n = 23) and conventional PTX (n = 28), in combination with a platinum agent, for the treatment of gastroesophageal cancer. The OS was 22 months for the Nanoxel® group and 12 months for the conventional PTX group, but the difference was not statistically significant [108]. The 3-week cycle with Nanoxel® was cost-effective when compared with conventional SB-PTX (at the same dosage and schedule regimen) regarding drug administration, necessity for premedication, and incidence and severity of AEs [108].

A more recent single center retrospective analysis suggested that a Nanoxel®–gemcitabine regimen was effective in advanced pancreatic cancer patients (n = 78) in routine clinical practice, with efficacy and toxicity similar to that of Abraxane®–gemcitabine at the same dosage (125 mg/m$^2$ of Abraxane® or Nanoxel® followed by 1000 mg/m$^2$ gemcitabine infusion on days 1, 8, and 15, every four weeks) [112]. Another longitudinal observational pharmacovigilance study conducted in a medical oncology ward in India over 18 months demonstrated that the adverse drug reaction profile of Nanoxel® (n = 10) was statistically comparable to conventional PTX (n = 10) but suggested a better tolerability since a significantly higher dose (330 mg/m$^2$ versus 260 mg/m$^2$) was employed [113]. Common AEs included myalgia, nausea, anemia, paresthesia, alopecia, diarrhea, and vomiting while hypersensitivity reactions were not observed despite no premedication in the case of Nanoxel® [113].

#### 4.1.4. Nanoxel®-M

Nanoxel®-M is a DTX polymeric micellar formulation developed by Samyang Biopharmaceutics Corporation (Seoul, South Korea) using the same amphiphilic diblock copolymer, mPEG-*b*-PDLLA, of their PTX micellar formulation, Genexol®-PM [81,83], similarly devoid of surfactant to prevent side effects commonly associated with Tween® 80 used to solubilize DTX in the conventional formulation Taxotere® that requires corticosteroid premedication.

In vitro cytotoxicity studies of Nanoxel®-PM in different human cancer cell lines, including H-460 (NSCLC), MCF-7 (breast cancer), and SKOV-3 (ovarian cancer), showed $IC_{50}$ values comparable to the ones obtained for Taxotere® (2.33 versus 4.66 ng/mL in H-460 cells, 1.73 versus 1.83 in MCF-7 cells, and 2.19 versus 3.25 ng/mL in SKOV-3 cells) [81]. In nude mice bearing human lung cancer (H-460) xenografts, IV administration of Nanoxel®-PM (13 mg/kg on days 0, 1, and 2) significantly delayed tumor growth and reduced tumor volume, showing comparable antitumor efficacy to Taxotere® [81]. The dose of Nanoxel®-PM chosen, 13 mg/kg, corresponded to 117 mg/m$^2$/cycle, close to the highest recommended single-agent dose of Taxotere® (100 mg/m$^2$) in humans [81].

Pharmacokinetic studies in mice, rats, and beagle dogs revealed similar pharmacokinetic profiles between Nanoxel®-PM and Taxotere®. Moreover, the relative magnitudes of $AUC_{0\to\infty}$ and $C_{max}$ of Nanoxel®-PM compared to those of Taxotere® were within 100% $\pm$ 20%, demonstrating bioequivalence [81]. The similarity in the pharmacokinetic profile of both formulations was attributed to DTX release from the micelles to bind albumin plasma protein after IV administration [81].

However, Nanoxel®-M enhanced collagen-induced (but not thrombin-induced) rat platelet aggregation in vitro while Taxotere® inhibited it, suggesting that the micellar formulation altered the toxicological profile of DTX [114]. Toxicity studies showed that a single IV infusion (30 min) of Nanoxel®-PM or Taxotere® to rats or three daily IV (bolus) administrations to mice at low (10 mg/kg), intermediate (13 mg/kg), and high (15 mg/kg) doses produced no significant differences in body weight changes or white blood cell (WBC) counts between the two treated groups at all tested doses [81]. A dose-escalating single IV toxicity study of Nanoxel®-PM in beagle dogs with three ascending doses (0.25, 0.50, and 0.75 mg/kg) did not detect any hypersensitivity reactions or fluid retention, contrary to Taxotere® administration, which was accompanied by severe anaphylactic-type reactions (e.g., erythema, facial swelling, and dyspnea) at all dose levels despite premedication with dexamethasone [81]. Furthermore, plasma histamine levels were related to the onset and duration of hypersensitivity reactions in the Taxotere® group, which showed a much higher peak level compared with Nanoxel®-PM (75–132 ng/mL versus 0.4–2.2 ng/mL). The infusion reactions to Taxotere® were attributed to the presence of Tween® 80 and suggest an improved safety profile for the surfactant-free Nanoxel®-PM formulation.

A multicenter trial to evaluate the safety and toxicity of Nanoxel®-M as adjuvant therapy, alone or in combination with cyclophosphamide, after surgery for early breast cancer in Korean patients (n = 55) showed that the micellar formulation reduced the incidence of taxane-induced peripheral neuropathy and thrombocytopenia compared with Taxotere® without vehicle-associated hypersensitivity reactions [115]. The most common side effects were grade 3/4 neutropenia (61.8%) followed by febrile neutropenia (4.5%) and mucositis (1.4%) [115].

A phase 2 multicenter study of Nanoxel®-PM and trastuzumab-pkrb (biosimilar to trastuzumab, a mAb against HER2) combination therapy in HER2-positive advanced salivary duct carcinoma demonstrated promising antitumor activity with a manageable toxicity profile [116]. Patients (n = 43) treated with Nanoxel®-PM (75 mg/m$^2$) and trastuzumab-pkrb (8 mg/kg in the first cycle and 6 mg/kg in subsequent cycles) every 3 weeks showed an ORR of 69.8%, DCR of 93.0%, median PFS of 7.9 months, and median OS of 23.3 months [116]. The most common treatment-related AEs were peripheral edema, myalgia, stomatitis, and alopecia while grade 3/4 AEs included neutropenia, febrile neutropenia, anemia, and decreased left ventricular ejection fraction, the latter related to trastuzumab-pkrb [116].

A multicenter, prospective observational study (NCT04066335) is currently ongoing to evaluate the safety of Nanoxel®-M injection in patients with breast cancer, NSCLC, and prostate, ovarian, head and neck, gastric, or esophageal cancers.

#### 4.1.5. NK105

NK105 is another freeze-dried PTX polymeric micellar formulation developed by NanoCarrier Co., Ltd. (Chiba, Japan) and licensed to Nippon Kayaku Co., Ltd. (Tokyo, Japan), composed of the amphiphilic block copolymers PEG and poly(aspartate), the latter modified by esterification with 4-phenyl-1-butanol to increase hydrophobicity of the core [117]. The PMs, with a size around 85 nm, allowed high drug loading (23% *w*/*w* PTX) through passive entrapment of the drug in the micellar core via hydrophobic interactions and provided effective drug retention following IV administration [117].

A preclinical pharmacokinetic study on colon 26 tumor-bearing CDF1 mice found that the plasma and tumor AUC values were around 90- and 25-fold higher, respectively, for NK105 than for free PTX after a single IV injection (100 mg/kg) of the drugs, due to prolonged circulation in the bloodstream and the EPR effect associated with the micellar formulation [117]. Moreover, at 72 h after the IV injection, the tumor PTX concentration was above 10 μg/g in the NK105 group but less than 0.1 μg/g in the free PTX group.

Although NK105 and conventional PTX formulation showed equivalent cytotoxic activity in vitro, exhibiting similar dose–response curves and $IC_{50}$ values on several human cancer cell lines derived from lung, gastric, esophagus, colon, breast, and ovarian tumors, NK105 showed improved in vivo antitumor efficacy in nude mice bearing human colorectal cancer (CRC) HT-29 xenografts due to enhanced tumor exposure via the EPR effect and sustained release from the micellar NPs [117]. Furthermore, repeated administration of NK105 to rats at 7-day intervals showed attenuated peripheral neurotoxicity when compared with free PTX [117], which was attributed to NK105 exclusion from the rat dorsal root ganglion (DRG) due to particle size (around 85 nm), while albumin-bound PTX particles of around 8 nm formed after injection of SB-PTX formulation can extravasate into DRG parenchyma, consistent with subsequent pharmacokinetic and histopathological studies [118].

NK105 (45 mg/kg single IV injection) was also a more potent radiosensitizing agent compared to free PTX at the same dosage in Lewis-lung-carcinoma-bearing mice due to more severe cell cycle arrest at the $G_2$/M phase induced by NK105 [119]. Histopathological examination of the mice lung sections revealed inflammatory cell infiltration, the presence of intra-alveolar macrophages, and destruction of the alveolar architecture, which were due to thoracic radiation and not to NK105 accumulation in the lung [119].

A phase 1 and pharmacokinetic study of NK105 (10–180 mg/m$^2$), administered to cancer patients (n = 19) as a 1 h IV infusion, every 3 weeks, without antiallergic premedication showed that NK105 was well tolerated, and the RD for the phase 2 study was established as 150 mg/m$^2$ every 3 weeks [57]. The DLTs included grade 4 neutropenia and grade 3 fever at the 180 mg/m$^2$ dose, which was designated as the MTD. NK105 exhibited a linear pharmacokinetic profile and its plasma AUC at 150 mg/m$^2$ was nearly 15-fold higher compared with that of the conventional PTX formulation at 210 mg/m$^2$ (conventional dose for a 3-week regimen in Japanese patients), consistent with the stability of the micelle formulation in plasma [57].

A phase 2 study to evaluate the efficacy and safety of NK105 (150 mg/m$^2$ IV infusion for 30 min every 3 weeks) in patients with advanced or recurrent gastric cancer (n = 57) after the failure of first-line chemotherapy showed modest antitumor activity, with an ORR of 25% and median PFS and OS of 3.0 and 14.4 months, respectively [120]. The most common AEs were alopecia, peripheral neuropathy, fatigue, myalgia, anorexia, rash, arthralgia, stomatitis, diarrhea, and nausea. Grade 4 toxicities included neutropenia (64.9%), leukocytopenia (17.5%), anemia (12.3%), lymphopenia (8.8%), and peripheral neuropathy (1.8%) but no grade 3/4 hypersensitive reactions were observed [120].

However, a phase 3 clinical trial (NCT01644890) comparing NK105 (65 mg/m$^2$ on days 1, 8, and 15 of a 28-day cycle) and PTX (80 mg/m$^2$, same schedule) in metastatic or recurrent breast cancer (n = 436) missed its primary endpoint (PFS with a non-inferiority margin of 1.215) [121]. The micellar formulation provided an ORR of 31.6% and median OS of 31.2 months compared with 39.0% and 36.3 months for PTX, respectively, although NK105 exhibited a more favorable toxicity profile, with lower incidence of grade 3/4 peripheral sensory neuropathy (1.4% versus 7.5% for PTX) [121].

Another phase 1 study to determine the RD of weekly administered NK105 (50–100 mg/m$^2$ IV infusion over 30 min) for 3 consecutive weeks in each 4-week cycle in patients with solid tumors (n = 16) found DLTs at 100 mg/m$^2$ due to neutropenia and the RD was established as 80 mg/m$^2$ [58]. In the subsequent exploratory dose-expansion phase, six out of ten patients treated with weekly NK105 at the RD achieved partial response and four reached stable disease status [58]. Neutropenia of grade $\geq$ 3 occurred in eight patients, requiring dose reduction or dose delay. On the other hand, non-hematological events, namely peripheral sensory neuropathy, were mostly grade 1, and no hypersensitivity reactions were observed. Based on these results, an initial NK105 dose of 65 mg/m$^2$, lower than the RD (80 mg/m$^2$) determined in the dose-escalation phase, was selected for the ensuing phase 3 study.

A phase 2 study comparing NK105 and PTX in advanced or recurrent breast cancer (n = 123), with both drugs being intravenously administered at 80 mg/m$^2$ on days 1, 8, and 15 of a 28-day cycle, revealed no significant difference in ORR, median PFS, and OS between the two groups [122]. The incidence of hematologic AEs was higher in the NK105 group, namely neutropenia (79.0% versus 55.7%), with several patients requiring treatment with granulocyte-colony-stimulating factor (G-CSF). However, the incidence of peripheral sensory neuropathy was lower in the NK105 group (64.5% versus 82.0%) with no grade 3/4 non-hematologic events [122].

A recent systematic review and meta-analysis comparing the efficacy and peripheral neuropathy of SB-PTX with NK105 monochemotherapy revealed no significant differences between the incidence of all-grade peripheral neuropathy among both groups [123]. However, the incidence of high-grade peripheral neuropathy was lower in the NK105 group, which also showed longer OS in cancer patients [123].

#### 4.1.6. CriPec® Docetaxel

CriPec® Docetaxel (CPC634), developed by Cristal Therapeutics (Maastricht, Netherlands), is a DTX-incorporating core-crosslinked PM with 65 nm size composed of mPEG$_{5k}$ and thermosensitive *N*-(2-hydroxypropyl)methacrylamide-oligolactate block copolymers (mPEG$_{5k}$-*b*-pHPMA-Lac$_n$) based on CriPec® technology, with DTX covalently bound to the crosslinked core through a hydrolyzable ester linker [124].

The CriPec® platform (Cristal Therapeutics, Netherlands) is based on amphiphilic block copolymers made of hydrophilic mPEG and thermosensitive *N*-(2-hydroxypropyl) methacrylamide (HPMA) derivatized with lactate side chains, designed to covalently entrap active pharmaceutical ingredients in CCPMs upon self-assembly [124]. Partial esterification of the lactate side chains of the hydrophobic segment with methacrylic acid allows covalent crosslinking of the hydrophobic blocks forming the micellar core by free radical polymerization, resulting in improved micelle stability and avoiding premature drug leakage. Furthermore, covalent attachment of the drug to the micellar core by free radical polymerization upon drug functionalization by covalent conjugation with a biodegradable linker containing a polymerizable moiety allows control of the site and rate of drug release by appropriate choice of the linker and enables higher encapsulation efficiency compared with physical loading [124]. The reactive block copolymers and the drug-linkers self-assemble into a micellar structure with the drug physically encapsulated in the micellar core, and the hydrophobic core-forming block copolymers and drug-linker are cocrosslinked by free radical polymerization, forming a 3D network [124]. Tunable size, within the range 35–100 nm, is dependent on the MW of the block copolymers [124]. The stealth effect of the hydrophilic dense PEG shell provides prolonged circulation while core-crosslinking, by preventing the reorganization of micelles, further contributes to reducing the interaction with plasma proteins. Neglectable protein corona was observed for CPC634 when incubated in human blood plasma [125].

CPC634 is manufactured as an aqueous dispersion stable for at least 5 years when stored at −80 °C to prevent premature drug release and hydrolysis of the core-crosslinks [124]. To overcome cold chain supply problems, a lyophilization methodology using trehalose as a cryoprotectant yielded a stable CPC634 freeze-dried cake with a moisture content lower than 0.1 wt% [126]. The trehalose-cryoprotected CPC634 could be reconstituted in less than 5 min at room temperature, with size, morphology, drug retention, and release kinetics identical to those of the non-freeze-dried formulation, and the methodology is readily translatable to large-scale manufacturing [126].

The covalent conjugation of DTX to the crosslinked core of CPC634 micelles allowed for in vitro sustained drug release under physiological conditions (PBS pH 7.4, 37 °C) upon hydrolysis of the ester linker and followed first-order kinetics [127]. A similar in vitro drug release profile was also observed in whole human blood at 37 °C, corroborating that DTX release from CPC634 is driven by chemical hydrolysis, since the crosslinked micellar core prevents enzyme access [127].

In mice bearing human breast (MDA-MB-231) tumor xenografts, administration of CPC634 (30 or 60 mg/kg single injection in tail vein) showed superior therapeutic efficacy compared to the marketed DTX formulation (Taxotere®) at the same dose [127]. Furthermore, a single IV injection of CPC634 at 125 mg/kg was enough to achieve complete regression of both small (150 $mm^3$) and established (550 $mm^3$) tumors, resulting in 100% survival of the animals. The potent antitumor effects of the nanoformulation were attributed to enhanced tumor accumulation and antistromal activity [127]. CPC634 also displayed better tolerability in healthy rats compared to Taxotere® [127].

A study of empty CPC634 CCPMs decorated with the cyclic RGD (cRGD) peptide targeting $\alpha_v\beta_3$ integrins has also been performed, showing higher in vitro uptake in cell lines expressing high levels of $\alpha_v\beta_3$ (e.g., A431 epidermoid carcinoma cells) [128]. In these cells, the cRGD-CPPMs were more efficiently internalized than the non-functionalized CPPMs (control), being found in the perinuclear region while peptide-free CCPMs colocalized with endosomes/lysosomes [128]. The uptake of cRGD-CCPM was not proportional to the increase in cRGD decoration, suggesting that relatively low decoration densities (1 mol% cRGD) may be enough for CCPM targeting and uptake in vivo without affecting their pharmacokinetic and biodistribution profiles [128].

A first-in-human phase 1, dose-escalation, and pharmacokinetic study (NCT02442531, NAPOLY trial) of CPC634 in patients with advanced solid tumors (n = 33) receiving CPC634 intravenously every 3 weeks (15–100 mg/$m^2$), every 2 weeks (45 mg/$m^2$) or every 3 weeks (60 mg/$m^2$) with dexamethasone premedication showed that cumulative skin toxicity at doses $\geq$ 60 mg/$m^2$ was the main DLT, which was absent in the corticosteroid-pretreated group [59]. Thus, the recommended phase 2 dose was determined at 60 mg/$m^2$ every 3 weeks with dexamethasone premedication. The formulation exhibited a dose-proportional pharmacokinetic profile with prolonged systemic exposure to DTX, in accordance with preclinical studies [59]. The development and validation of a bioanalytical method for the determination of both total and released DTX from CPC634 in human plasma and tumor tissue using sensitive and selective liquid chromatography–tandem mass spectroscopy (LC-MS/MS) were successfully applied in the pharmacokinetic analysis of serum and tissue samples from cancer patients treated with CPC634 [129].

A two-arm pharmacokinetic study (CriTax study) in patients with solid tumors (n = 24) randomized to receive CPC634 (75 mg/$m^2$, 1 h IV infusion) in cycle 1 and conventional DTX (75 mg/$m^2$, 1-h IV infusion) in cycle 2 (arm A) or vice versa (arm B) revealed that the plasma AUC was 27% higher for CPC634-released DTX while $C_{max}$ was 91% lower compared with conventional DTX, which contributed to a lower incidence of neutropenia during CPC634 treatment [60]. Tumor biopsies showed that CPC634 administration enhanced the intratumoral DTX exposure, resulting in 4.6-fold higher total DTX concentration in the metastatic lesions compared with conventional DTX but comparable released DTX concentration [60].

Additionally, CPC634 administration resulted in a 3.7-fold higher total skin DTX concentration compared with conventional DTX while the released DTX concentrations were not statistically different [130]. Histopathological examination of skin biopsies taken at baseline and at day 8 of both cycles revealed increased apoptosis and micronucleation after treatment with either CPC634 or conventional DTX, which could induce inflammatory reactions leading to skin toxicity, often associated with DTX treatment [130].

A phase 2 study (NCT03742713, CINOVA trial) of CPC634 in 24 patients with platinum-resistant recurrent ovarian cancer showed disappointing clinical activity of the formulation [131]. None of the patients had an objective response, and the trial was prematurely stopped due to futility [131]. The most common AEs were mainly gastrointestinal (96%) but also fatigue (44%), dyspnea (40%), and infections (40%) [131].

A first-in-human imaging study (NCT03712423, PICCOLO trial) with zirconium-89-radiolabeled CPC634 was performed to enable visualization and quantification of NP accumulation in human solid tumors [132]. In seven patients with solid tumors administered $^{89}$Zr-CPC634 at a high therapeutic dose (60 mg/m$^2$ DTX) or a low diagnostic dose (1–2 mg DTX), positron emission tomography–computed tomography (PET/CT) imaging showed accumulation in 46% and 41% of tumor lesions, respectively, and pharmacokinetic mean half-life of 97.0 $\pm$ 14.4 h for the therapeutic dose and 62.4 $\pm$ 12.9 h for the diagnostic dose [132]. Thus, PET/CT imaging with a diagnostic dose of $^{89}$Zr-CPC634 accurately reflects tumor accumulation of the therapeutic dose without causing any AEs, showing potential for patient stratification in clinical practice [132].

### *4.2. Irinotecan-Based Micelle Formulations*

Irinotecan (CPT-11) is a water-soluble semi-synthetic derivative of the natural alkaloid camptothecin isolated from the bark and stem of the Chinese tree *Camptotheca acuminata*, which is frequently used in the chemotherapy of advanced or metastatic CRC [133]. In vivo, the CPT-11 prodrug is hydrolyzed by carboxylesterases into the pharmacologically active metabolite 7-ethyl-10-hydroxycamptothecin (SN-38), which is metabolized in the liver into the inactive glucuronide by hepatic uridine 5′-diphosphoglucuronosyl transferase 1A1 (UGT1A1) and 1A7 isomorphs (UGT1A7) and mainly excreted in the bile [133]. In the intestine, SN-38G suffers deglucuronidation by bacterial β-glucuronidases, regenerating SN-38, which can be reabsorbed, resulting in the enterohepatic recirculation of SN-38. Late-onset diarrhea experienced by a vast majority of cancer patients on irinotecan-based chemotherapy has been attributed to intestinal overexposure to SN-38, the major active metabolite of irinotecan [133]. Additionally, polymorphisms of the UGT1A1 gene (e.g., *UGT1A1*6* and *UGT1A1*28*), have been associated with a higher risk of severe neutropenia and irinotecan-induced delayed diarrhea [134].

SN-38, like camptothecin and its derivatives, is an inhibitor of DNA topoisomerase I (Top1), a nuclear enzyme involved in DNA replication and transcription highly expressed in cancer tissues, forming a stable drug–enzyme–DNA ternary complex that hinders DNA replication, ultimately resulting in apoptosis and cell death [133]. Contrary to CPT-11, SN-38 is poorly water-soluble (<5 μg/mL) and unstable at pH > 6 due to spontaneous and reversible hydrolysis of its lactone ring to the inactive carboxylate open-ring form [133].

#### *NK012*

NK012, developed by NanoCarrier Co., Ltd. (Chiba, Japan) and licensed to Nippon Kayaku, Co., Ltd. (Tokyo, Japan), is a freeze-dried polymeric micellar formulation of SN-38, the pharmacologically active metabolite of CPT-11. NK012 micelles, with a 20 nm diameter, are prepared by self-assembly of amphiphilic diblock copolymers made of

$PEG_{12k}$ and $p(Glu)_{7k}$ bearing 20% (*w*/*w*) SN-38 covalently attached to the carboxylate groups of the hydrophobic amino acid segment by ester bonds [133,135]. Unlike CPT-11, NK012 can release SN-38 through chemical hydrolysis of the phenyl ester bond at physiological pH (pH 7.4), thus its therapeutic effect is independent of carboxylesterase enzymatic activity, which varies among the population [133,135]. In vitro release studies showed that the amount of SN-38 released from NK012 in PBS (pH 7.3) at 37 °C achieved 57% at 24 h and 74% at 48 h and that these values decreased to 1% and 3%, respectively, in 5% glucose solution at pH 4.6, demonstrating the stability of the formulation in weak acidic media [135].

Extensive preclinical studies demonstrated the potent antitumoral activity of NK012 in vivo, particularly against solid tumors, being more effective than the SN-38 prodrug CPT-11 by selectively accumulating in the tumor tissue via the EPR effect and exhibiting a safer intestinal toxicity profile in several human tumor xenografts [133,135]. Moreover, the small size (20 nm) of NK012 also allowed effective penetration and distribution within hypovascular and stroma-rich tumors, like pancreatic cancer [136,137] and scirrhous stomach cancer [138], often intractable due to inefficient penetration of anticancer agents. In this regard, orthotopic tumor xenografts provide a better model compared with subcutaneous xenografts in terms of tumor vascularity and intersticium [137].

NK012 (30 mg/kg/day) efficacy in mice bearing orthotopic human pancreatic cancer cell (SUIT-2) xenografts was superior to that of CPT-11 (66.7 mg/kg/day) and gemcitabine (16.5 mg/kg/day), reducing the number of metastatic nodules in the peritoneal cavity, due to enhanced accumulation within the tumor tissue and sustained release of SN-38 from NK012 [137]. In mice orthotopically transplanted with scirrhous gastric cancer cells, NK012 showed enhanced distribution with prolonged SN-38 release when compared with CPT-11 and was effective against peritoneal nodules [138].

In mice bearing metastasis to the liver, colonized 7 days after portal vein administration of human colon cancer HT-29 cells, NK012 administration (30 mg/kg) eradicated the liver metastasis and improved survival rate compared with CPT-11 (66.7 mg/kg) [139]. Prolonged accumulation of NK012 and free SN-38 released from the PMs was observed in the tumors, liver, and spleen, lasting for 6 weeks after NK012 administration, while accumulation of free SN-38 converted from the CPT-11 prodrug rapidly decreased within 24 h [139]. Similarly, NK012 displayed a stronger antitumor effect compared with CPT-11 against liver metastasis produced by injecting human gastric cancer HSC-57 cells into the portal vein of mice, with a survival rate of 100% on day 131 versus 0% in the CPT-11-treated group [140].

NK012 showed significantly higher antitumor activity in nude mice with human CRC HT-29 cell xenografts subcutaneously implanted when compared with CPT-11 [141]. Pharmacokinetic analysis revealed that the plasma AUC of NK012 (30 mg/kg) was nearly 200-fold higher than that of CPT-11 (66.7 mg/kg) while the AUC of free SN-38 released from NK012 was 14-fold higher than that obtained from CPT-11 [141]. Moreover, the tumor concentration of free SN-38 reached 90.4 ng/g and 4.5 ng/g at 24 h after administration of NK012 or CPT-11, respectively, suggesting that prolonged circulation of NK012 in the bloodstream enhances tumor distribution due to the EPR effect, resulting in potent antitumor activity of NK012 in vivo [141]. Similarly, in combination therapy regimens with 5-fluorouracil, the replacement of CPT-11 by NK012 resulted in a higher synergistic antitumor effect in this experimental model of human CRC [142].

In the subcutaneous murine syngeneic renal adenocarcinoma (Renca) model, used as a hypervascular tumor model mimicking human renal cell carcinoma, NK012 (20 mg/kg/day on days 0, 4, and 8) was able to eradicate fast-growing Renca tumors in 60% of mice [143]. Injection of Renca cells into the tail vein of mice resulted in lung metastases, but treatment with NK012 significantly reduced the number of metastatic nodules and improved survival [143]. Biodistribution studies revealed an enhanced and prolonged distribution of free SN-38 in metastatic lung tissues, but not in healthy (non-metastatic) lung tissue, after NK012 administration [143].

In mice subcutaneously injected with VEGF-secreting human small-cell lung cancer cells (SBC-3/VEGF), NK012 markedly enhanced SN-38 distribution and accumulation in tumors due to the EPR effect, promoted by the hypervascularity and hyperpermeability induced by VEGF, resulting in remarkably higher antitumor activity when compared with CPT-11 [141]. Similarly, combination therapy with NK012 and cisplatin provided superior efficacy in relative tumor volume reduction compared with CPT-11/cisplatin and was not associated with severe diarrhea [144]. The higher concentration of CPT-11 found in the small intestine epithelium, which can be reabsorbed and converted to SN-38 that damages the intestinal mucosa and provokes diarrhea, was responsible for intestinal toxicity in the CPT-11/cisplatin-treated group [144]. NK012 in combination with S-1, an oral dihydropyrimidine dehydrogenase inhibitory fluoropyrimidine, also displayed a synergistic efficacy superior to that of CPT-11/S-1 and reduced intestinal toxicity, including lower incidence of diarrhea, in mice subcutaneously implanted with NSCLC (PC-14 or EBC-1 cell) xenografts [145].

Therapeutic combination of NK012 (5 or 30 mg/kg) with bevacizumab (5 mg/kg), an anti-VEGF humanized mAb, was more efficient than NK012 (5 or 30 mg/kg) at inhibiting tumor growth in nude mice subcutaneously implanted with human lung cancer (PC-14 or A549) xenografts [146]. Pharmacokinetic data revealed that the concentrations of NK012 and free SN-38 after administration of NK012 alone were not significantly different from those obtained for the combination of NK012 plus bevacizumab, suggesting that VEGF-induced angiogenesis inhibition by bevacizumab does not disturb NK012 tumor accumulation and produces an additional antitumor effect by reducing the area of proliferating vascular endothelial cells in the tumors [146].

Glioma is another type of hypervascular tumor with irregular vascular architecture and high expression levels of VEGF. NK012 was more effective than CPT-11 at reducing tumor volume and increasing survival rate in mice bearing glioblastoma (U87MG) orthotopic xenografts, which was attributed to enhanced intratumoral accumulation of NK012 with prolonged and sustained release of SN-38, since SN-38 antitumor activity is time-dependent [147]. However, free SN-38 was not detected in normal brain tissues after IV injection of either NK012 or CPT-11, suggesting that both NK012 and CPT-11 are unable to cross the BBB in the normal brain but extravasate from the brain tumor blood vessels, with the NPs preferentially accumulating in the tumor tissue [147]. Further studies showed that NK012 monotherapy was even more effective against orthotopic tumors than CPT-11 combined with bevacizumab [148]. Moreover, convection-enhanced delivery (CED) of NK012 enabled consistent distribution of SN-38 with minimum brain tissue damage in healthy rat brains after delivery of 40 μg NK012 while severe damage was observed with SN-38 at the same dose [149]. CED circumvents the BBB by delivering agents directly into the tumor or surrounding brain parenchyma based on continuous positive-pressure infusion, resulting in large volumes of distribution and high local drug concentrations with reduced potential systemic toxicity [149]. Local delivery of NK012 via CED significantly prolonged survival in rats with human U87MG brain tumor orthotopic xenografts [149].

In a mouse model of orthotopic multiple myeloma created using CD138-positive U2661B1 cells, which produce human IgE lambda light chain (monoclonal protein), IV administration of NK012 was able to suppress plasma elevation of human monoclonal protein levels and proliferation of CD138-positive myeloma cells in mouse bone marrow in a dose-dependent manner [150]. NK012 monotherapy and in combination with the proteasome inhibitor bortezomib prolonged the median survival time compared with the control (untreated) group and bortezomib alone, respectively [150].

A first-in-human phase 1, dose-escalating study in Japan, enrolling patients with solid tumors refractory to standard therapy (n = 24), showed that administration of NK012 (2–28 mg/m$^2$ as a 30 min IV infusion every 3 weeks) was well tolerated and objective responses were observed in patients with refractory esophageal cancer and lung carcinoma [62]. The most common DLT was neutropenia, observed in two out of nine patients at the 28 mg/m$^2$ dose level during cycle 1. Non-hematologic toxicity, namely diarrhea, was mostly grade 1/2. A subsequent phase 2 study evaluating the efficacy and safety of NK012 (28 mg/m$^2$ IV infusion over 30 min, every 3 weeks) in Japanese patients with unresectable metastatic CRC (n = 58) previously treated with an oxaliplatin-based chemotherapy regimen found similar ORRs between NK012 monotherapy and irinotecan (CPT-11) monotherapy (3.8% versus 4.2%, respectively) reported in the phase 3 EPIC trial but with low incidence of grade $\geq$ 3 diarrhea [151]. The study included cancer patients homozygous or heterozygous for *UGT1A1*28* or *UGT1A1*6* originally excluded in the phase 1 trial. Based on the incidence and severity of grade $\geq$ 3 neutropenia and febrile neutropenia, the initial dose of 28 mg/m$^2$ NK012 was considered too high for these patients.

Another phase 1 dose escalation study was independently conducted in the USA [63]. Administration of NK012 (9–37 mg/m$^2$ as a 30 min infusion, every 21 or 28 days, without premedication) to patients with previously treated advanced solid tumors (n = 38) showed promising antitumor activity, with partial responses in triple-negative breast cancer (n = 3), SCLC (n = 1), endometrial cancer (n = 1), and pancreatic neuroendocrine tumor (n = 1). The recommended phase 2 dose was set as 20 mg/m$^2$ every 28 days, which was also identified as the MTD in the 21-day schedule, with myelosuppression as the main DLT [63]. Gastrointestinal toxicity was mild, including grade < 3 diarrhea. Pharmacokinetic analysis showed that NK012 (28 mg/m$^2$) had a higher plasma AUC compared to that of CPT-11 (250 mg/m$^2$) and that the half-life of SN-38 was significantly prolonged in NK012 when compared to CPT-11, demonstrating a sustained high systemic concentration of SN-38 in the micellar formulation [63].

A phase 1/2 study of NK012 (12–24 mg/m$^2$) in patients with relapsed or refractory multiple myeloma (n = 16) established 20 mg/m$^2$ as the RD of NK012, with grade 4 neutropenia being responsible for the majority of DLTs at a dose of 24 mg/m$^2$ [152]. However, the study was terminated at the end of the phase 1 stage since all patients failed to achieve an objective response [152].

### 4.3. Anthracycline Micellar Formulations

Anthracyclines are antibiotics produced by *Streptomyces* spp. with a broad spectrum of antitumoral activity. Chemically, anthracyclines are glycoside drugs consisting of an anthraquinone aglycone coupled with an amino sugar (daunosamine), and the intercalation of the planar aromatic anthraquinone moiety between adjacent DNA base pairs contributes to their cytotoxic effects. Although anthracyclines are DNA-intercalating agents, inhibition of eukaryotic topoisomerase II (Top2) in proliferating cancer cells is considered the primary mode of action responsible for the potent cytotoxic activity of the drugs [153]. Anthracycline antibiotics are Top2 poisons that trap the enzyme–DNA cleavage complexes by stacking between DNA base pairs at the DNA/protein interface, interacting with both nucleotides as well as amino acid residues to form stable ternary complexes, which inhibits DNA re-ligation, generating DNA double-strand breaks and triggering apoptotic cell death [153].

Doxorubicin (DOX) is a cytotoxic anthracycline antibiotic produced by *Streptomyces peucetius* subsp. *caesius* (ATCC 27952) with a characteristic red color and natural fluorescence due to the anthraquinone chromophore. DOX is used alone or in combination with other chemotherapeutic agents as first-line therapy for several types of cancer, including breast, ovarian, thyroid, bladder, SCLC, bone sarcomas, neuroblastoma, acute lymphoblastic/myeloblastic leukemia, and Hodgkin lymphoma [153,154]. However, the therapeutic effect of DOX is limited by severe AEs, namely myelosuppression, nephrotoxicity, and dose-dependent acute and chronic cardiotoxicity. Among those, the most deleterious side effect is cardiomyopathy, potentially leading to congestive heart failure [153,154].

Besides being a Top2 poison and a DNA-intercalating agent, DOX-induced intracellular ROS generation also contributes to the drug cytotoxicity. At physiological pH, the amine sugar moiety of DOX is positively charged and binds with high affinity to negatively charged cardiolipin present in the inner mitochondrial membrane of metabolically active cells (e.g., cardiomyocytes and hepatocytes), promoting DOX accumulation in these organelles. DOX is reduced by microsomal (NADPH-cytochrome P450) and mitochondrial

(Complex I) oxidoreductases to a semiquinone radical species, which can complex with $Fe^{2+}$. The free radical complex can spontaneously reduce oxygen to superoxide anion radical, regenerating DOX in the process and reinitiating the cycle [153]. Increased levels of superoxide and other ROS and RNS generated in the process, including hydroxyl radicals and peroxynitrite, contribute to oxidative and nitrosative stress, mitochondrial dysfunction, DNA damage, and lipid peroxidation-dependent ferroptosis [153]. Although ROS detoxification can be achieved by endogenous antioxidative enzymes, such as superoxide dismutase (SOD), catalase, and glutathione peroxidase, the lower levels of these free-radical-scavenging systems expressed in cancer and myocardial cells contribute to DOX antitumor activity and associated cardiotoxicity [153]. Doxorubicinol (DOXol), a cytotoxic metabolite formed by the reduction of DOX catalyzed by cytosolic NADPH-dependent carbonyl and aldo-keto reductases located in erythrocytes, heart, liver, and kidney cells, disrupts calcium homeostasis by interfering with the sarcoendoplasmic reticulum calcium ATPase (SERCA) and the cardiac ryanodine receptor (RyR2) and is a relevant contributor to DOX-induced cardiomyopathy [153].

DOX is available in the form of a water-soluble salt, DOX hydrochloride (Adriamycin®, Farmitalia-Carlo Erba, Milan, Italy), for IV administration, usually with a cardioprotective agent, such as dexrazoxane, an iron chelator [154]. Liposomal formulations for injection (e.g., Doxil®/Caelyx®, Myocet®) are also available with lower incidence of cardiotoxicity but more expensive [154]. Furthermore, the pegylated liposomal formulation of DOX (Doxil®/Caelyx®) is associated with dose-limiting palmar plantar erythrodysthesia [154].

Several anthracycline analogs have been synthesized in attempts to improve therapeutic efficacy and reduce off-target toxicity. Among the few that reached the market was epirubicin (4′-epidoxorubicin), the 4′-epimer of DOX. Epirubicin (EPI) and DOX have similar potency, but EPR exhibits reduced cardiotoxicity, which is reflected in their maximum recommended cumulative doses, 1000 $mg/m^2$ for EPR and 550 $mg/m^2$ for DOX [83].

#### 4.3.1. NK911

NK911, developed by NanoCarrier Co., Ltd. (Chiba, Japan) and licensed to Nippon Kayaku (Tokyo, Japan), is a polymeric micellar formulation of DOX with a 40 nm size composed of amphiphilic diblock copolymers made of $PEG_{5k}$ and $p(Asp)_{4k}$, made more hydrophobic by partial conjugation (near 45%) of the drug to the carboxylic groups of the amino acid side chains through amide bonds, and containing physically entrapped DOX stabilized via $\pi$–$\pi$-stacking interactions with the conjugated drug [155]. Contrary to the ester bonds in NK012, the amide bond is hydrolytically stable, and it is the physically encapsulated free drug rather than conjugated DOX that is responsible for the cytotoxic activity [64].

A preclinical study showed that the PMs accumulated in solid tumors in mice by the EPR effect and DOX released from the inner core by diffusion exerted significantly higher antitumor activity than free DOX [155]. Concerning the release of DOX from the conjugated block copolymer, administration of a DOX-conjugated polymer to dogs showed that DOX concentration in plasma was 100-fold less than that of NK911 containing the same amount of DOX-conjugated polymer. Thus, conjugated DOX does not influence plasma DOX concentrations after IV injection of NK911 [64].

NK911 was the first polymeric micellar formulation to proceed into clinical trials, in 2001. In a phase 1 clinical trial enrolling 23 patients with metastatic or recurrent solid tumors refractory to conventional chemotherapy, IV administration of NK911 (6–67 $mg/m^2$) every 3 weeks showed that the formulation was well tolerated, without any infusion-related reactions [64]. A partial response was obtained in one patient with metastatic pancreatic cancer and eight patients exhibited stable disease for longer than 4 weeks. Neutropenia was the main hematological toxicity, with DLTs observed at a dose of 67 $mg/m^2$ (grade 4 neutropenia lasting more than 5 days), which was determined as the MTD. Common non-hematological toxicities included mild alopecia, stomatitis, and anorexia. The recommended phase 2 dose was established as 50 $mg/m^2$ every 3 weeks [64]. At this dose level, the plasma AUC of NK911 was 2-fold higher than that of free DOX but more than 100-fold lower than that of Doxil® (PEGylated liposomes), indicating that NK911 is less stable in plasma than the liposomal formulation. However, the volume of distribution at a steady state of NK911 was nearly 180-fold higher than that of Doxil® at the same dose level, suggesting that the distribution of DOX in tumor tissue may be wider in the case of the PMs when compared to the nanoliposomes upon extravasation from the tumor vessels [64].

#### 4.3.2. SP1049C

SP1049C, developed by Supratek Pharma Inc. (Montreal, QC, Canada), is a P-gp-targeting polymeric micellar formulation of DOX, which is non-covalently incorporated in mixed micelles (22–27 nm) made from a blend of triblock copolymers, Pluronic® L61 and Pluronic® F127 (1:8 *w*/*w*) [83,156,157]. Pluronic® L61 was shown to sensitize DOX-resistant cancer cells through an interplay between ATP depletion, membrane fluidization, and inhibition of P-gp ATPase activity, while Pluronic® F127 provided micellar stabilization [156,157]. SP1049C was effective in vitro against MDR cells normally not susceptible to DOX, which was attributed to an increase in drug uptake, energy-dependent drug efflux inhibition, and changes in intracellular drug trafficking [64]. SP1049C also exhibited improved antitumor efficacy in vivo against drug-resistant tumors due to enhanced tumor accumulation through the EPR effect while distribution in liver, kidney, heart, and lung was similar to conventional DOX but with higher brain levels for SP1049C [156].

A phase 1 dose-escalation trial in patients with advanced cancer (n = 26) administered SP1049C (5–90 mg/m$^2$) as an IV infusion once every 3 weeks for up to six cycles showed myelosuppression as a DLT at 90 mg/m$^2$ [66]. The MTD was 70 mg/m$^2$ and was also the RD for phase 2 studies [66]. The pharmacokinetic profile of SP1049C showed a slower clearance when compared with conventional DOX [66]. Antitumor activity following SP1049C administration was observed in three patients with advanced resistant solid tumors (Ewing's sarcoma, carcinosarcoma, and esophageal adenocarcinoma) that had received prior therapy [66]. Nausea, vomiting, fatigue, and alopecia were common side effects but palmar plantar erythrodysthesia was not observed [66].

A subsequent phase 2 study in 21 patients with metastatic or locally advanced unresectable adenocarcinoma of the esophagus or gastroesophageal junction (chemotherapy naïve) treated with SP1049C (75 mg/m$^2$, IV infusion) every 3 weeks showed an ORR of 47%, median OS of 10 months, and PFS of 6.6 months. Grade 3/4 neutropenia (61.9%) was the main drug-related AE [158]. Non-hematological AEs included alopecia (66.7%), mucositis (47.6%), anorexia (19%), vomiting (19%), nausea (14.3%), and lethargy (14.3%) [158]. Asymptomatic and small decrements (grade 1) in left ventricular ejection fraction were observed in four patients, which discontinued treatment [158]. A phase 3 clinical study of SP1049C in metastatic adenocarcinoma of the upper gastrointestinal tract was started but no results have been reported, although SP1049C was granted orphan drug status by the FDA for esophageal carcinoma in 2005 and for gastric cancer in 2008 [83,159].

#### 4.3.3. NC-6300

NC-6300, developed by NanoCarrier Co., Ltd. (Chiba, Japan), is a pH-sensitive polymeric micellar formulation with a particle size of 40–80 nm composed of PEG$_{12k}$ and poly(α,β-aspartic acid) block copolymers, the latter partially modified with benzyl groups for stabilization of the micellar structure, and conjugated with EPI via an acid-labile hydrazone bond [160].

NC-6300 accumulates in tumor tissue due to the EPR effect and selectively releases the drug in the acidic TME [160]. In vitro drug release studies showed that at pH 3.0, 80% of EPI was released from NC-6300 within 1 h while at pH 7.0 or 7.4 only 20% of the drug was released within 24 h [160]. Pharmacokinetic studies in rats showed highly enhanced plasma retention of NC-6300 compared with native EPI (AUC 116.7 versus 0.053 μg·h/mL, respectively, both intravenously administered at 1 mg/kg dose) [160]. NC-6300 (15 and 20 mg/kg three times with a 4-day interval between doses) was able to regress a Hep3B human hepatic tumor and to inhibit the growth of MDA-MB-231 human breast tumor in xenografted mice while EPI (7 mg/kg at the same schedule) only slowed tumor growth [160]). Tissue distribution studies of NC-6300 (20 mg/kg) showed efficient release of EPI in the tumor, with a release ratio of 74% against 20–46% in healthy tissues. The AUC value of released EPI in the tumor and in the heart was 4.3-fold higher and 0.28-fold lower, respectively, compared with the native free EPI solution at the same dose, resulting in a 15-fold higher therapeutic index for the polymeric micellar formulation [160].

Preclinical evaluation of NC-6300 (10 or 15 mg/kg weekly, for 3 weeks) in mice bearing subcutaneous or orthotopic xenografts of human hepatocellular carcinoma Hep3B cells showed that the formulation improved drug antitumoral activity and survival rate when compared with conventional EPI (10 mg/kg, at the same schedule), with no significant cardiotoxic effects [161]. NC-6300 increased EPI concentrations in the plasma, liver, spleen, and tumor and decreased drug levels in the kidney, lung, and heart compared with the native drug [161].

NC-6300 has also been conjugated with an antitissue factor mAb (clone 1849) for targeted cancer therapy, since tissue factor (TF), an initiator of the extrinsic blood coagulation cascade, is frequently overexpressed in cancer cells and tumor vascular endothelium [162]. The antitumoral activity of anti-TF-NC-6300 was higher in mice bearing tumor xenografts with high TF expression (human gastric cancer 44As3 cells and human pancreatic cancer BxPC3 cells) compared with NC-6300 but in low-TF-expressing xenografts (human pancreatic cancer SUIT2 cells) both formulations showed similar activity, although with higher tumor accumulation of anti-TF-NC-6300.

However, clone 1849 antibody was found to inhibit TF-associated blood coagulation activity and was replaced by clone 1859 in a subsequent study, which had no effect on blood coagulation [163]. The novel anti-TF-NC-6300 formulation showed higher in vitro cytocidal effects in BxPC3 cells compared with NC-6300 but not in the SUIT2 cell line. Similarly, the in vivo tumor growth inhibition efficacy of anti-TF-NC-6300 was superior to NC-6300 in BxPC3 xenografts, but not in the SUIT2 xenograft model, demonstrating the enhanced antitumor effect of anti-TF-NC-6300 in the high-TF-expressing tumor [163].

Targeted immunotherapy with NC-6300 in combination with anti-PD-L1 antibody was found to potentiate immune checkpoint inhibition in mouse models of osteosarcoma and fibrosarcoma, and NC-6300 was even more effective than the MTD of DOX at increasing tumor growth delay induced by anti-PD-L1 antibody [164]. Further mechanistic studies showed that NC-6300 induced immunogenic cell death and normalized the TME, and the combination with anti-PD-L1 antibody increased the intratumoral density and proliferation of T cells [164].

The mechanisms underlying the antitumoral effects resulting from the combination of NC-6300 and high-intensity focused ultrasound (HIFU) were investigated in human pancreatic adenocarcinoma (BxPC-3) and human promyelocytic leukemia (HL-60) cell lines [165]. The sonodynamic therapy (SDT) system employed a specific HIFU irradiation sequence consisting of a short-duration high-intensity triggering pulse (2000 W/cm$^2$, 0.02 ms) to generate cavitation bubbles and a heating wave (10–1000 W/cm$^2$, 10 ms) for sustention of cavitation bubbles and bubble-enhanced heating [165]. The combination of NC-6300 with trigger-pulsed HIFU (TP-HIFU) was shown to increase ROS production in vitro without drug degradation due to the protective hydrophilic shell of the micelles [165]. Moreover, the generation of superoxide anions by TP-HIFU increased upon the addition of NC-6300, and the sonosensitizer potency of NC-6300 was superior to that of EPI.

SDT based on the combination of a low dose of NC-6300 (2.5 mg/kg, 24 h prior to HIFU irradiation) and low-energy HIFU (270 or 360 W/cm$^2$) showed improved efficacy in mouse models of colon cancer (Colon-26) and pancreatic cancer (MIA PaCa-2) compared with NC-6300 monotherapy or HIFU alone [166]. SDT with NC-6300 (7.5–30 mg/m$^2$) and HIFU (9–30 sequences) were effective in the treatment of canine cancer in four pet dogs with spontaneous tumors (chondrosarcoma, osteosarcoma, hepatocellular cancer, and prostate cancer) with no AEs after five SDT sessions [167].

A first-in-human phase 1, dose-escalation study of NC-6300 in patients with advanced or recurrent solid tumors (n = 19) administered NC-6300 (15–225 mg/m$^2$) as 10 min IV infusion every 3 weeks showed a partial response in one patient with breast cancer and stable disease in ten patients [168]. The recommended phase 2 dose was set as 170 mg/m$^2$, which was also the MTD. The human pharmacokinetic profile of NC-6300 was linear and consistent with preclinical studies in rats and monkeys.

A phase 1b, dose-escalation trial of NC-6300 monotherapy (125–215 mg/m$^2$, IV, every 3 weeks) in patients (n = 29) with advanced, metastatic, or unresectable solid tumors, including soft-tissue sarcomas (n = 11), showed an ORR of 11%, with partial responses in angiosarcoma and endometrial stromal sarcoma. DLTs included grade 3/4 neutropenia, thrombocytopenia, anemia, febrile neutropenia, stomatitis, and lung infection [67]. The MTD and RD for phase 2 studies were determined to be 185 mg/m$^2$ and 150 mg/m$^2$, respectively. Based on the promising antitumor activity against angiosarcoma, an expansion cohort was undertaken (NCT03168061) which enrolled 10 patients [169]. Administration of NC-6300 at the RD (150 mg/m$^2$, IV), once every 3 weeks, resulted in a median PFS of 5.4 months (3.8 months and 8.2 months in patients with and without prior anthracycline treatment, respectively) [169]. The most common AEs were neutropenia, thrombocytopenia, leukopenia, anemia, fatigue, and nausea [169].

### *4.4. Platinum-Based Micelle Formulations*

Cisplatin (CDDP) is a platinum coordination complex with a broad spectrum of antitumor activity used as first-line therapy for several solid tumors, including breast, ovarian, testicular, bladder, head and neck, liver, and small-cell and non-small-cell lung cancers, either alone or in combination with radiation and/or other chemotherapeutic drugs [170,171].

The potent genotoxicity of cisplatin, activated intracellularly by the aquation of the two chloride leaving groups, results from the formation of mainly intrastrand but also interstrand DNA crosslinks through coordination bonds between the platinum atoms and the purine nucleobases [170,171]. However, non-selective distribution of the drug results in acute dose-related severe AEs, namely nephrotoxicity, myelosuppression, neurotoxicity, and ototoxicity, and the therapeutic effect is further limited by intrinsic or acquired drug resistance [171].

Platinum complexes like cisplatin undergo stepwise aquation reactions in which the chloride ions are replaced by water molecules leading to the pharmacologically active cationic mono- and diaqua complexes [170,171]. The rates of aquation of platinum complexes depend on the concentration of chloride ions in the media, thus the drugs are relatively stable in plasma due to the high chloride concentration (100 mM). On the other hand, the low intracellular chloride concentration (4–12 mM) promotes the formation of the cationic aqua forms of the platinum complexes, which do not readily diffuse out of the cell since their charge hinders crossing of the lipophilic cellular membrane, becoming trapped within the cell and binding to intracellular targets, mainly DNA but also RNA and proteins [170].

Carboplatin is a second-generation platinum designed to reduce cisplatin DLT by replacing the readily exchangeable chloride ligands with a bidentate 1,1-cyclobutanedicarboxylic acid ligand, thus slowing down the rate of aquation reactions, which also reduces the drug potency [170,171]. However, the lower excretion rate of carboplatin results in higher retention (half-life of 30 h versus 1.5–3.6 h for cisplatin) and longer-lasting effects [170]. Carboplatin has reduced nephrotoxic side effects compared with cisplatin but is associated with severe myelosuppression.

Oxaliplatin is a third-generation platinum complex developed to overcome cellular resistance to cisplatin and carboplatin. The parent compound, cis-dichloro(1,2-diamminocyclohexane)platinum(II) (DACHPt), is a potent anticancer agent with a broader spectrum of activity and no crossresistance with cisplatin and carboplatin, obtained by replacing the two amine groups of cisplatin by 1,2-diamminocyclohexane (DACH) [171]. However,

DACHPt lacks water solubility (0.25 mg/mL compared with 1.2 mg/mL for cisplatin), which was enhanced in oxaliplatin by replacing both chloride ligands with a bidentate oxalate ligand [170]. Oxaliplatin undergoes rapid non-enzymatic biotransformation due to displacement of the labile oxalate group by water and nucleophiles, namely chloride ions, present in biological media to form cytotoxic mono- and diaqua/chloro platinum complexes, which complicates the drug pharmacokinetics. The higher cytotoxic activity of oxaliplatin compared with cisplatin and carboplatin has been attributed to the bulky DACH ligand, which induces DNA lesions that are poorly recognized and/or prevent binding by DNA repair enzymes [170]. Moreover, oxaliplatin can induce ribosome biogenesis stress and enable immunogenic cell death by promoting a T-cell-dependent immune response, and these differing modes of action further contribute to the efficacy of oxaliplatin in cisplatin-resistant cell lines [171].

Oxaliplatin (Eloxatin®, Sanofi-Aventis) is indicated as the first-line treatment of metastatic CRC, in combination with 5-fluorouracil and leuvocorin, known as the FOLFOX regimen, and as adjunctive therapy after resection of the primary tumor. Oxaliplatin lacks the nephrotoxicity of cisplatin and the severe myelosuppression of carboplatin but induces severe peripheral neuropathy, often the DLT, characterized by acute neuropathy that includes acral paresthesia and dysesthesia triggered or enhanced by exposure to cold, and chronic neuropathy, with loss of sensory and motor function after long-term treatment [170,171].

#### 4.4.1. NC-6004 (Nanoplatin™)

NC-6004 (Nanoplatin™), developed by NanoCarrier Co., Ltd. (Chiba, Japan) and licensed to Orient Europharma Co., Ltd. (Taiwan), is a cisplatin polymeric micellar formulation comprising amphiphilic diblock copolymers made of PEG and p(Glu) with a micelle size around 30 nm prepared through polymer–metal complex formation between cisplatin and the carboxylate groups of the hydrophobic segment [83,172]. In physiological media, NC-6004 is expected to release cisplatin through an exchange reaction between the carboxylate groups of p(Glu) and chloride ions present in the media [172].

NC-6004 was stable in distilled water in long-time storage but in physiological saline a sustained drug release was observed, lasting longer than 150 h, which was accompanied by the decay of the carrier micelles [172]. The micelles had remarkably prolonged blood circulation and showed high selectivity towards cancer cells in Lewis-lung-carcinoma-bearing mice, effectively accumulating in solid tumors by passive targeting through the EPR effect and showing reduced accumulation in normal tissues (kidney, liver, spleen, and muscle) [172]. Both NC-6004 and free cisplatin, at the same dose regimen (4 mg/kg, five 2-day cycles), had significant antitumor activity in murine colon adenocarcinoma 26 (C 26)-bearing mice compared with a non-treated control group, but only NC-6004-treated mice showed complete tumor regression without significant body weight loss [172].

Further studies showed that the secondary structure in the polypeptide segment of the PEG-*b*-p(Glu) copolymer, characterized by $\alpha$-helix bundles in the micellar core, was critical for stabilization of micellar structure against dilution in physiological media, prolonging blood circulation and achieving sustained drug release in the TME through surface erosion of the bundled core by chloride ions and disassembly of the micelles [173]. The formulation accomplished selective tumor accumulation after IV injection (4 mg/kg, three times at 2-day interval) in mice bearing subcutaneous human pancreatic adenocarcinoma (BxPC3) xenografts, with reduced non-specific distribution to the liver and spleen, and effectively suppressed tumor growth [173].

The in vitro growth inhibitory effect of NC-6004 against human oral squamous cell carcinoma cell lines (OSC-19, OSC-20, HSC-3, and HSC-4) was inferior to that of cisplatin [174]. However, both formulations showed comparable in vivo antitumor effects in an orthotopic tongue cancer (OSC-19) mouse model, with the micellar formulation providing a better safety profile, with minimal renal cell damage [174]. Moreover, NC-6004 showed prolonged blood and lymphatic circulation, reducing the incidence of lymphatic metastasis compared with cisplatin [174].

The antitumor effect of NC-6004 (0.5, 2.5, or 5.0 mg/kg IV, every 3 days, for a total of three injections) in nude mice implanted with the human gastric cancer cell line MKN-45 was comparable to or higher than that of cisplatin at the same dose schedule, with tumor concentrations of platinum peaking at 10 min and 48 h after administration of cisplatin and NC-6004, respectively [175]. Additionally, combined treatment with NC-6004 and S-1 in mice bearing human gastric cancer (44As3Luc) xenografts showed significantly lower body weight loss compared with cisplatin plus S-1 while retaining similar antitumor activity.

In healthy rats, a single IV injection of NC-6004 significantly inhibited the nephrotoxicity and neurotoxicity of cisplatin, according to data from histopathological and biochemical studies [175]. Renal platinum concentrations at 10 min and 1 h after administration of NC-6004 (5 mg/kg) were 11.6- and 3.1-fold lower, respectively, compared with the cisplatin (5 mg/kg) group [175]. Rats treated with cisplatin (10 mg/kg) also showed higher plasma concentrations of blood urea nitrogen (BUN) and creatinine compared with animals given NC-6004 (10 and 15 mg/kg). Thus, NC-6004 may facilitate treatment on an outpatient basis due to decreased renal toxicity since it does not require hospitalization for hydration to prevent cisplatin nephrotoxicity [175,176]. The neurophysiological examination was performed after 11 IV administrations of NC-6004 or cisplatin, both at 2 mg/kg, twice a week [175]. Contrary to NC-6004-treated rats, the cisplatin-treated rats showed a significant delay in sensory nerve conduction velocity in their hind paws and degeneration of the sciatic nerve, which was attributed to significantly reduced accumulation of platinum in nerve tissue following NC-6004 administration [175].

NC-6004 also prevented ototoxicity, a common side effect of high-dose cisplatin therapy, in healthy guinea pigs. Treatment with NC-6004 (8 or 12 mg/kg bolus IV injection) resulted in no apparent auditory brainstem responses (ABRs) while treatment with cisplatin (8 or 12 mg/kg bolus IV injection plus subcutaneous hydration with 20 mL normal saline to avoid renal damage) lead to dose-dependent threshold shifts and significant hair-cell loss [177]. Platinum distribution and concentration in the organ of Corti were significantly reduced in NC-6004-treated guinea pigs compared with the cisplatin-treated group, indicating that NC-6004 prevented cisplatin-induced ototoxicity by circumventing the vulnerable hair cells in the inner ear due to the micelle's size (around 30 nm), which does not allow crossing the blood–cochlear barrier through the intrastrial space (around 15 nm) [177].

The first-in-human phase 1, dose-escalation study of NC-6004 (10–120 mg/m$^2$, IV, every 3 weeks) in patients with solid tumors (n = 17) conducted in the UK revealed renal impairment and hypersensitivity reactions at a dose of 120 mg/m$^2$, despite implementation of a premedication regimen and posthydration, which was established as the MTD [69]. Only one DLT occurred in a patient treated with 90 mg/m$^2$ of NC-6004, which was determined as the RD. Seven patients showed stable disease. Pharmacokinetic analysis showed that IV administration of NC-6004 reduced $C_{max}$ and increased AUC compared with cisplatin at the same dose (120 mg/m$^2$), indicating that the delayed and sustained release of cisplatin following IV administration of NC-6004 contributed to its lower toxicity and better safety profile compared to conventional cisplatin [69].

Results from a phase 1/2 study (NCT00910741) conducted in Asia (Taiwan and Singapore) enrolling patients with pancreatic cancer (n = 19) treated with NC-6004 (30, 60, 90, and 120 mg/m$^2$ every 3 weeks on day 1) plus gemcitabine (1000 mg/m$^2$ twice every 3 weeks, on days 1 and 8) registered two DLTs at 120 mg/m$^2$, which was determined as the MTD, while the RD was established as 90 mg/m$^2$. These values were identical to the ones obtained for the monotherapy regimen in the UK study [178]. However, the combination regimen showed modest efficacy, with one partial response and ten patients experiencing stable disease among the seventeen in the evaluable population. A prophylactic two-dose oral steroid regimen was implemented to reduce the risk of hypersensitivity reactions, which were not observed [178]. Nevertheless, NC-6004 entered and completed a phase 3 clinical trial (NCT02043288) for evaluation of the impact of NC-6004 addition to gemcitabine in the treatment of locally advanced or metastatic pancreatic cancer in Asian patients, but no results have been posted yet.

An open-label phase 1 study of NC-6004 (60 or 90 mg/m$^2$, IV, on day 1, in every 3-week cycle) in combination with gemcitabine (1000 mg/m$^2$, IV, on days 1 and 8 starting on the second cycle) in Japanese patients with advanced solid tumors (n = 12) established both the MTD and the RD at 90 mg/m$^2$ [179]. One patient showed partial response while eight patients had stable disease. The most frequent drug-related AEs were neutrophil decrease (66.7%) and WBC count decrease (41.7%). Prophylactic hydration therapy before and after treatment with NC-6004 was necessary to prevent renal toxicity [179].

In a phase 1b/2 study (NCT02240238) conducted in the US and Europe, patients with advanced solid tumors (n = 22) were treated with NC-6004 (60–180 mg/m$^2$ on day 1) and gemcitabine (1250 mg/m$^2$ on days 1 and 8) every 3 weeks [180]. The most common grade 3/4 hematologic AEs were leukopenia (68%) and thrombocytopenia (59%), and the MTD and phase 2 RD were both determined to be 135 mg/m$^2$, higher than the corresponding values reported in the UK study [69] and the Asian study [178]. The inconsistency may be due to different study designs since the latter studies used a 3 + 3 modified Fibonacci dose escalation design while the US study adopted the Bayesian continual reassessment model. No clinically significant nephro-, neuro-, or ototoxicity was observed. Among 20 evaluable patients, 3 showed partial responses (15%), 14 had stable disease (70%), and tumor shrinkage was detected in 11 patients (55%) [180].

The expansion phase 2 study (NCT02240238) of NC-6004 (135 mg/m$^2$ on day 1) plus gemcitabine (1250 mg/m$^2$ on days 1 and 8) in patients with squamous NSCLC (n = 34), biliary tract cancer (n = 50), or bladder cancer (n = 13) showed a median PFS of 3.9, 4.3, and 6.8 months, respectively [68]. The most common grade 3 treatment-emergent AEs were nausea, anemia, neutropenia, and hyponatremia, independently of the type of cancer [68].

A phase 2a/2b clinical trial (NCT03771820) of NC-6004 plus the checkpoint inhibitor pembrolizumab in patients with HNSCC refractory to platinum or platinum-containing regimens (n = 16) treated with the recommended phase 2 dose (135 mg/m$^2$) demonstrated that the formulation was safe and well tolerated [181]. No grade 3/4 toxicity or clinically significant nephro-, neuro-, or ototoxicity was observed, despite the RD being higher than conventional cisplatin therapeutic doses, and the most common side effect was hypomagnesemia (31%). Three patients showed partial response (21%) while tumor shrinkage occurred in eight patients (57%) [181].

Based on the promising therapeutic efficacy and safety of the NC-6004 cisplatin formulation, NC-4016 was developed for the delivery of oxaliplatin in order to modify its pharmacokinetics, improve antitumor activity, and decrease drug-related toxicity, as discussed in the next section.

#### 4.4.2. NC-4016

NC-4016, developed by NanoCarrier Co., Ltd. (Chiba, Japan), is a polymeric micellar formulation of DACHPt, the oxaliplatin parent complex, composed of $PEG_{12k}$-$p(Glu)_{6k}$ diblock copolymers [182,183]. The PMs, with 30–40 nm size, were prepared through polymer–metal complexation between DACHPt and the carboxylic groups of the hydrophobic copolymer [182,183]. The platinum complexes are released from the micelle core by exchange reaction between chloride ions present in the media and carboxylic groups of the p(Glu) copolymer complexed with DACHPt. Drug release studies performed in PBS (pH 7.4) at 37 °C, mimicking physiological conditions, demonstrated the in vitro sustained release of platinum from NC-4016 after an induction period of 12 h [183].

The growth inhibitory effect of NC-4016 in a human cervical adenocarcinoma (KB) cell line was weaker than that of oxaliplatin in vitro, presumably due to the slow-release behavior of DACHPt complexes from the micelles [184]. However, the in vivo antitumoral efficacy of the micellar formulation was superior to that of oxaliplatin at equivalent Pt doses in nude mice bearing subcutaneous KB xenografts, which was attributed to higher Pt concentrations in tumor [184]. A 74% reduction in tumor weight was achieved after administration of NC-4016 compared with only 33% in the oxaliplatin-treated group [184]. Additionally, in a rat model of oxaliplatin-induced neuropathic pain, no acute cold hypersensitivity was observed in the NC-4016-treated group, contrary to the oxaliplatin group [184]

NC-4016 was shown to maintain micelle form during blood circulation, extravasating from blood vessels into tumor tissues and selectively dissociating within late endosomes, thus enhancing drug delivery to the nucleus of cancer cells compared with free oxaliplatin [185]. The high intratumoral accumulation of NC-4016 micelles, combined with their subcellular drug targeting, avoiding cytoplasmic detoxification systems and improving intracellular delivery, allowed the formulation to overcome oxaliplatin resistance in vivo in a human CRC model (HT29 and HT29/ox xenografts) [185].

In a mouse model of multiple liver metastases from murine colon adenocarcinoma (C26 cells), mice treated with NC-4016 showed significant reduction in metastatic nodules and liver weight compared with mice treated with oxaliplatin [186]. High levels of NC-4016 were found to accumulate in metastatic livers, producing a strong antitumor effect without severe AEs, which was attributed to significantly higher accumulation of the micellar formulation in the metastatic liver compared with oxaliplatin [186]. On the other hand, distribution of the PMs in healthy livers was limited, demonstrating their selectivity for tumor tissue [186].

The NC-4016 micelles, due to their small size, were able to penetrate poorly permeable pancreatic tumors in mice [187] and to accumulate in orthotopic scirrhous gastric tumors, inhibiting tumor growth and their lymph node metastasis [188]. Repeated systemic administration of NC-4016 (2 mg/kg weekly, for 8 weeks) in a transgenic mouse model of spontaneous murine pancreatic cancer inhibited the growth of primary tumors due to efficient accumulation and penetration in tumor tissue and reduced the development of metastases and ascites, preventing peritoneal metastasis and prolonging the survival of mice [189]. The model used elastase-1-promoted luciferase and simian virus 40 T and t antigens (EL1-luc/TAg) transgenic mice, which continuously express SV40 T oncogene, and can gradually develop cancer and metastasis under viable immunity, angiogenesis, and inflammation processes, consistent with the evolution of human pancreatic cancer, thus avoiding altered microenvironment features present in allograft and xenograft tumor models that may affect the behavior of nanocarriers [189].

Combination therapy with NC-4016 and NC-6300 (EPI micelles) provided higher synergistic activity in mice bearing human gastric (44As3Luc cells) xenografts, exhibiting higher antitumoral activity against the subcutaneous xenografts and improving OS in the orthotopic tumor model compared with the combination EPI plus oxaliplatin, with lower cardiotoxicity and neurotoxicity [190]. The intratumoral concentrations of EPI and platinum were significantly higher upon administration of the PMs in comparison with the conventional drug combination [190].

Functionalization of NC-4016 with the cRGD peptide has been performed based on the peptide inhibitory activity against the development of metastasis and the cytotoxic activity of the DACHPt-loaded PMs, and the capability of cRGD-installed NC-4016 PMs for cooperatively inhibiting the formation and progression of lymph node metastasis was assessed in a syngeneic melanoma model [191]. Both conjugated and non-conjugated micelles showed comparable antitumor activity against the primary tumors and the established metastatic foci in lymph nodes [191]. On the other hand, the conjugated micelles significantly enhanced the efficacy against lymph node metastasis draining from primary tumors through improved inhibition of melanoma cell migration due to the synergistic effect [191].

Additional loading of NC-4016 PMs with gadolinium-diethylenetriaminpentaacetic acid (Gd-DTPA), a magnetic resonance imaging contrast agent, was performed to obtain a formulation suitable for simultaneous imaging and therapy in an orthotopic rat model of hepatocellular carcinoma (N1-S1 rat hepatoma cells) [192]. The incorporation of drug and contrast agent in the micelles corresponded to 45% and 5% of the carboxylic groups in PEG-*b*-p(Glu) copolymers, respectively, and the double-loaded nanocarrier had a size of 33 nm. After a single injection of Gd-DTPA/DACHPt-loaded micelles into the hepatic artery, the micelles achieved strong and specific tumor contrast enhancement, induced high levels of tumor apoptosis, and significantly suppressed tumor size and growth without severe AEs [192]. Survival rate was significantly improved compared with oxaliplatin and saline control groups [192].

A phase 1 dose-escalation and pharmacokinetic study (NCT03168035) of NC-4016 (15–80 $mg/m^2$ IV infusion over 2 h, every 3 weeks) in 34 patients with advanced solid tumors or lymphoma was completed in 2017 but no results have been published yet.

## 5. Polymeric Micelles for Cancer Immunotherapy

Cancer immunotherapies, involving stimulation of innate and adaptive immune responses crucial to antitumor immunity, are mainly based on immune checkpoint inhibitors (ICIs), such as antiprogrammed cell death protein 1 (PD-1) and antiprogrammed death-ligand 1 (PD-L1) antibodies, cell-based therapies like engineered chimeric antigen receptor T cells (CAR-T), and cancer vaccines [193]. However, in many solid tumors the success of immunotherapy is often hampered by primary and acquired resistance. NP-based approaches to improve immune cell infiltration into the immunosuppressive TME have the potential to enhance drug efficacy and overcome therapy resistance [193].

The cytosolic DNA sensing cyclic GMP-AMP synthase (cGAS)-stimulator of interferon genes (STING) pathway represents a promising target for cancer immunotherapy. STING is endogenously activated by 2′,3′-cyclic GMP-AMP (cGAMP), a cyclic dinucleotide synthesized by cGAS in response to cytosolic DNA as a danger signal. Acute genomic stressors induced by radiation, cisplatin, and intrinsic DNA damage are known to generate cytosolic DNA responsible for cGAS-STING activation in cancer cells [194]. Activation of STING by endogenous cGAMP or cGAMP agonists mediates a type-I interferon (IFN-I) response that promotes the maturation and migration of dendritic cells, which in turn presents tumor-associated antigens on major histocompatibility complexes to activate $CD8^+$ T cells for tumor-specific cell killing [194,195].

*ONM-501*

ONM-501, developed by OncoNano Medicine (TX, Southlake, USA), is a dual-activating polyvalent STING agonist comprising cGAMP loaded into PMs made from a STING-activating, pH-sensitive diblock copolymer, $(PEG)_{114}$-*b*-poly $[2\text{-(hexamethyleneimino)ethyl methacrylate}]_{90}$ (PC7A), based on OncoNano OMNI™ proprietary polymer technology, part of the company's proprietary pH-activated micelle platform (ON-BOARD™).

The ultrapH-sensitive (UPS) PC7A copolymers ($pK_a$ 6.9), comprising ionizable seven-membered ring heterocyclic tertiary amine side chains in the hydrophobic segment, exhibit a highly cooperative protonation process upon pH-triggered self-assembly at a critical micellization protonation degree (CMPD) of 0.85 [196]. Below the pH transition threshold (pH < 6.9), the tertiary amine groups become highly protonated, and the micelles dissociate into water-soluble cationic unimers (hydrodynamic diameters < 10 nm) while above the threshold (pH > 6.9) the unimers are deprotonated and become hydrophobic, driving the formation of core–shell PMs (hydrodynamic diameters around 30 nm) [196]. The protonation cooperativity driven by the phase transition of PC7A copolymers occurs at a sharp pH and turns the copolymers into pH-triggered "on–off" switchable nanocarriers due to the bimodal proton distribution between highly protonated unimer ("on") and neutral micelle ("off") states [196]. Thus, PC7A micelles are stable at physiological pH of 7.4, preventing drug leakage and prolonging blood circulation while achieving instantaneous payload release upon exposure to acidic microenvironments [196]. PC7A micelles have been used in tumor vaccines to target early endosomal pH (6.5–7.0) for enhanced cytosolic delivery of tumor antigens and crosspresentation to antigen-presenting cells (APCs) in draining lymph nodes [197].

Furthermore, the ability of PC7A copolymers to bind and activate STING through polyvalent phase condensation led to elevated expressions of costimulatory molecules (CD86) on dendritic cells and rapid release of type-I IFNs, boosting antitumor immunity for cancer immunotherapy [197]. Thus, PC7A is a potent vaccine adjuvant, and PC7A nanovaccines (0.5 μg antigen, 30 μg polymer) showed robust cytotoxic T cell response with low systemic cytokine expression, significantly inhibiting tumor growth in multiple tumor mouse models, including B16-F10 melanoma, colon cancer MC38, and human papillomavirus (HPV)-E6/E7 TC-1 tumors upon subcutaneous injection 5 days after tumor inoculation, followed by a booster shot 5 days later [197]. Combination of the STING-activating PC7A nanovaccine with anti-PD-1 mAb, an immune checkpoint inhibitor, displayed a synergistic effect with 100% survival over 60 days in a TC-1 tumor model. Rechallenging of the tumor-free animals with TC-1 cells led to complete inhibition of tumor growth, suggesting that nanovaccine-induced activation of memory T cells is responsible for the generation of a long-term antitumor response [197]. Interestingly, intratumoral delivery of PC7A nanovaccine achieved stronger antitumor immunity and efficacy compared with subcutaneous delivery [198].

Further studies demonstrated the polyvalent PC7A-induced phase condensation mechanism for STING activation and revealed that PC7A binds to a non-competitive surface-binding site on the protein distinct from the cGAMP-binding pocket (or other cyclic dinucleotides), resulting in prolonged expression of interferon-stimulated genes (*Ifnb1* and *Cxcl10*) compared with the endogenous ligand, with PC7A retaining immune activity in several cGAMP-resistant STING variants [199]. Moreover, cGAMP-loaded PC7A micelles (2.5 μg/50 μg polymer), i.e., ONM-501, showed a synergistic antitumor immune response in tumor-bearing mice, significantly improving long-term survival compared with either free cGAMP (2.5 μg) or empty PC7A micelles (50 μg), upon intratumoral injection [199], as well as in vitro synergistic STING activation in resected human tumors and lymph nodes [199].

At physiological pH, ONM-501 micelles protect cGAMP from enzymatic degradation, prevent drug leakage and systemic toxicity, and enable targeted endolysosome delivery in the acidic pH of the TME through micelle dissociation, releasing both the endogenous ligand and the STING-activating polymer, which produces dual "burst" and "sustained" STING activation, observed across different species [195,200]. Increased IFNB1 and CXCL10 mRNA levels have been found in peripheral blood mononuclear cells (PBMCs) of rats, mice, beagle dogs, cynomolgus monkeys, and humans after 24 h treatment with ONM-501, consistent with STING activation [200].

Single- and multiple-dose toxicology studies in healthy rats and cynomolgus monkeys showed that ONM-501 (7.5–30 mg/kg, subcutaneously) was well tolerated without severe systemic AEs [201]. Dose-dependent increases in lymphocytes and cytokines were observed, consistent with STING activation [202]. Pharmacokinetic and biodistribution studies (in vivo and ex vivo) revealed that systemic exposure of mice to ONM-501 (2.5 μg/50 μg polymer) was lower after intratumoral administration than after subcutaneous administration to healthy mice, consistent with increased retention of both active moieties of ONM-501 (cGAMP and PC7A) within tumors [202].

The combination of cGAMP canonical binding and PC7A polymer non-canonical binding results in synergistic STING activation and provides potent antitumor efficacy in multiple murine syngeneic tumor models, which was further enhanced by combination with the anti-PD1 checkpoint inhibitor [201]. The combination regimen improved therapeutic outcomes compared with monotherapies, in both anti-PD1-sensitive ("hot") and -resistant ("cold") models, and prolonged long-term survival over 100 days in 30%, 40%, 50%, and 80% of animals in MC38, CT26, B16-F10, and A20 tumor models, respectively. Pharmacodynamic analysis showed enhanced tumor T cell infiltration and ONM-501-upregulated PD-L1 expression in tumor tissue [201]. Moreover, tumor inhibition was observed in both primary and distal MC38 tumors in the same animal after treatment with ONM-501 (three intratumoral injections with 3-day interval), the systemic abscopal effect being confirmed by the reduction of lung metastasis in an immune "cold" triple-negative orthotopic breast cancer 4T1 model [200]. ONM-501 has recently entered a first-in-human multicenter phase 1, dose-escalation and dose-expansion study (NCT06022029) in patients with advanced solid tumors and lymphomas, as intratumorally delivered monotherapy and in combination with intravenous cemiplimab-rwlc (Libtayo®, Regeneron), an anti-PD1 mAb [196].

## 6. Polymeric Micelles for Cancer Diagnosis

Polymeric micellar formulations offer several advantages compared with small-molecule contrast agents, including long blood-pool residence times, tumor accumulation by the EPR effect, potential for cancer active targeting and triggered release of payloads, and tunable biodistribution for enhanced contrast specificity between tumor and healthy tissues [28].

In cancer imaging-based diagnosis and monitoring, X-ray computed tomography (CT), single-photon emission computed tomography (SPECT), magnetic resonance imaging (MRI), positron emission tomography (PET), optical imaging, and ultrasonography play important roles [22]. Tumor, node, metastasis (TNM) staging, objective response, and left ventricular ejection fraction (LVEF) are relevant imaging biomarkers in clinical oncology [22].

Moreover, these non-invasive and real-time imaging technologies provide valuable information regarding nanomedicines' pharmacokinetics and biodistribution, tumor accumulation and penetration, and drug release profile, once the appropriate formulation for incorporation of imaging agents and the suitable imaging modality are chosen [28]. In this context, PMs are especially suited since these nanocarriers are able to incorporate both chemotherapeutic drugs and imaging agents, providing a theranostic platform for simultaneous diagnostic/imaging and therapeutic purposes in order to achieve customized and personalized cancer therapy that maximizes drug specificity and efficacy [28].

*Pegsitacianine*

Pegsitacianine (ONM-100) is a pH-activable fluorescent PM made from amphiphilic block copolymers from the proprietary ON-BOARD™ polymeric micelle platform (OncoNano Medicine, Inc., Texas, USA), encapsulating indocyanine green (ICG), an FDA-approved NIR fluorophore [203]. The ON-BOARD™ platform uses UPS block copolymers based on PEG-*b*-PR, where PR is a hydrophobic polymer containing ionizable linear or cyclic tertiary amine groups/side chains [203]. The payloads can be physically entrapped or chemically bound to the polymeric micellar core, protected from systemic exposure [203].

The UPS block copolymers show positive cooperativity resulting from pH-triggered hydrophobic micellization above a sharp pH threshold while at lower pH values the neutral micelles dissociate into protonated dimers, releasing their payloads [204]. These binary on/off switchable systems with a transistor-like response to pH, which allow fine tuning of $pK_a$ and pH transition sharpness by changing the hydrophobic chain length and/or alkyl substituents in the ionizable amino groups, provide useful probes for chemical and biological sensing [204].

The UPS nanoprobe pegsitacianine is an optimized pH-activatable ICG-encoded nanosensor (PINS) with a hydrodynamic diameter of 26.0 $\pm$ 1.1 nm, consisting of block copolymers of hydrophilic PEG and a hydrophobic block of ethylpropylaminoethyl (EPA) methacrylate and 2-aminoethyl methacrylate (AMA) random copolymers, p($EPA_{100}$-r-AMA-ICG), synthesized using the atom transfer radical polymerization (ATRP) method, and covalently conjugated to ICG via an amidation reaction between the AMA primary amine groups and the *N*-hydroxysuccinimide (NHS) ester derivative of ICG [203]. The PM is stable at physiological pH 7.4 and the fluorescence of ICG, sequestered within the hydrophobic segments of the micellar core, is quenched during circulation in the bloodstream due to homo-Förster resonance energy transfer (homo-FRET) between the dye molecules [203]. However, at pH 6.9 the cooperative dissociation of the micelles into the protonated unimers activates the fluorescent dye [203]. Thus, the nanoprobe allows the targeting of the acidic extracellular TME (pH 6.5–6.9), a metabolic hallmark common to most solid tumors regardless of their histology or anatomic location, avoiding the use of specific surface biomarkers with limited therapeutic utility due to genetic or phenotypic heterogeneity [203]. The pH nanotransistor, with binary off/on response at a transition pH of 6.9, amplifies the fluorescence signal in the tumor over that in the surrounding normal tissues, with suppression of signal in blood (pH 7.4) [203].

Pegsitacianine (2.5 mg/kg IV injection 24 h prior to imaging) was able to detect a broad range of human tumors (head and neck, breast, peritoneal metastasis, kidney, brain, and pancreatic tumors) in mouse models using existing clinical cameras [203]. Furthermore, pegsitacianine administration (2.5 mg/kg IV injection 12–24 h before surgery) to mice bearing human head and neck HN5 or triple-negative 4T1 breast orthotopic tumors allowed real-time tumor-acidosis-guided surgery (TAGS) of occult nodules (<1 $mm^3$), significantly improving mice survival [203]. In murine flank xenograft models of lung cancer, the probe selectively labeled human adenocarcinoma (A549) as well as human squamous cell carcinoma (H1264) xenografts, with mean tumor-to-background ratio (TBR) > 2.0 for both histologic subtypes of lung cancer, according to NIR images 24 h after injection of 2 mg/kg pegsitacianine and further confirmed by microscopic analysis of tumor sections [205]. Pegsitacianine (1 mg/kg, IV) was administered to patients undergoing lung cancer surgery as part of an ongoing phase 2 trial (NCT05048082), now completed, and in the human pilot study the nanoprobe localized pulmonary adenocarcinoma (TBR 2.7) and pulmonary squamous cell carcinoma (TBR 2.4) in real time, corroborating successful clinical translation as an IMI probe to label human lung cancer [205].

A phase 1 clinical trial in the Netherlands (EudraCT 2017-003543-38, the SHINE study) exploiting metabolic acidosis in solid cancers using pegsitacianine for fluorescence-guided surgery reported that a 1.2 mg/kg single IV infusion of the nanoprobe 24 h ± 8 h prior to oncologic surgery was well tolerated and allowed visualization of four solid tumor types (HNSCC, breast cancer, esophageal cancer, and CRC) in 30 patients, both in vivo and ex vivo [206]. Among these patients, 13 subjects with HNSCC demonstrated that a fluorescent lesion on the surgical specimen with a TBR > 1.5 was correlated to a tumor-positive resection margin, detected directly after excision by fluorescence-guided intraoperative imaging [207].

During intraoperative fluorescence imaging, pegsitacianine enabled visualization of all the tumor-positive resection margins undetected during standard of care (SOC) surgery, which correlated with the final histopathological evaluation, yielding 100% sensitivity and no false negatives [206]. Moreover, additional occult lesions were identified via pegsitacianine fluorescence in five patients that would have been missed in SOC surgery [206]. This phase 1 study was the first to report a systemically administered probe displaying nanoscale cooperativity to overcome metabolic and phenotypic variability between different patients and tumors, with no overlap between tumor and background fluorescence [206].

In a non-randomized, open-label, phase 2 study (NCT04950166), administration of a single IV dose of pegsitacianine (1 mg/kg) to 50 patients 24–72 h before cytoreductive surgery and re-examination of the peritoneal cavity under NIR illumination following surgery allowed identification of eventual fluorescent tissue, which was excised and evaluated by histopathology [208]. Among the 40 patients evaluable for clinically significant events across six primary tumor types, residual disease was detected with pegsitacianine in 20 (50%) of them, and the high rate of occult residual disease detected suggests that the use of the probe can improve surgeon assessment and performance during cytoreductive surgery [208]. The probe showed high sensitivity and the absence of serious AEs, with only transient non-anaphylactic infusion reactions reported in 28% of patients [208]. Pegsitacianine has received Breakthrough Therapy Designation by the FDA as an adjunct for the visualization of metastatic disease in the peritoneal cavity in patients undergoing cytoreductive surgery in 2022 and is ready for phase 3 clinical evaluation.

## 7. Conclusions

Despite advancements in early detection and therapies, cancer remains a significant global health issue with a high incidence and mortality rate. Conventional chemotherapy is recognized as an effective and extensively used therapeutic option for most types of cancers. However, lack of selectivity, side effects, toxicity, and drug resistance are the main concerns, which can be potentially overcome by nanotechnology. Among nanoparticulate systems targeted to cancer cells, PMs stand out, efficiently encapsulating poorly water-soluble chemotherapeutic drugs, with their size, morphology, and solubility impacting circulation. They are simple to manufacture, increase the efficiency of drug loading, and can be easily customized and tailored to meet specific needs, which constitutes a distinct advantage over other nanoparticulate DDSs. PEGylation, decoration with targeting moieties, charge conversion, crosslinking of the core, and development of stimuli-responsive PMs have been employed to avoid MPS uptake, ameliorate pharmacokinetic properties, improve cellular internalization, and enhance selectivity of drug delivery towards cancer cells.

However, instability and a lack of economically viable production strategies restrict clinical translation, which will require better management of the partnership between the in vivo behavior and the physicochemical properties of PMs requiring an interplay between various domains of knowledge like chemistry, physics, biology, and nanomedicine. Nevertheless, several polymeric micellar formulations have entered clinical trials, and a few have obtained regulatory approval, such as Genexol®-PM and Nanoxel®, which have been in the clinic for almost twenty years.

Clinical failures of PMs may involve the payload, deficient tumor accumulation, the selection of individuals with diverse demographics, and more advanced tumor progression. Additionally, passive targeting by the EPR effect can differ significantly over time between patients and different tumor types, as well as within the same patient population, which could justify its publicized failure in the clinic. On the other hand, no animal model can accurately replicate all the features of human malignancy. Another major concern is the sustainable manufacture of high-quality clinical-grade PMs that adhere to Good Manufacturing Practice (GMP) standards, and the clinical safety issues related to toxicity.

Future directions for a successful translational from preclinical demonstrations to the multifunctional PMs loaded with anticancer drugs in the clinical setting may entail (i) stratification of patients; (ii) improved target-driven design; (iii) combined applications in the form of both multidrug nanomaterials and multimodal treatments; and (iv) advice from regulators who can identify any potential problems affecting the approval of the nanoformulation.

**Author Contributions:** Conceptualization, writing, review and editing, A.S., C.F. and L.P. All authors have read and agreed to the published version of the manuscript.

**Funding:** This research received no external funding.

**Institutional Review Board Statement:** Not applicable.

**Informed Consent Statement:** Not applicable.

**Data Availability Statement:** Not applicable.

**Conflicts of Interest:** The authors declare no conflicts of interest.

## References

1. Avramović, N.; Mandić, B.; Savić-Radojević, A.; Simić, T. Polymeric Nanocarriers of Drug Delivery Systems in Cancer Therapy. *Pharmaceutics* **2020**, *12*, 298. [CrossRef] [PubMed]
2. Cordani, M.; Dando, I.; Ambrosini, G.; González-Menéndez, P. Signaling, Cancer Cell Plasticity, and Intratumor Heterogeneity. *Cell Commun. Signal.* **2024**, *22*, 255. [CrossRef] [PubMed]
3. Negut, I.; Bita, B. Polymeric Micellar Systems—A Special Emphasis on "Smart" Drug Delivery. *Pharmaceutics* **2023**, *15*, 976. [CrossRef] [PubMed]

4. WHO Global Cancer Burden Growing, Amidst Mounting Need for Services. Available online: https://www.who.int/news/item/01-02-2024-global-cancer-burden-growing--amidst-mounting-need-for-services (accessed on 28 July 2024).
5. Wu, S.; Zhu, W.; Thompson, P.; Hannun, Y.A. Evaluating Intrinsic and Non-Intrinsic Cancer Risk Factors. *Nat. Commun.* **2018**, *9*, 3490. [CrossRef] [PubMed]
6. Vaghari-Tabari, M.; Ferns, G.A.; Qujeq, D.; Andevari, A.N.; Sabahi, Z.; Moein, S. Signaling, Metabolism, and Cancer: An Important Relationship for Therapeutic Intervention. *J. Cell. Physiol.* **2021**, *236*, 5512–5532. [CrossRef] [PubMed]
7. Institute for Health Metrics and Evaluation (IHME) Global Burden of Disease Collaborative Network. Available online: https://www.healthdata.org/gbd/2019 (accessed on 5 July 2024).
8. de Visser, K.E.; Joyce, J.A. The Evolving Tumor Microenvironment: From Cancer Initiation to Metastatic Outgrowth. *Cancer Cell* **2023**, *41*, 374–403. [CrossRef] [PubMed]
9. Tilsed, C.M.; Fisher, S.A.; Nowak, A.K.; Lake, R.A.; Lesterhuis, W.J. Cancer Chemotherapy: Insights into Cellular and Tumor Microenvironmental Mechanisms of Action. *Front. Oncol.* **2022**, *12*, 960317. [CrossRef] [PubMed]
10. Bajracharya, R.; Song, J.G.; Patil, B.R.; Lee, S.H.; Noh, H.M.; Kim, D.H.; Kim, G.L.; Seo, S.H.; Park, J.W.; Jeong, S.H.; et al. Functional Ligands for Improving Anticancer Drug Therapy: Current Status and Applications to Drug Delivery Systems. *Drug Deliv.* **2022**, *29*, 1959–1970. [CrossRef] [PubMed]
11. Hong, L.; Li, W.; Li, Y.; Yin, S. Nanoparticle-Based Drug Delivery Systems Targeting Cancer Cell Surfaces. *RSC Adv.* **2023**, *13*, 21365–21382. [CrossRef]
12. Barba, I.; Carrillo-Bosch, L.; Seoane, J. Targeting the Warburg Effect in Cancer: Where Do We Stand? *Int. J. Mol. Sci.* **2024**, *25*, 3142. [CrossRef]
13. Dickens, E.; Ahmed, S. Principles of Cancer Treatment by Chemotherapy. *Surgery* **2018**, *36*, 134–138. [CrossRef]
14. Liu, J.; Wang, H.; Yi, X.; Chao, Y.; Geng, Y.; Xu, L.; Yang, K.; Liu, Z. PH-Sensitive Dissociable Nanoscale Coordination Polymers with Drug Loading for Synergistically Enhanced Chemoradiotherapy. *Adv. Funct. Mater.* **2017**, *27*, 1703832. [CrossRef]
15. Behranvand, N.; Nasri, F.; Zolfaghari Emameh, R.; Khani, P.; Hosseini, A.; Garssen, J.; Falak, R. Chemotherapy: A Double-Edged Sword in Cancer Treatment. *Cancer Immunol. Immunother.* **2022**, *71*, 507–526. [CrossRef] [PubMed]
16. Bholakant, R.; Dong, B.; Zhou, X.; Huang, X.; Zhao, C.; Huang, D.; Zhong, Y.; Qian, H.; Chen, W.; Feijen, J. Multi-Functional Polymeric Micelles for Chemotherapy-Based Combined Cancer Therapy. *J. Mater. Chem. B* **2021**, *9*, 8718–8738. [CrossRef]
17. Wan, Z.; Zheng, R.; Moharil, P.; Liu, Y.; Chen, J.; Sun, R.; Song, X.; Ao, Q. Polymeric Micelles in Cancer Immunotherapy. *Molecules* **2021**, *26*, 1220. [CrossRef]
18. Wei, J.; Long, Y.; Guo, R.; Liu, X.; Tang, X.; Rao, J.; Yin, S.; Zhang, Z.; Li, M.; He, Q. Multifunctional Polymeric Micelle-Based Chemo-Immunotherapy with Immune Checkpoint Blockade for Efficient Treatment of Orthotopic and Metastatic Breast Cancer. *Acta Pharm. Sin. B* **2019**, *9*, 819–831. [CrossRef]
19. Roma-Rodrigues, C.; Mendes, R.; Baptista, P.V.; Fernandes, A.R. Targeting Tumor Microenvironment for Cancer Therapy. *Int. J. Mol. Sci.* **2019**, *20*, 840. [CrossRef] [PubMed]
20. Parodi, A.; Kolesova, E.P.; Voronina, M.V.; Frolova, A.S.; Kostyushev, D.; Trushina, D.B.; Akasov, R.; Pallaeva, T.; Zamyatnin, A.A. Anticancer Nanotherapeutics in Clinical Trials: The Work behind Clinical Translation of Nanomedicine. *Int. J. Mol. Sci.* **2022**, *23*, 13368. [CrossRef]
21. Ghosh, B.; Biswas, S. Polymeric Micelles in Cancer Therapy: State of the Art. *J. Control. Release* **2021**, *332*, 127–147. [CrossRef]
22. Hossen, S.; Hossain, M.K.; Basher, M.K.; Mia, M.N.H.; Rahman, M.T.; Uddin, M.J. Smart Nanocarrier-Based Drug Delivery Systems for Cancer Therapy and Toxicity Studies: A Review. *J. Adv. Res.* **2019**, *15*, 1–18. [CrossRef]
23. Augustine, R.; Hasan, A.; Primavera, R.; Wilson, R.J.; Thakor, A.S.; Kevadiya, B.D. Cellular Uptake and Retention of Nanoparticles: Insights on Particle Properties and Interaction with Cellular Components. *Mater. Today Commun.* **2020**, *25*, 101692. [CrossRef]
24. Maboudi, A.H.; Lotfipour, M.H.; Rasouli, M.; Azhdari, M.H.; MacLoughlin, R.; Bekeschus, S.; Doroudian, M. Micelle-Based Nanoparticles with Stimuli-Responsive Properties for Drug Delivery. *Nanotechnol. Rev.* **2024**, *13*, 20230218. [CrossRef]
25. Postovalova, A.S.; Tishchenko, Y.A.; Istomina, M.S.; Karpov, T.E.; Shipilovskikh, S.A.; Akhmetova, D.; Rogova, A.; Gavrilova, N.V.; Timin, A.S. Comparison of Passive Targeted Delivery of Inorganic and Organic Nanocarriers among Different Types of Tumors. *Nanomedicine* **2024**, *59*, 102753. [CrossRef] [PubMed]
26. Wang, Q.; Atluri, K.; Tiwari, A.K.; Babu, R.J. Exploring the Application of Micellar Drug Delivery Systems in Cancer Nanomedicine. *Pharmaceuticals* **2023**, *16*, 433. [CrossRef] [PubMed]
27. Su, C.; Liu, Y.; Li, R.; Wu, W.; Fawcett, J.P.; Gu, J. Absorption, Distribution, Metabolism and Excretion of the Biomaterials Used in Nanocarrier Drug Delivery Systems. *Adv. Drug Deliv. Rev.* **2019**, *143*, 97–114. [CrossRef] [PubMed]
28. Movassaghian, S.; Merkel, O.M.; Torchilin, V.P. Applications of Polymer Micelles for Imaging and Drug Delivery. *Wiley Interdiscip. Rev. Nanomed. Nanobiotechnol.* **2015**, *7*, 691–707. [CrossRef] [PubMed]
29. Chaudhuri, A.; Ramesh, K.; Kumar, D.N.; Dehari, D.; Singh, S.; Kumar, D.; Agrawal, A.K. Polymeric Micelles: A Novel Drug Delivery System for the Treatment of Breast Cancer. *J. Drug Deliv. Sci. Technol.* **2022**, *77*, 103886. [CrossRef]
30. Nasr, M.; Hashem, F.; Teiama, M.; Tantawy, N.; Abdelmoniem, R. Folic Acid Grafted Mixed Polymeric Micelles as a Targeted Delivery Strategy for Tamoxifen Citrate in Treatment of Breast Cancer. *Drug Deliv. Transl. Res.* **2024**, *14*, 945–958. [CrossRef] [PubMed]
31. Fu, Z.; Xiang, J. Aptamer-Functionalized Nanoparticles in Targeted Delivery and Cancer Therapy. *Int. J. Mol. Sci.* **2020**, *21*, 9123. [CrossRef]

32. Cao, Z.; Zuo, X.; Liu, X.; Xu, G.; Yong, K.T. Recent Progress in Stimuli-Responsive Polymeric Micelles for Targeted Delivery of Functional Nanoparticles. *Adv. Colloid Interface Sci.* **2024**, *330*, 103206. [CrossRef]
33. Zhou, Q.; Zhang, L.; Yang, T.H.; Wu, H. Stimuli-Responsive Polymeric Micelles for Drug Delivery and Cancer Therapy. *Int. J. Nanomed.* **2018**, *13*, 2921–2942. [CrossRef] [PubMed]
34. Khan, S.; Vahdani, Y.; Hussain, A.; Haghighat, S.; Heidari, F.; Nouri, M.; Bloukh, S.H.; Edis, Z.; Babadaei, M.M.N.; Ale-Ebrahim, M.; et al. Polymeric Micelles Functionalized with Cell Penetrating Peptides as Potential PH-Sensitive Platforms in Drug Delivery for Cancer Therapy: A Review. *Arab. J. Chem.* **2021**, *14*, 103264. [CrossRef]
35. Zhang, Z.; Wang, L.; Guo, Z.; Sun, Y.; Yan, J. A PH-Sensitive Imidazole Grafted Polymeric Micelles Nanoplatform Based on ROS Amplification for Ferroptosis-Enhanced Chemodynamic Therapy. *Colloids Surf. B Biointerfaces* **2024**, *237*, 113871. [CrossRef] [PubMed]
36. Slor, G.; Tevet, S.; Amir, R.J. Stimuli-Induced Architectural Transition as a Tool for Controlling the Enzymatic Degradability of Polymeric Micelles. *ACS Polym. Au* **2022**, *2*, 380–386. [CrossRef]
37. Liu, J.; Jia, B.; Li, Z.; Li, W. Reactive Oxygen Species-Responsive Polymer Drug Delivery Systems. *Front. Bioeng. Biotechnol.* **2023**, *11*, 1115603. [CrossRef] [PubMed]
38. Long, M.; Liu, X.; Huang, X.; Lu, M.; Wu, X.; Weng, L.; Chen, Q.; Wang, X.; Zhu, L.; Chen, Z. Alendronate-Functionalized Hypoxia-Responsive Polymeric Micelles for Targeted Therapy of Bone Metastatic Prostate Cancer. *J. Control. Release* **2021**, *334*, 303–317. [CrossRef]
39. Van Der Vlies, A.J.; Xu, J.; Ghasemi, M.; Bator, C.; Bell, A.; Rosoff-Verbit, B.; Liu, B.; Gomez, E.D.; Hasegawa, U. Thioether-Based Polymeric Micelles with Fine-Tuned Oxidation Sensitivities for Chemotherapeutic Drug Delivery. *Biomacromolecules* **2022**, *23*, 77–88. [CrossRef] [PubMed]
40. Nishimura, S.; Nishida, K.; Ueda, T.; Shiomoto, S.; Tanaka, M. Biocompatible Poly(*N* -(ω-Acryloyloxy- *n* -Alkyl)-2-Pyrrolidone)s with Widely-Tunable Lower Critical Solution Temperatures (LCSTs): A Promising Alternative to Poly(*N* -Isopropylacrylamide). *Polym. Chem.* **2022**, *13*, 2519–2530. [CrossRef]
41. Miranda, M.S.; Almeida, A.F.; Gomes, M.E.; Rodrigues, M.T. Magnetic Micellar Nanovehicles: Prospects of Multifunctional Hybrid Systems for Precision Theranostics. *Int. J. Mol. Sci.* **2022**, *23*, 11793. [CrossRef]
42. Guzmán Rodríguez, A.; Sablón Carrazana, M.; Rodríguez Tanty, C.; Malessy, M.J.A.; Fuentes, G.; Cruz, L.J. Smart Polymeric Micelles for Anticancer Hydrophobic Drugs. *Cancers* **2023**, *15*, 4. [CrossRef]
43. Farjadian, F.; Ghasemi, S.; Akbarian, M.; Hoseini-Ghahfarokhi, M.; Moghoofei, M.; Doroudian, M. Physically Stimulus-Responsive Nanoparticles for Therapy and Diagnosis. *Front. Chem.* **2022**, *10*, 952675. [CrossRef] [PubMed]
44. Overchuk, M.; Weersink, R.A.; Wilson, B.C.; Zheng, G. Photodynamic and Photothermal Therapies: Synergy Opportunities for Nanomedicine. *ACS Nano* **2023**, *17*, 7979–8003. [CrossRef] [PubMed]
45. Wei, P.; Cornel, E.J.; Du, J. Ultrasound-Responsive Polymer-Based Drug Delivery Systems. *Drug Deliv. Transl. Res.* **2021**, *11*, 1323–1339. [CrossRef] [PubMed]
46. Zhang, X.; He, N.; Zhang, L.; Dai, T.; Sun, Z.; Shi, Y.; Li, S.; Yu, N. Application of High Intensity Focused Ultrasound Combined with Nanomaterials in Anti-Tumor Therapy. *Drug Deliv.* **2024**, *31*, 2342844. [CrossRef] [PubMed]
47. Kolosnjaj-Tabi, J.; Gibot, L.; Fourquaux, I.; Golzio, M.; Rols, M.P. Electric Field-Responsive Nanoparticles and Electric Fields: Physical, Chemical, Biological Mechanisms and Therapeutic Prospects. *Adv. Drug Deliv. Rev.* **2019**, *138*, 56–67. [CrossRef] [PubMed]
48. Kuperkar, K.; Patel, D.; Atanase, L.I.; Bahadur, P. Amphiphilic Block Copolymers: Their Structures, and Self-Assembly to Polymeric Micelles and Polymersomes as Drug Delivery Vehicles. *Polymers* **2022**, *14*, 4702. [CrossRef] [PubMed]
49. Raval, N.; Maheshwari, R.; Shukla, H.; Kalia, K.; Torchilin, V.P.; Tekade, R.K. Multifunctional Polymeric Micellar Nanomedicine in the Diagnosis and Treatment of Cancer. *Mater. Sci. Eng. C* **2021**, *126*, 112186. [CrossRef]
50. Talelli, M.; Barz, M.; Rijcken, C.J.F.; Kiessling, F.; Hennink, W.E.; Lammers, T. Core-Crosslinked Polymeric Micelles: Principles, Preparation, Biomedical Applications and Clinical Translation. *Nano Today* **2015**, *10*, 93–117. [CrossRef] [PubMed]
51. Kim, T.-Y.; Kim, D.-W.; Chung, J.-Y.; Shin, S.G.; Kim, S.-C.; Heo, D.S.; Kim, N.K.; Bang, Y.-J. Phase I and Pharmacokinetic Study of Genexol-PM, a Cremophor-Free, Polymeric Micelle-Formulated Paclitaxel, in Patients with Advanced Malignancies. *Clin. Cancer Res.* **2004**, *10*, 3708–3716. [CrossRef]
52. Lim, W.T.; Tan, E.H.; Toh, C.K.; Hee, S.W.; Leong, S.S.; Ang, P.C.S.; Wong, N.S.; Chowbay, B. Phase I Pharmacokinetic Study of a Weekly Liposomal Paclitaxel Formulation (Genexol®-PM) in Patients with Solid Tumors. *Ann. Oncol.* **2009**, *21*, 382–388. [CrossRef]
53. Ibrahim, N.K.; Desai, N.; Legha, S.; Soon-Shiong, P.; Theriault, R.L.; Rivera, E.; Esmaeli, B.; Ring, S.E.; Bedikian, A.; Hortobagyi, G.N.; et al. Phase I and Pharmacokinetic Study of ABI-007, a Cremophor-Free, Protein-Stabilized, Nanoparticle Formulation of Paclitaxel 1. *Clin. Cancer Res.* **2002**, *8*, 1038–1044. [PubMed]
54. Mross, K.; Hollaè, N.; Hauns, B.; Schumacher, M.; Maier-Lenz, H. The Pharmacokinetics of a 1-h Paclitaxel Infusion. *Cancer Chemother. Pharmacol.* **2000**, *45*, 463–470. [CrossRef] [PubMed]
55. Shi, M.; Sun, J.; Zhou, J.; Yu, H.; Yu, S.; Xia, G.; Wang, L.; Teng, Y.; Liu, G.; Yu, C.; et al. Phase I Dose Escalation and Pharmacokinetic Study on the Nanoparticle Formulation of Polymeric Micellar Paclitaxel for Injection in Patients with Advanced Solid Malignancies. *Investig. New Drugs* **2018**, *36*, 269–277. [CrossRef] [PubMed]

56. Bapsy, P.; Raghunadharao, D.; Majumdar, A.; Ganguly, S.; Roy, A.; Uppal, G.; Mukherjee, R.; Burman, A.; Saha, N. DO/NDR/02 a Novel Polymeric Nanoparticle Paclitaxel: Results of a Phase I Dose Escalation Study. *J. Clin. Oncol.* **2004**, *22*, 2026. [CrossRef]
57. Hamaguchi, T.; Kato, K.; Yasui, H.; Morizane, C.; Ikeda, M.; Ueno, H.; Muro, K.; Yamada, Y.; Okusaka, T.; Shirao, K.; et al. A Phase I and Pharmacokinetic Study of NK105, a Paclitaxel-Incorporating Micellar Nanoparticle Formulation. *Br. J. Cancer* **2007**, *97*, 170–176. [CrossRef] [PubMed]
58. Mukai, H.; Kato, K.; Esaki, T.; Ohsumi, S.; Hozomi, Y.; Matsubara, N.; Hamaguchi, T.; Matsumura, Y.; Goda, R.; Hirai, T.; et al. Phase I Study of NK105, a Nanomicellar Paclitaxel Formulation, Administered on a Weekly Schedule in Patients with Solid Tumors. *Investig. New Drugs* **2016**, *34*, 750–759. [CrossRef] [PubMed]
59. Atrafi, F.; Dumez, H.; Mathijssen, R.H.J.; van der Houven van Oordt, C.W.M.; Rijcken, C.J.F.; Hanssen, R.; Eskens, F.A.L.M. Schöffski, P. A Phase I Dose-Escalation and Pharmacokinetic Study of a Micellar Nanoparticle with Entrapped Docetaxel (CPC634) in Patients with Advanced Solid Tumours. *J. Control. Release* **2020**, *325*, 191–197. [CrossRef] [PubMed]
60. Atrafi, F.; van Eerden, R.A.G.; van Hylckama Vlieg, M.A.M.; Hoop, E.O.; de Bruijn, P.; Lolkema, M.P.; Moelker, A.; Rijcken, C.J. Hanssen, R.; Sparreboom, A.; et al. Intratumoral Comparison of Nanoparticle Entrapped Docetaxel (CPC634) with Conventional Docetaxel in Patients with Solid Tumors. *Clin. Cancer Res.* **2020**, *26*, 3537–3545. [CrossRef]
61. Extra, J.-M.; Rousseau, F.; Bruno, R.; Clavel, M.; Le Bail, N.; Marty, M. Phase I and Pharmacokinetic Study of Taxotere (RP 56976, NSC 628503) Given as a Short Intravenous Infusion. *Cancer Res.* **1993**, *53*, 1037–1042.
62. Hamaguchi, T.; Doi, T.; Eguchi-Nakajima, T.; Kato, K.; Yamada, Y.; Shimada, Y.; Fuse, N.; Ohtsu, A.; Matsumoto, S.I.; Takanashi, M.; et al. Phase I Study of NK012, a Novel SN-38-Incorporating Micellar Nanoparticle, in Adult Patients with Solid Tumors. *Clin. Cancer Res.* **2010**, *16*, 5058–5066. [CrossRef]
63. Burris, H.A.; Infante, J.R.; Anthony Greco, F.; Thompson, D.S.; Barton, J.H.; Bendell, J.C.; Nambu, Y.; Watanabe, N.; Jones, S.F. A Phase I Dose Escalation Study of NK012, an SN-38 Incorporating Macromolecular Polymeric Micelle. *Cancer Chemother. Pharmacol.* **2016**, *77*, 1079–1086. [CrossRef] [PubMed]
64. Matsumura, Y.; Hamaguchi, T.; Ura, T.; Muro, K.; Yamada, Y.; Shimada, Y.; Shirao, K.; Okusaka, T.; Ueno, H.; Ikeda, M.; et al. Phase I Clinical Trial and Pharmacokinetic Evaluation of NK911, a Micelle-Encapsulated Doxorubicin. *Br. J. Cancer* **2004**, *91*, 1775–1781. [CrossRef]
65. Gabizon, A.; Catane, R.; Uziely, B.; Kaufman, B.; Safra, T.; Cohen, R.; Martin, F.; Huang, A.; Barenholz, Y. Prolonged Circulation Time and Enhanced Accumulation in Malignant Exudates of Doxorubicin Encapsulated in Polyethylene-Glycol Coated Liposomes. *Cancer* **1994**, *154*, 987–992.
66. Danson, S.; Ferry, D.; Alakhov, V.; Margison, J.; Kerr, D.; Jowle, D.; Brampton, M.; Halbert, G.; Ranson, M. Phase I Dose Escalation and Pharmacokinetic Study of Pluronic Polymer-Bound Doxorubicin (SP1049C) in Patients with Advanced Cancer. *Br. J. Cancer* **2004**, *90*, 2085–2091. [CrossRef]
67. Chawla, S.P.; Goel, S.; Chow, W.; Braiteh, F.; Singh, A.S.; Olson, J.E.G.; Osada, A.; Bobe, I.; Riedel, R.F. A Phase 1b Dose Escalation Trial of NC-6300 (Nanoparticle Epirubicin) in Patients with Advanced Solid Tumors or Advanced, Metastatic, or Unresectable Soft-Tissue Sarcoma. *Clin. Cancer Res.* **2020**, *26*, 4225–4232. [CrossRef]
68. Volovat, S.R.; Ciuleanu, T.-E.; Koralewski, P.; Olson, J.E.G.; Croitoru, A.; Koynov, K.; Stabile, S.; Cerea, G.; Osada, A.; Bobe, I.; et al. A Multicenter, Single-Arm, Basket Design, Phase II Study of NC-6004 plus Gemcitabine in Patients with Advanced Unresectable Lung, Biliary Tract, or Bladder Cancer. *Oncotarget* **2020**, *11*, 3105–3117. [CrossRef]
69. Plummer, R.; Wilson, R.H.; Calvert, H.; Boddy, A.V.; Griffin, M.; Sludden, J.; Tilby, M.J.; Eatock, M.; Pearson, D.G.; Ottley, C.J.; et al. A Phase i Clinical Study of Cisplatin-Incorporated Polymeric Micelles (NC-6004) in Patients with Solid Tumours. *Br. J. Cancer* **2011**, *104*, 593–598. [CrossRef]
70. Guo, Y.; Yang, X.; Zhang, Y.; Luo, F.; Yang, J.; Zhang, X.; Mi, J.; Xie, Y. Hyaluronic Acid/Dextran-Based Polymeric Micelles Co-Delivering Ursolic Acid and Doxorubicin to Mitochondria for Potentiating Chemotherapy in MDR Cancer. *Carbohydr. Polym.* **2024**, *332*, 121897. [CrossRef] [PubMed]
71. Jin, G.W.; Rejinold, N.S.; Choy, J.H. Multifunctional Polymeric Micelles for Cancer Therapy. *Polymers* **2022**, *14*, 4839. [CrossRef]
72. Yang, Y.; Yun, K.; Li, Y.; Zhang, L.; Zhao, W.; Zhu, Z.; Tian, B.; Chen, F.; Pan, W. Self-Assembled Multifunctional Polymeric Micelles for Tumor-Specific Bioimaging and Synergistic Chemo-Phototherapy of Cancer. *Int. J. Pharm.* **2021**, *602*, 120651. [CrossRef]
73. Hasenstein, J.R.; Shin, H.C.; Kasmerchak, K.; Buehler, D.; Kwon, G.S.; Kozak, K.R. Antitumor Activity of Triolimus: A Novel Multidrug-Loaded Micelle Containing Paclitaxel, Rapamycin, and 17-AAG. *Mol. Cancer Ther.* **2012**, *11*, 2233–2242. [CrossRef] [PubMed]
74. Cho, H.; Kwon, G.S. Polymeric Micelles for Neoadjuvant Cancer Therapy and Tumor-Primed Optical Imaging. *ACS Nano* **2011**, *5*, 8721–8729. [CrossRef] [PubMed]
75. Sofias, A.M.; Dunne, M.; Storm, G.; Allen, C. The Battle of "Nano" Paclitaxel. *Adv. Drug Deliv. Rev.* **2017**, *122*, 20–30. [CrossRef] [PubMed]
76. Le, B.; Powers, G.L.; Tam, Y.T.; Schumacher, N.; Malinowski, R.L.; Steinke, L.; Kwon, G.; Marker, P.C. Multi-Drug Loaded Micelles Delivering Chemotherapy and Targeted Therapies Directed against HSP90 and the PI3K/AKT/MTOR Pathway in Prostate Cancer. *PLoS ONE* **2017**, *12*, e0174658. [CrossRef]
77. Hosseini, S.M.; Mohammadnejad, J.; Salamat, S.; Beiram Zadeh, Z.; Tanhaei, M.; Ramakrishna, S. Theranostic Polymeric Nanoparticles as a New Approach in Cancer Therapy and Diagnosis: A Review. *Mater. Today Chem.* **2023**, *29*, 101400. [CrossRef]

78. Bernabeu, E.; Cagel, M.; Lagomarsino, E.; Moretton, M.; Chiappetta, D.A. Paclitaxel: What Has Been Done and the Challenges Remain Ahead. *Int. J. Pharm.* **2017**, *526*, 474–495. [CrossRef] [PubMed]
79. Gong, J.; Chen, M.; Zheng, Y.; Wang, S.; Wang, Y. Polymeric Micelles Drug Delivery System in Oncology. *J. Control. Release* **2012**, *159*, 312–323. [CrossRef]
80. Gelderblom, H.; Verweij, J.; Nooter, K.; Sparreboom, A. Cremophor EL: The Drawbacks and Advantages of Vehicle Selection for Drug Formulation. *Eur. J. Cancer* **2001**, *37*, 1590–1598. [CrossRef]
81. Lee, S.W.; Yun, M.H.; Jeong, S.W.; In, C.H.; Kim, J.Y.; Seo, M.H.; Pai, C.M.; Kim, S.O. Development of Docetaxel-Loaded Intravenous Formulation, Nanoxel-PM$^{TM}$ Using Polymer-Based Delivery System. *J. Control. Release* **2011**, *155*, 262–271. [CrossRef]
82. Jia, Y.; Jiang, Y.; He, Y.; Zhang, W.; Zou, J.; Magar, K.T.; Boucetta, H.; Teng, C.; He, W. Approved Nanomedicine against Diseases. *Pharmaceutics* **2023**, *15*, 774. [CrossRef]
83. Zheng, X.; Xie, J.; Zhang, X.; Sun, W.; Zhao, H.; Li, Y.; Wang, C. An Overview of Polymeric Nanomicelles in Clinical Trials and on the Market. *Chin. Chem. Lett.* **2021**, *32*, 243–257. [CrossRef]
84. Schwartzberg, L.S.; Navari, R.M. Safety of Polysorbate 80 in the Oncology Setting. *Adv. Ther.* **2018**, *35*, 754–767. [CrossRef] [PubMed]
85. Kim, S.C.; Kim, D.W.; Shim, Y.H.; Seok Bang, J.; Oh, H.S.; Kim, S.W.; Seo, M.H. In Vivo Evaluation of Polymeric Micellar Paclitaxel Formulation: Toxicity and Efficacy. *J. Control. Release* **2001**, *72*, 191–202. [CrossRef] [PubMed]
86. Werner, M.E.; Cummings, N.D.; Sethi, M.; Wang, E.C.; Sukumar, R.; Moore, D.T.; Wang, A.Z. Preclinical Evaluation of Genexol-Pm, a Nanoparticle Formulation of Paclitaxel, as a Novel Radiosensitizer for the Treatment of Non-Small Cell Lung Cancer. *Int. J. Radiat. Oncol. Biol. Phys.* **2013**, *86*, 463–468. [CrossRef] [PubMed]
87. Van Zuylen, L.; Karlsson, M.O.; Verweij, J.; Brouwer, E.; De Bruijn, P.; Nooter, K.; Stoter, G.; Sparreboom, A. Pharmacokinetic Modeling of Paclitaxel Encapsulation in Cremophor EL Micelles. *Cancer Chemother. Pharmacol.* **2001**, *47*, 309–318. [CrossRef] [PubMed]
88. Lee, K.S.; Chung, H.C.; Im, S.A.; Park, Y.H.; Kim, C.S.; Kim, S.B.; Rha, S.Y.; Lee, M.Y.; Ro, J. Multicenter Phase II Trial of Genexol-PM, a Cremophor-Free, Polymeric Micelle Formulation of Paclitaxel, in Patients with Metastatic Breast Cancer. *Breast Cancer Res. Treat.* **2008**, *108*, 241–250. [CrossRef] [PubMed]
89. Saif, M.W.; Podoltsev, N.A.; Rubin, M.S.; Figueroa, J.A.; Lee, M.Y.; Kwon, J.; Rowen, E.; Yu, J.; Kerr, R.O. Phase II Clinical Trial of Paclitaxel Loaded Polymeric Micelle in Patients with Advanced Pancreatic Cancer. *Cancer Investig.* **2010**, *28*, 186–194. [CrossRef] [PubMed]
90. Kim, D.W.; Kim, S.Y.; Kim, H.K.; Kim, S.W.; Shin, S.W.; Kim, J.S.; Park, K.; Lee, M.Y.; Heo, D.S. Multicenter Phase II Trial of Genexol-PM, a Novel Cremophor-Free, Polymeric Micelle Formulation of Paclitaxel, with Cisplatin in Patients with Advanced Non-Small-Cell Lung Cancer. *Ann. Oncol.* **2007**, *18*, 2009–2014. [CrossRef]
91. Nam, S.H.; Lee, S.W.; Lee, Y.J.; Kim, Y.M. Safety and Tolerability of Weekly Genexol-PM, a Cremophor-Free Polymeric Micelle Formulation of Paclitaxel, with Carboplatin in Gynecologic Cancer: A Phase I Study. *Cancer Res. Treat.* **2023**, *55*, 1346–1354. [CrossRef]
92. Lee, S.W.; Kim, Y.M.; Cho, C.H.; Kim, Y.T.; Kim, S.M.; Hur, S.Y.; Kim, J.H.; Kim, B.G.; Kim, S.C.; Ryu, H.S.; et al. An Open-Label, Randomized, Parallel, Phase Ii Trial to Evaluate the Efficacy and Safety of a Cremophor-Free Polymeric Micelle Formulation of Paclitaxel as First-Line Treatment for Ovarian Cancer: A Korean Gynecologic Oncology Group Study (KGOG-3021). *Cancer Res. Treat.* **2018**, *50*, 195–203. [CrossRef]
93. Ahn, H.K.; Jung, M.; Sym, S.J.; Shin, D.B.; Kang, S.M.; Kyung, S.Y.; Park, J.W.; Jeong, S.H.; Cho, E.K. A Phase II Trial of Cremorphor EL-Free Paclitaxel (Genexol-PM) and Gemcitabine in Patients with Advanced Non-Small Cell Lung Cancer. *Cancer Chemother. Pharmacol.* **2014**, *74*, 277–282. [CrossRef] [PubMed]
94. Kim, J.Y.; Do, Y.R.; Song, H.S.; Cho, Y.Y.; Ryoo, H.M.; Bae, S.H.; Kim, J.G.; Chae, Y.S.; Kang, B.W.; Baek, J.H.; et al. Multicenter Phase II Clinical Trial of Genexol-Pm® with Gemcitabine in Advanced Biliary Tract Cancer. *Anticancer Res.* **2017**, *37*, 1467–1473. [CrossRef] [PubMed]
95. Kim, H.S.; Lee, J.Y.; Lim, S.H.; Sun, J.M.; Lee, S.H.; Ahn, J.S.; Park, K.; Moon, S.H.; Ahn, M.J. A Prospective Phase II Study of Cisplatin and Cremophor EL-Free Paclitaxel (Genexol-PM) in Patients with Unresectable Thymic Epithelial Tumors. *J. Thorac. Oncol.* **2015**, *10*, 1800–1806. [CrossRef]
96. Keam, B.; Lee, K.-W.; Lee, S.-H.; Kim, J.-S.; Kim, J.H.; Wu, H.-G.; Eom, K.-Y.; Kim, S.; Ahn, S.-H.; Chung, E.-J.; et al. A Phase II Study of Genexol-PM and Cisplatin as Induction Chemotherapy in Locally Advanced Head and Neck Squamous Cell Carcinoma. *Oncologist* **2019**, *24*, 751-e231. [CrossRef] [PubMed]
97. Lee, J.L.; Ahn, J.H.; Park, S.H.; Lim, H.Y.; Kwon, J.H.; Ahn, S.; Song, C.; Hong, J.H.; Kim, C.S.; Ahn, H. Phase II Study of a Cremophor-Free, Polymeric Micelle Formulation of Paclitaxel for Patients with Advanced Urothelial Cancer Previously Treated with Gemcitabine and Platinum. *Investig. New Drugs* **2012**, *30*, 1984–1990. [CrossRef] [PubMed]
98. Joly, F.; Houédé, N.; Noal, S.; Chevreau, C.; Priou, F.; Chinet-Charrot, P.; Rolland, F.; Fléchon, A.; Henry-Amar, M.; Culine, S. Do Patients with Advanced Urothelial Carcinoma Benefit from Weekly Paclitaxel Chemotherapy? A GETUG Phase II Study. *Clin. Genitourin. Cancer* **2009**, *7*, E28–E33. [CrossRef]
99. Lee, S.Y.; Park, H.S.; Lee, K.Y.; Kim, H.J.; Jeon, Y.J.; Jang, T.W.; Lee, K.H.; Kim, Y.C.; Kim, K.S.; Oh, I.J.; et al. Paclitaxel-Loaded Polymeric Micelle (230 Mg/M2) and Cisplatin (60 Mg/M2) vs. Paclitaxel (175 Mg/M2) and Cisplatin (60 Mg/M2) in Advanced Non-Small-Cell Lung Cancer: A Multicenter Randomized Phase IIB Trial. *Clin. Lung Cancer* **2013**, *14*, 275–282. [CrossRef]

100. Lee, S.W.; Kim, Y.M.; Kim, Y.T.; Kang, S.B. An Open-Label, Multicenter, Phase i Trial of a Cremophor-Free, Polymeric Micelle Formulation of Paclitaxel Combined with Carboplatin as a First-Line Treatment for Advanced Ovarian Cancer: A Korean Gynecologic Oncology Group Study (KGOG-3016). *J. Gynecol. Oncol.* **2017**, *28*, e26. [CrossRef]
101. Park, I.H.; Sohn, J.H.; Kim, S.B.; Lee, K.S.; Chung, J.S.; Lee, S.H.; Kim, T.Y.; Jung, K.H.; Cho, E.K.; Kim, Y.S.; et al. An Open-Label, Randomized, Parallel, Phase III Trial Evaluating the Efficacy and Safety of Polymeric Micelle-Formulated Paclitaxel Compared to Conventional Cremophor EL-Based Paclitaxel for Recurrent or Metastatic HER2-Negative Breast Cancer. *Cancer Res. Treat.* **2017**, *49*, 569–577. [CrossRef]
102. Park, S.J.; Son, J.H.; Kong, T.W.; Chang, S.J.; Kim, H.S. Effect of High-Dose Polymeric Nanoparticle Micellar Paclitaxel on Improved Progression-Free Survival in Patients with Optimally Resected Stage III or IV High-Grade Carcinoma of the Ovary: A Prospective Cohort Study with Historical Controls. *Front. Oncol.* **2024**, *14*, 1203129. [CrossRef]
103. Lu, J.; Lou, Y.; Zhang, Y.; Zhong, R.; Zhang, W.; Zhang, X.; Wang, H.; Chu, T.; Han, B.; Zhong, H. Paclitaxel Has a Reduced Toxicity Profile in Healthy Rats After Polymeric Micellar Nanoparticle Delivery. *Int. J. Nanomed.* **2023**, *18*, 263–276. [CrossRef] [PubMed]
104. Socinski, M.A.; Bondarenko, I.; Karaseva, N.A.; Makhson, A.M.; Vynnychenko, I.; Okamoto, I.; Hon, J.K.; Hirsh, V.; Bhar, P.; Zhang, H.; et al. Weekly Nab-Paclitaxel in Combination with Carboplatin versus Solvent-Based Paclitaxel plus Carboplatin as First-Line Therapy in Patients with Advanced Non-Small-Cell Lung Cancer: Final Results of a Phase III Trial. *J. Clin. Oncol.* **2012**, *30*, 2055–2062. [CrossRef] [PubMed]
105. Shi, M.; Gu, A.; Tu, H.; Huang, C.; Wang, H.; Yu, Z.; Wang, X.; Cao, L.; Shu, Y.; Yang, R.; et al. Comparing Nanoparticle Polymeric Micellar Paclitaxel and Solvent-Based Paclitaxel as First-Line Treatment of Advanced Non-Small-Cell Lung Cancer: An Open-Label, Randomized, Multicenter, Phase III Trial. *Ann. Oncol.* **2021**, *32*, 85–96. [CrossRef]
106. Lu, J.; Gu, A.; Wang, W.; Huang, A.; Han, B.; Zhong, H. Polymeric Micellar Paclitaxel (Pm-Pac) Prolonged Overall Survival for NSCLC Patients without Pleural Metastasis. *Int. J. Pharm.* **2022**, *623*, 121961. [CrossRef]
107. Wang, F.Y.; Huang, X.M.; Cao, Y.Q.; Cao, J.; Ni, J.; Li, K.; Lu, M.; Huang, X.E. Nanoparticle Polymeric Micellar Paclitaxel Versus Paclitaxel for Patients with Advanced Gastric Cancer. *J. Gastrointest. Cancer* **2024**. [CrossRef]
108. Ranade, A.A.; Joshi, D.A.; Phadke, G.K.; Patil, P.P.; Kasbekar, R.B.; Apte, T.G.; Dasare, R.R.; Mengde, S.D.; Parikh, P.M.; Bhattacharyya, G.S.; et al. Clinical and Economic Implications of the Use of Nanoparticle Paclitaxel (Nanoxel) in India. *Ann. Oncol.* **2013**, *24*, v6–v12. [CrossRef]
109. Giodini, L.; Re, F.L.; Campagnol, D.; Marangon, E.; Posocco, B.; Dreussi, E.; Toffoli, G. Nanocarriers in Cancer Clinical Practice: A Pharmacokinetic Issue. *Nanomedicine* **2017**, *13*, 583–599. [CrossRef] [PubMed]
110. Madaan, A.; Singh, P.; Awasthi, A.; Verma, R.; Singh, A.T.; Jaggi, M.; Mishra, S.K.; Kulkarni, S.; Kulkarni, H. Efficiency and Mechanism of Intracellular Paclitaxel Delivery by Novel Nanopolymer-Based Tumor-Targeted Delivery System, Nanoxel™. *Clin. Transl. Oncol.* **2013**, *15*, 26–32. [CrossRef]
111. Ranade, A.A.; Bapsy, P.P.; Nag, S.; Raghunadharao, D.; Raina, V.; Advani, S.H.; Patil, S.; Maru, A.; Gangadharan, V.P.; Goswami, C.; et al. A Multicenter Phase II Randomized Study of Cremophor-Free Polymeric Nanoparticle Formulation of Paclitaxel in Women with Locally Advanced and/or Metastatic Breast Cancer after Failure of Anthracycline. *Asia Pac. J. Clin. Oncol.* **2013**, *9*, 176–181. [CrossRef]
112. Ostwal, V.; Sahu, A.; Zanwar, S.; Nayak, L.; Shrikhande, S.V.; Shetty, N.; Gupta, S.; Ramaswamy, A. Experience with Non-Cremophor-Based Paclitaxel-Gemcitabine Regimen in Advanced Pancreatic Cancer: Results from a Single Tertiary Cancer Centre. *Indian J. Med. Res.* **2018**, *148*, 284–290. [CrossRef]
113. Brahmachari, B.; Hazra, A.; Majumdar, A. Adverse Drug Reaction Profile of Nanoparticle versus Conventional Formulation of Paclitaxel: An Observational Study. *Indian J. Pharmacol.* **2011**, *43*, 126–130. [CrossRef] [PubMed]
114. Do, V.Q.; Park, K.H.; Park, J.M.; Lee, M.Y. Comparative in Vitro Toxicity Study of Docetaxel and Nanoxel, a Docetaxel-Loaded Micellar Formulation Using Cultured and Blood Cells. *Toxicol. Res.* **2019**, *35*, 201–207. [CrossRef] [PubMed]
115. Gwak, G.; Chung, M.; Kim, T.H.; Park, I.; Kim, J.; Um, E.; Lee, A.; Kim, J. Il A Multi-Center Trial to Evaluate the Safety and Toxicity of Nanoxel<Sup>®</Sup>-M in Breast Cancer Patients. *J. Breast Dis.* **2021**, *9*, 45–55. [CrossRef]
116. Lee, J.; Park, S.; Jung, H.A.; Lee, S.H.; Seo, S.; Kim, S.B.; Kim, J.W.; Lee, K.W.; Kang, E.J.; Kim, J.W.; et al. A Phase 2 Multicenter Study of Docetaxel-PM and Trastuzumab-Pkrb Combination Therapy in Recurrent or Metastatic Salivary Gland Carcinomas. *Cancer* **2023**, *129*, 2966–2974. [CrossRef] [PubMed]
117. Hamaguchi, T.; Matsumura, Y.; Suzuki, M.; Shimizu, K.; Goda, R.; Nakamura, I.; Nakatomi, I.; Yokoyama, M.; Kataoka, K.; Kakizoe, T. NK105, a Paclitaxel-Incorporating Micellar Nanoparticle Formulation, Can Extend in Vivo Antitumour Activity and Reduce the Neurotoxicity of Paclitaxel. *Br. J. Cancer* **2005**, *92*, 1240–1246. [CrossRef]
118. Nakamura, I.; Ichimura, E.; Goda, R.; Hayashi, H.; Mashiba, H.; Nagai, D.; Yokoyama, H.; Onda, T.; Masuda, A. An in Vivo Mechanism for the Reduced Peripheral Neurotoxicity of NK105: A Paclitaxel-Incorporating Polymeric Micellar Nanoparticle Formulation. *Int. J. Nanomed.* **2017**, *12*, 1293–1304. [CrossRef] [PubMed]
119. Negishi, T.; Koizumi, F.; Uchino, H.; Kuroda, J.; Kawaguchi, T.; Naito, S.; Matsumura, Y. NK105, a Paclitaxel-Incorporating Micellar Nanoparticle, Is a More Potent Radiosensitising Agent Compared to Free Paclitaxel. *Br. J. Cancer* **2006**, *95*, 601–606. [CrossRef]

120. Kato, K.; Chin, K.; Yoshikawa, T.; Yamaguchi, K.; Tsuji, Y.; Esaki, T.; Sakai, K.; Kimura, M.; Hamaguchi, T.; Shimada, Y.; et al. Phase II Study of NK105, a Paclitaxel-Incorporating Micellar Nanoparticle, for Previously Treated Advanced or Recurrent Gastric Cancer. *Investig. New Drugs* **2012**, *30*, 1621–1627. [CrossRef]
121. Fujiwara, Y.; Mukai, H.; Saeki, T.; Ro, J.; Lin, Y.C.; Nagai, S.E.; Lee, K.S.; Watanabe, J.; Ohtani, S.; Kim, S.B.; et al. A Multi-National, Randomised, Open-Label, Parallel, Phase III Non-Inferiority Study Comparing NK105 and Paclitaxel in Metastatic or Recurrent Breast Cancer Patients. *Br. J. Cancer* **2019**, *120*, 475–480. [CrossRef]
122. Kosaka, Y.; Saeki, T.; Takano, T.; Aruga, T.; Yamashita, T.; Masuda, N.; Koibuchi, Y.; Osaki, A.; Watanabe, J.; Suzuki, R. Multicenter Randomized Open-Label Phase II Clinical Study Comparing Outcomes of NK105 and Paclitaxel in Advanced or Recurrent Breast Cancer. *Int. J. Nanomed.* **2022**, *17*, 4567–4578. [CrossRef]
123. Taheri, A.; Rad, A.; Sadeghi, E.; Varshosaz, J. Comparison of Efficacy and Peripheral Neuropathy of Solvent-Based Paclitaxel with Paclitaxel Poliglumex and NK105: A Systematic Review and Metaanalysis. *Curr. Pharm. Des.* **2021**, *27*, 2041–2055. [CrossRef] [PubMed]
124. Rijcken, C.J.F.; De Lorenzi, F.; Biancacci, I.; Hanssen, R.G.J.M.; Thewissen, M.; Hu, Q.; Atrafi, F.; Liskamp, R.M.J.; Mathijssen, R.H.J.; Miedema, I.H.C.; et al. Design, Development and Clinical Translation of CriPec®-Based Core-Crosslinked Polymeric Micelles. *Adv. Drug Deliv. Rev.* **2022**, *191*, 114613. [CrossRef] [PubMed]
125. Alberg, I.; Kramer, S.; Schinnerer, M.; Hu, Q.; Seidl, C.; Leps, C.; Drude, N.; Möckel, D.; Rijcken, C.; Lammers, T.; et al. Polymeric Nanoparticles with Neglectable Protein Corona. *Small* **2020**, *16*, 1907574. [CrossRef] [PubMed]
126. Ojha, T.; Hu, Q.; Colombo, C.; Wit, J.; van Geijn, M.; van Steenbergen, M.J.; Bagheri, M.; Königs-Werner, H.; Buhl, E.M.; Bansal, R.; et al. Lyophilization Stabilizes Clinical-Stage Core-Crosslinked Polymeric Micelles to Overcome Cold Chain Supply Challenges. *Biotechnol. J.* **2021**, *16*, 2000212. [CrossRef]
127. Hu, Q.; Rijcken, C.J.; Bansal, R.; Hennink, W.E.; Storm, G.; Prakash, J. Complete Regression of Breast Tumour with a Single Dose of Docetaxel-Entrapped Core-Cross-Linked Polymeric Micelles. *Biomaterials* **2015**, *53*, 370–378. [CrossRef] [PubMed]
128. De Lorenzi, F.; Rizzo, L.Y.; Daware, R.; Motta, A.; Baues, M.; Bartneck, M.; Vogt, M.; van Zandvoort, M.; Kaps, L.; Hu, Q.; et al. Profiling Target Engagement and Cellular Uptake of CRGD-Decorated Clinical-Stage Core-Crosslinked Polymeric Micelles. *Drug Deliv. Transl. Res.* **2023**, *13*, 1195–1211. [CrossRef] [PubMed]
129. Braal, C.L.; de Bruijn, P.; Atrafi, F.; van Geijn, M.; Rijcken, C.J.F.; Mathijssen, R.H.J.; Koolen, S.L.W. A New Method for the Determination of Total and Released Docetaxel from Docetaxel-Entrapped Core-Crosslinked Polymeric Micelles (CriPec®) by LC–MS/MS and Its Clinical Application in Plasma and Tissues in Patients with Various Tumours. *J. Pharm. Biomed. Anal.* **2018**, *161*, 168–174. [CrossRef] [PubMed]
130. Atrafi, F.; van Eerden, R.A.G.; Koolen, S.L.W.; de Bruijn, P.; Rijcken, C.J.F.; Hanssen, R.; Eskens, F.A.L.M.; Lolkema, M.P.; Hoop, E.O.-D.; Damman, J.; et al. Docetaxel Skin Exposure and Micronucleation Contributes to Skin Toxicity Caused by Cpc634. *Cancers* **2021**, *13*, 3741. [CrossRef]
131. Boere, I.; Vergote, I.; Hanssen, R.; Jalving, M.; Gennigens, C.; Ottevanger, P.; van de Wouw, Y.J.; Rijcken, C.J.F.; Mathijssen, R.H.J.; Ledermann, J. CINOVA: A Phase II Study of CPC634 (Nanoparticulate Docetaxel) in Patients with Platinum Resistant Recurrent Ovarian Cancer. *Int. J. Gynecol. Cancer* **2023**, *33*, 1247–1252. [CrossRef]
132. Miedema, I.H.C.; Zwezerijnen, G.J.C.; Huisman, M.C.; Doeleman, E.; Mathijssen, R.H.J.; Lammers, T.; Hu, Q.; van Dongen, G.A.M.S.; Rijcken, C.J.F.; Vugts, D.J.; et al. PET-CT Imaging of Polymeric Nanoparticle Tumor Accumulation in Patients. *Adv. Mater.* **2022**, *34*, 2201043. [CrossRef]
133. Si, J.; Zhao, X.; Gao, S.; Huang, D.; Sui, M. Advances in Delivery of Irinotecan (CPT-11) Active Metabolite 7-Ethyl-10-Hydroxycamptothecin. *Int. J. Pharm.* **2019**, *568*, 118499. [CrossRef]
134. Atasilp, C.; Biswas, M.; Jinda, P.; Nuntharadthanaphong, N.; Rachanakul, J.; Hongkaew, Y.; Vanwong, N.; Saokaew, S.; Sukasem, C. Association of *UGT1A1*6*, *UGT1A1*28*, or *ABCC2 c.3972C>T* Genetic Polymorphisms with Irinotecan-Induced Toxicity in Asian Cancer Patients: Meta-Analysis. *Clin. Transl. Sci.* **2022**, *15*, 1613–1633. [CrossRef] [PubMed]
135. Matsumura, Y. Preclinical and Clinical Studies of NK012, an SN-38-Incorporating Polymeric Micelles, Which Is Designed Based on EPR Effect. *Adv. Drug Deliv. Rev.* **2011**, *63*, 184–192. [CrossRef]
136. Saito, Y.; Yasunaga, M.; Kuroda, J.; Koga, Y.; Matsumura, Y. Enhanced Distribution of NK012, a Polymeric Micelle-Encapsulated SN-38, and Sustained Release of SN-38 within Tumors Can Beat a Hypovascular Tumor. *Cancer Sci.* **2008**, *99*, 1258–1264. [CrossRef] [PubMed]
137. Saito, Y.; Yasunaga, M.; Kuroda, J.-I.; Koga, Y.; Matsumura, Y. Antitumour Activity of NK012, SN-38-Incorporating Polymeric Micelles, in Hypovascular Orthotopic Pancreatic Tumour. *Eur. J. Cancer* **2010**, *46*, 650–658. [CrossRef]
138. Nakajima, T.E.; Yanagihara, K.; Takigahira, M.; Yasunaga, M.; Kato, K.; Hamaguchi, T.; Yamada, Y.; Shimada, Y.; Mihara, K.; Ochiya, T.; et al. Antitumor Effect of SN-38-Releasing Polymeric Micelles, NK012, on Spontaneous Peritoneal Metastases from Orthotopic Gastric Cancer in Mice Compared with Irinotecan. *Cancer Res.* **2008**, *68*, 9318–9322. [CrossRef]
139. Takahashi, A.; Ohkohchi, N.; Yasunaga, M.; Kuroda, J.I.; Koga, Y.; Kenmotsu, H.; Kinoshita, T.; Matsumura, Y. Detailed Distribution of NK012, an SN-38-Incorporating Micelle, in the Liver and Its Potent Antitumor Effects in Mice Bearing Liver Metastases. *Clin. Cancer Res.* **2010**, *16*, 4822–4831. [CrossRef]
140. Yanagihara, K.; Takigahira, M.; Kubo, T.; Ochiya, T.; Hamaguchi, T.; Matsumura, Y. Marked Antitumor Effect of NK012, a SN-38-Incorporating Micelle Formulation, in a Newly Developed Mouse Model of Liver Metastasis Resulting from Gastric Cancer. *Ther. Deliv.* **2014**, *5*, 129–138. [CrossRef] [PubMed]

141. Koizumi, F.; Kitagawa, M.; Negishi, T.; Onda, T.; Matsumoto, S.I.; Hamaguchi, T.; Matsumura, Y. Novel SN-38-Incorporating Polymeric Micelles, NK012, Eradicate Vascular Endothelial Growth Factor-Secreting Bulky Tumors. *Cancer Res.* **2006**, *66* 10048–10056. [CrossRef]
142. Nakajima, T.E.; Yasunaga, M.; Kano, Y.; Koizumi, F.; Kato, K.; Hamaguchi, T.; Yamada, Y.; Shirao, K.; Shimada, Y.; Matsumura, Y. Synergistic Antitumor Activity of the Novel SN-38-Incorporating Polymeric Micelles, NK012, Combined with 5-Fluorouracil in a Mouse Model of Colorectal Cancer, as Compared with That of Irinotecan plus 5-Fluorouracil. *Int. J. Cancer* **2008**, *122*, 2148–2153. [CrossRef]
143. Sumitomo, M.; Koizumi, F.; Asano, T.; Horiguchi, A.; Ito, K.; Asano, T.; Kakizoe, T.; Hayakawa, M.; Matsumura, Y. Novel SN-38-Incorporated Polymeric Micelle, NK012, Strongly Suppresses Renal Cancer Progression. *Cancer Res.* **2008**, *68*, 1631–1635. [CrossRef] [PubMed]
144. Nagano, T.; Yasunaga, M.; Goto, K.; Kenmotsu, H.; Koga, Y.; Kuroda, J.I.; Nishimura, Y.; Sugino, T.; Nishiwaki, Y.; Matsumura Y. Antitumor Activity of NK012 Combined with Cisplatin against Small Cell Lung Cancer and Intestinal Mucosal Changes in Tumor-Bearing Mouse after Treatment. *Clin. Cancer Res.* **2009**, *15*, 4348–4355. [CrossRef] [PubMed]
145. Nagano, T.; Yasunaga, M.; Goto, K.; Kenmotsu, H.; Koga, Y.; Kuroda, J.; Nishimura, Y.; Sugino, T.; Nishiwaki, Y.; Matsumura, Y. Synergistic Antitumor Activity of the SN-38-incorporating Polymeric Micelles NK012 with S-1 in a Mouse Model of Non-small Cell Lung Cancer. *Int. J. Cancer* **2010**, *127*, 2699–2706. [CrossRef] [PubMed]
146. Kenmotsu, H.; Yasunaga, M.; Goto, K.; Nagano, T.; Kuroda, J.I.; Koga, Y.; Takahashi, A.; Nishiwaki, Y.; Matsumura, Y. The Antitumor Activity of NK012, an SN-38-Incorporating Micelle, in Combination with Bevacizumab against Lung Cancer Xenografts *Cancer* **2010**, *116*, 4597–4604. [CrossRef] [PubMed]
147. Kuroda, J.I.; Kuratsu, J.I.; Yasunaga, M.; Koga, Y.; Saito, Y.; Matsumura, Y. Potent Antitumor Effect of SN-38-Incorporating Polymeric Micelle, NK012, against Malignant Glioma. *Int. J. Cancer* **2009**, *124*, 2505–2511. [CrossRef] [PubMed]
148. Kuroda, J.I.; Kuratsu, J.I.; Yasunaga, M.; Koga, Y.; Kenmotsu, H.; Sugino, T.; Matsumura, Y. Antitumor Effect of NK012, a 7-Ethyl-10-Hydroxycamptothecin-Incorporating Polymeric Micelle, on U87MG Orthotopic Glioblastoma in Mice Compared with Irinotecan Hydrochloride in Combination with Bevacizumab. *Clin. Cancer Res.* **2010**, *16*, 521–529. [CrossRef] [PubMed]
149. Zhang, R.; Saito, R.; Mano, Y.; Sumiyoshi, A.; Kanamori, M.; Sonoda, Y.; Kawashima, R.; Tominaga, T. Convection-Enhanced Delivery of SN-38-Loaded Polymeric Micelles (NK012) Enables Consistent Distribution of SN-38 and Is Effective against Rodent Intracranial Brain Tumor Models. *Drug Deliv.* **2016**, *23*, 2780–2786. [CrossRef] [PubMed]
150. Miyazaki, O.; Sekine, K.; Nakajima, N.; Ichimura, E.; Ebara, K.; Nagai, D.; Onda, T.; Miyakawa, Y.; Okamoto, K.; Morino, T. Antimyeloma Activity of NK012, a Micelle-Forming Macromolecular Prodrug of SN-38, in an Orthotopic Model. *Int. J. Cancer* **2014**, *134*, 218–223. [CrossRef] [PubMed]
151. Hamaguchi, T.; Tsuji, A.; Yamaguchi, K.; Takeda, K.; Uetake, H.; Esaki, T.; Amagai, K.; Sakai, D.; Baba, H.; Kimura, M.; et al. A Phase II Study of NK012, a Polymeric Micelle Formulation of SN-38, in Unresectable, Metastatic or Recurrent Colorectal Cancer Patients. *Cancer Chemother. Pharmacol.* **2018**, *82*, 1021–1029. [CrossRef]
152. Ri, M.; Suzuki, K.; Iida, S.; Hatake, K.; Chou, T.; Taniwaki, M.; Watanabe, N.; Tsukamoto, T. A Phase I/II Study for Dose-Finding, and to Investigate the Safety, Pharmacokinetics and Preliminary Efficacy of NK012, an SN-38-Incorporating Macromolecular Polymeric Micelle, in Patients with Multiple Myeloma. *Intern. Med.* **2018**, *57*, 939–946. [CrossRef]
153. Kciuk, M.; Gielecińska, A.; Mujwar, S.; Kołat, D.; Kałuzińska-Kołat, Ż.; Celik, I.; Kontek, R. Doxorubicin—An Agent with Multiple Mechanisms of Anticancer Activity. *Cells* **2023**, *12*, 659. [CrossRef]
154. D'Angelo, N.A.; Noronha, M.A.; Câmara, M.C.C.; Kurnik, I.S.; Feng, C.; Araujo, V.H.S.; Santos, J.H.P.M.; Feitosa, V.; Molino, J.V.D.; Rangel-Yagui, C.O.; et al. Doxorubicin Nanoformulations on Therapy against Cancer: An Overview from the Last 10 Years. *Biomater. Adv.* **2022**, *133*, 112623. [CrossRef] [PubMed]
155. Nakanishi, T.; Fukushima, S.; Okamoto, K.; Suzuki, M.; Matsumura, Y.; Yokoyama, M.; Okano, T.; Sakurai, Y.; Kataoka, K. Development of the Polymer Micelle Carrier System for Doxorubicin. *J. Control. Release* **2001**, *74*, 295–302. [CrossRef] [PubMed]
156. Alakhov, V.; Klinski, E.; Li, S.; Pietrzynski, G.; Venne, A.; Batrakova, E.; Bronitch, T.; Kabanov, A. Block Copolymer-Based Formulation of Doxorubicin. From Cell Screen to Clinical Trials. *Colloids Surf. B Biointerfaces* **1999**, *16*, 113–134. [CrossRef]
157. Kabanov, A.V.; Batrakova, E.V.; Alakhov, V.Y. Pluronic Block Copolymers for Overcoming Drug Resistance in Cancer. *Adv. Drug Deliv. Rev.* **2002**, *54*, 759–779. [CrossRef] [PubMed]
158. Valle, J.W.; Armstrong, A.; Newman, C.; Alakhov, V.; Pietrzynski, G.; Brewer, J.; Campbell, S.; Corrie, P.; Rowinsky, E.K.; Ranson, M. A Phase 2 Study of SP1049C, Doxorubicin in P-Glycoprotein-Targeting Pluronics, in Patients with Advanced Adenocarcinoma of the Esophagus and Gastroesophageal Junction. *Investig. New Drugs* **2011**, *29*, 1029–1037. [CrossRef] [PubMed]
159. Kaur, J.; Gulati, M.; Jha, N.K.; Disouza, J.; Patravale, V.; Dua, K.; Singh, S.K. Recent Advances in Developing Polymeric Micelles for Treating Cancer: Breakthroughs and Bottlenecks in Their Clinical Translation. *Drug Discov. Today* **2022**, *27*, 1495–1512. [CrossRef] [PubMed]
160. Harada, M.; Bobe, I.; Saito, H.; Shibata, N.; Tanaka, R.; Hayashi, T.; Kato, Y. Improved Anti-Tumor Activity of Stabilized Anthracycline Polymeric Micelle Formulation, NC-6300. *Cancer Sci.* **2011**, *102*, 192–199. [CrossRef]
161. Takahashi, A.; Yamamoto, Y.; Yasunaga, M.; Koga, Y.; Kuroda, J.I.; Takigahira, M.; Harada, M.; Saito, H.; Hayashi, T.; Kato, Y.; et al. NC-6300, an Epirubicin-Incorporating Micelle, Extends the Antitumor Effect and Reduces the Cardiotoxicity of Epirubicin. *Cancer Sci.* **2013**, *104*, 920–925. [CrossRef]

162. Yamamoto, Y.; Hyodo, I.; Koga, Y.; Tsumura, R.; Sato, R.; Obonai, T.; Fuchigami, H.; Furuya, F.; Yasunaga, M.; Harada, M.; et al. Enhanced Antitumor Effect of Anti-Tissue Factor Antibody-Conjugated Epirubicin-Incorporating Micelles in Xenograft Models. *Cancer Sci.* **2015**, *106*, 627–634. [CrossRef]
163. Sugaya, A.; Hyodo, I.; Koga, Y.; Yamamoto, Y.; Takashima, H.; Sato, R.; Tsumura, R.; Furuya, F.; Yasunaga, M.; Harada, M.; et al. Utility of Epirubicin-Incorporating Micelles Tagged with Anti-Tissue Factor Antibody Clone with No Anticoagulant Effect. *Cancer Sci.* **2016**, *107*, 335–340. [CrossRef] [PubMed]
164. Mpekris, F.; Panagi, M.; Michael, C.; Voutouri, C.; Tsuchiya, M.; Wagatsuma, C.; Kinoh, H.; Osada, A.; Akinaga, S.; Yoshida, S.; et al. Translational Nanomedicine Potentiates Immunotherapy in Sarcoma by Normalizing the Microenvironment. *J. Control. Release* **2023**, *353*, 956–964. [CrossRef] [PubMed]
165. Takemae, K.; Okamoto, J.; Horise, Y.; Masamune, K.; Muragaki, Y. Function of Epirubicin-Conjugated Polymeric Micelles in Sonodynamic Therapy. *Front. Pharmacol.* **2019**, *10*, 546. [CrossRef]
166. Maeda, M.; Muragaki, Y.; Okamoto, J.; Yoshizawa, S.; Abe, N.; Nakamoto, H.; Ishii, H.; Kawabata, K.; Umemura, S.; Nishiyama, N.; et al. Sonodynamic Therapy Based on Combined Use of Low Dose Administration of Epirubicin-Incorporating Drug Delivery System and Focused Ultrasound. *Ultrasound Med. Biol.* **2017**, *43*, 2295–2301. [CrossRef]
167. Horise, Y.; Maeda, M.; Konishi, Y.; Okamoto, J.; Ikuta, S.; Okamoto, Y.; Ishii, H.; Yoshizawa, S.; Umemura, S.; Ueyama, T.; et al. Sonodynamic Therapy with Anticancer Micelles and High-Intensity Focused Ultrasound in Treatment of Canine Cancer. *Front. Pharmacol.* **2019**, *10*, 447834. [CrossRef]
168. Mukai, H.; Kogawa, T.; Matsubara, N.; Naito, Y.; Sasaki, M.; Hosono, A. A First-in-Human Phase 1 Study of Epirubicin-Conjugated Polymer Micelles (K-912/NC-6300) in Patients with Advanced or Recurrent Solid Tumors. *Investig. New Drugs* **2017**, *35*, 307–314. [CrossRef]
169. Riedel, R.F.; Chua, V.; Moradkhani, A.; Krkyan, N.; Ahari, A.; Osada, A.; Chawla, S.P. Results of NC-6300 (Nanoparticle Epirubicin) in an Expansion Cohort of Patients with Angiosarcoma. *Oncologist* **2022**, *27*, 809-e765. [CrossRef]
170. Forgie, B.N.; Prakash, R.; Telleria, C.M. Revisiting the Anti-Cancer Toxicity of Clinically Approved Platinating Derivatives. *Int. J. Mol. Sci.* **2022**, *23*, 15410. [CrossRef]
171. Shahlaei, M.; Asl, S.M.; Derakhshani, A.; Kurek, L.; Karges, J.; Macgregor, R.; Saeidifar, M.; Kostova, I.; Saboury, A.A. Platinum-Based Drugs in Cancer Treatment: Expanding Horizons and Overcoming Resistance. *J. Mol. Struct.* **2024**, *1301*, 137366. [CrossRef]
172. Nishiyama, N.; Okazaki, S.; Cabral, H.; Miyamoto, M.; Kato, Y.; Sugiyama, Y.; Nishio, K.; Matsumura, Y.; Kataoka, K. Novel Cisplatin-Incorporated Polymeric Micelles Can Eradicate Solid Tumors in Mice. *Cancer Res.* **2003**, *63*, 8977–8983. [PubMed]
173. Mochida, Y.; Cabral, H.; Miura, Y.; Albertini, F.; Fukushima, S.; Osada, K.; Nishiyama, N.; Kataoka, K. Bundled Assembly of Helical Nanostructures in Polymeric Micelles Loaded with Platinum Drugs Enhancing Therapeutic Efficiency against Pancreatic Tumor. *ACS Nano* **2014**, *8*, 6724–6738. [CrossRef] [PubMed]
174. Endo, K.; Ueno, T.; Kondo, S.; Wakisaka, N.; Murono, S.; Ito, M.; Kataoka, K.; Kato, Y.; Yoshizaki, T. Tumor-Targeted Chemotherapy with the Nanopolymer-Based Drug NC-6004 for Oral Squamous Cell Carcinoma. *Cancer Sci.* **2013**, *104*, 369–374. [CrossRef] [PubMed]
175. Uchino, H.; Matsumura, Y.; Negishi, T.; Koizumi, F.; Hayashi, T.; Honda, T.; Nishiyama, N.; Kataoka, K.; Naito, S.; Kakizoe, T. Cisplatin-Incorporating Polymeric Micelles (NC-6004) Can Reduce Nephrotoxicity and Neurotoxicity of Cisplatin in Rats. *Br. J. Cancer* **2005**, *93*, 678–687. [CrossRef]
176. Kudo, M.; Yamamoto, Y.; Koga, Y.; Hamaguchi, T.; Akimoto, T.; Yasunaga, M.; Matsumura, Y. Effect of Combined Treatment with Micelle-Incorporated Cisplatin (NC-6004) and S-1 on Human Gastric Cancer Xenografts. *Mol. Clin. Oncol.* **2016**, *5*, 817–822. [CrossRef] [PubMed]
177. Baba, M.; Matsumoto, Y.; Kashio, A.; Cabral, H.; Nishiyama, N.; Kataoka, K.; Yamasoba, T. Micellization of Cisplatin (NC-6004) Reduces Its Ototoxicity in Guinea Pigs. *J. Control. Release* **2012**, *157*, 112–117. [CrossRef]
178. Su, W.; Chen, L.; Li, C.; Chen, J.; Lin, Y.; Choo, S.; Matsumura, Y. Phase I/II Study of NC-6004, A Novel Micellar Formulation of Cisplatin, In Combination with Gemcitabine in Patients with Pancreatic Cancer in Asia—Results of Phase I. *Ann. Oncol.* **2012**, *23*, ix247. [CrossRef]
179. Doi, T.; Hamaguchi, T.; Shitara, K.; Iwasa, S.; Shimada, Y.; Harada, M.; Naito, K.; Hayashi, N.; Masada, A.; Ohtsu, A. NC-6004 Phase I Study in Combination with Gemcitabine for Advanced Solid Tumors and Population PK/PD Analysis. *Cancer Chemother. Pharmacol.* **2017**, *79*, 569–578. [CrossRef]
180. Subbiah, V.; Grilley-Olson, J.E.; Combest, A.J.; Sharma, N.; Tran, R.H.; Bobe, I.; Osada, A.; Takahashi, K.; Balkissoon, J.; Camp, A.; et al. Phase Ib/II Trial of NC-6004 (Nanoparticle Cisplatin) plus Gemcitabine in Patients with Advanced Solid Tumors. *Clin. Cancer Res.* **2018**, *24*, 43–51. [CrossRef] [PubMed]
181. Osada, A.; Mangel, L.; Fijuth, J.; Żurawski, B.; Ursulovic, T.; Nikolin, B.; Djan, I.; Olson, J.G. Phase IIa/IIb Clinical Trial of NC-6004 (Nanoparticle Cisplatin) plus Pembrolizumab in Patients with Head and Neck Cancer (HNSCC) Who Have Failed Platinum or a Platinum-Containing Regimen. *Eur. J. Cancer* **2020**, *138*, S35. [CrossRef]
182. Cabral, H.; Nishiyama, N.; Kataoka, K. Optimization of (1,2-Diamino-Cyclohexane)Platinum(II)-Loaded Polymeric Micelles Directed to Improved Tumor Targeting and Enhanced Antitumor Activity. *J. Control. Release* **2007**, *121*, 146–155. [CrossRef]
183. Cabral, H.; Nishiyama, N.; Okazaki, S.; Koyama, H.; Kataoka, K. Preparation and Biological Properties of Dichloro(1,2-Diaminocyclohexane) Platinum(II) (DACHPt)-Loaded Polymeric Micelles. *J. Control. Release* **2005**, *101*, 223–232. [CrossRef] [PubMed]

184. Ueno, T.; Endo, K.; Hori, K.; Ozaki, N.; Tsuji, A.; Kondo, S.; Wakisaka, N.; Murono, S.; Kataoka, K.; Kato, Y.; et al. Assessment of Antitumor Activity and Acute Peripheral Neuropathy of 1,2-Diaminocyclohexane Platinum (II)-Incorporating Micelles (NC-4016). *Int. J. Nanomed.* **2014**, *9*, 3005–3012. [CrossRef] [PubMed]
185. Murakami, M.; Cabral, H.; Matsumoto, Y.; Wu, S.; Kano, M.R.; Yamori, T.; Nishiyama, N.; Kataoka, K. Improving Drug Potency and Efficacy by Nanocarrier-Mediated Subcellular Targeting. *Sci. Transl. Med.* **2011**, *3*, 64ra2. [CrossRef]
186. Nirei, T.; Ishihara, S.; Tanaka, T.; Kiyomatsu, T.; Kawai, K.; Hata, K.; Nozawa, H.; Watanabe, T. Polymeric Micelles Loaded with (1,2-Diaminocyclohexane)Platinum(II) against Colorectal Cancer. *J. Surg. Res.* **2017**, *218*, 334–340. [CrossRef] [PubMed]
187. Cabral, H.; Matsumoto, Y.; Mizuno, K.; Chen, Q.; Murakami, M.; Kimura, M.; Terada, Y.; Kano, M.R.; Miyazono, K.; Uesaka, M.; et al. Accumulation of Sub-100 Nm Polymeric Micelles in Poorly Permeable Tumours Depends on Size. *Nat. Nanotechnol.* **2011**, *6*, 815–823. [CrossRef] [PubMed]
188. Rafi, M.; Cabral, H.; Kano, M.R.; Mi, P.; Iwata, C.; Yashiro, M.; Hirakawa, K.; Miyazono, K.; Nishiyama, N.; Kataoka, K. Polymeric Micelles Incorporating (1,2-Diaminocyclohexane)Platinum (II) Suppress the Growth of Orthotopic Scirrhous Gastric Tumors and Their Lymph Node Metastasis. *J. Control. Release* **2012**, *159*, 189–196. [CrossRef]
189. Cabral, H.; Murakami, M.; Hojo, H.; Terada, Y.; Kano, M.R.; Chung, U.-I.; Nishiyama, N.; Kataoka, K. Targeted Therapy of Spontaneous Murine Pancreatic Tumors by Polymeric Micelles Prolongs Survival and Prevents Peritoneal Metastasis. *Proc. Natl. Acad. Sci. USA* **2013**, *110*, 11397–11402. [CrossRef] [PubMed]
190. Yamamoto, Y.; Hyodo, I.; Takigahira, M.; Koga, Y.; Yasunaga, M.; Harada, M.; Hayashi, T.; Kato, Y.; Matsumura, Y. Effect of Combined Treatment with the Epirubicin-Incorporating Micelles (NC-6300) and 1,2-Diaminocyclohexane Platinum (II)-Incorporating Micelles (NC-4016) on a Human Gastric Cancer Model. *Int. J. Cancer* **2014**, *135*, 214–223. [CrossRef] [PubMed]
191. Makino, J.; Cabral, H.; Miura, Y.; Matsumoto, Y.; Wang, M.; Kinoh, H.; Mochida, Y.; Nishiyama, N.; Kataoka, K. CRGD-Installed Polymeric Micelles Loading Platinum Anticancer Drugs Enable Cooperative Treatment against Lymph Node Metastasis. *J. Control. Release* **2015**, *220*, 783–791. [CrossRef]
192. Vinh, N.Q.; Naka, S.; Cabral, H.; Murayama, H.; Kaida, S.; Kataoka, K.; Morikawa, S.; Tani, T. MRI-Detectable Polymeric Micelles Incorporating Platinum Anticancer Drugs Enhance Survival in an Advanced Hepatocellular Carcinoma Model. *Int. J. Nanomed.* **2015**, *10*, 4137–4147. [CrossRef]
193. Emens, L.A.; Romero, P.J.; Anderson, A.C.; Bruno, T.C.; Capitini, C.M.; Collyar, D.; Gulley, J.L.; Hwu, P.; Posey, A.D.; Silk, A.W.; et al. Challenges and Opportunities in Cancer Immunotherapy: A Society for Immunotherapy of Cancer (SITC) Strategic Vision. *J. Immuno Ther. Cancer* **2024**, *12*, e009063. [CrossRef] [PubMed]
194. Won, J.K.; Bakhoum, S.F. The Cytosolic DNA-Sensing CGAS–Sting Pathway in Cancer. *Cancer Discov.* **2020**, *10*, 26–39. [CrossRef]
195. Bennett, Z.T.; Li, S.; Sumer, B.D.; Gao, J. Polyvalent Design in the CGAS-STING Pathway. *Semin. Immunol.* **2021**, *56*, 101580. [CrossRef] [PubMed]
196. Wang, M.; Bennett, Z.T.; Singh, P.; Feng, Q.; Wilhelm, J.; Huang, G.; Gao, J. Elucidation of Protonation Cooperativity of a STING-Activating Polymer. *Adv. Mater.* **2023**, *35*, 2305255. [CrossRef] [PubMed]
197. Luo, M.; Wang, H.; Wang, Z.; Cai, H.; Lu, Z.; Li, Y.; Du, M.; Huang, G.; Wang, C.; Chen, X.; et al. A STING-Activating Nanovaccine for Cancer Immunotherapy. *Nat. Nanotechnol.* **2017**, *12*, 648–654. [CrossRef] [PubMed]
198. Jiang, X.; Wang, J.; Zheng, X.; Liu, Z.; Zhang, X.; Li, Y.; Wilhelm, J.; Cao, J.; Huang, G.; Zhang, J.; et al. Intratumoral Administration of STING-Activating Nanovaccine Enhances T Cell Immunotherapy. *J. Immunother. Cancer* **2022**, *10*, e003960. [CrossRef] [PubMed]
199. Li, S.; Luo, M.; Wang, Z.; Feng, Q.; Wilhelm, J.; Wang, X.; Li, W.; Wang, J.; Cholka, A.; Fu, Y.; et al. Prolonged Activation of Innate Immune Pathways by a Polyvalent STING Agonist. *Nat. Biomed. Eng.* **2021**, *5*, 455–466. [CrossRef] [PubMed]
200. Li, S.; Wang, J.; Wilhelm, J.; Su, Q.; Bharadwaj, G.; Miller, J.; Li, W.; Torres, K.; Han, R.; Zhao, T.; et al. Abstract 4234: ONM-501: A Polyvalent STING Agonist for Oncology Immunotherapy. *Cancer Res.* **2022**, *82*, 4234. [CrossRef]
201. Chen, Z.; Miller, J.; Li, W.; Torres, K.; Su, Q.; Huang, G.; Saud O Albaroodi, Y.; Morsch, R.; McElvaney, T.; Stavros, F.; et al. 1155 ONM-501, a Polyvalent STING Agonist, Exhibits Anti-Tumor Efficacy with Increased Tumor T-Cell Infiltration in Mice and Is Well Tolerated in Rats and Non-Human Primates. *J. ImmunoTher. Cancer* **2022**, *10*, A1198. [CrossRef]
202. Chen, Z.; Huang, G.; Torres, K.; Stavros, F.; Ahmed, A.; Miller, J.; Zhao, T.; Gao, J.; Han, R. Abstract LB245: ONM-501, a Dual-Activating Polyvalent STING Agonist, Enhances Tumor Retention and Demonstrates Favorable Preclinical Safety Profile. *Cancer Res.* **2023**, *83*, LB245. [CrossRef]
203. Zhao, T.; Huang, G.; Li, Y.; Yang, S.; Ramezani, S.; Lin, Z.; Wang, Y.; Ma, X.; Zeng, Z.; Luo, M.; et al. A Transistor-like PH Nanoprobe for Tumour Detection and Image-Guided Surgery. *Nat. Biomed. Eng.* **2016**, *1*, 0006. [CrossRef] [PubMed]
204. Li, Y.; Zhao, T.; Wang, C.; Lin, Z.; Huang, G.; Sumer, B.D.; Gao, J. Molecular Basis of Cooperativity in PH-Triggered Supramolecular Self-Assembly. *Nat. Commun.* **2016**, *7*, 13214. [CrossRef] [PubMed]
205. Kennedy, G.T.; Azari, F.S.; Chang, A.; Chang, A.; Bou-Samra, P.; Desphande, C.; Delikatny, E.J.; Eruslanov, E.; Kucharczuk, J.C.; Rice, D.C.; et al. A PH-Activatable Nanoprobe Labels Diverse Histologic Subtypes of Human Lung Cancer During Resection. *Mol. Imaging Biol.* **2023**, *25*, 824–832. [CrossRef] [PubMed]
206. Voskuil, F.J.; Steinkamp, P.J.; Zhao, T.; van der Vegt, B.; Koller, M.; Doff, J.J.; Jayalakshmi, Y.; Hartung, J.P.; Gao, J.; Sumer, B.D.; et al. Exploiting Metabolic Acidosis in Solid Cancers Using a Tumor-Agnostic PH-Activatable Nanoprobe for Fluorescence-Guided Surgery. *Nat. Commun.* **2020**, *11*, 3257. [CrossRef]

207. Steinkamp, P.J.; Voskuil, F.J.; van der Vegt, B.; Doff, J.J.; Schepman, K.P.; de Visscher, S.A.H.J.; Kelder, W.; Jayalakshmi, Y.; Gao, J.; Sumer, B.D.; et al. A Standardized Framework for Fluorescence-Guided Margin Assessment for Head and Neck Cancer Using a Tumor Acidosis Sensitive Optical Imaging Agent. *Mol. Imaging Biol.* **2021**, *23*, 809–817. [CrossRef]
208. Wagner, P.; Levine, E.A.; Kim, A.C.; Shen, P.; Fleming, N.D.; Westin, S.N.; Berry, L.K.; Karakousis, G.C.; Tanyi, J.L.; Olson, M.T.; et al. Detection of Residual Peritoneal Metastases Following Cytoreductive Surgery Using Pegsitacianine, a PH-Sensitive Imaging Agent: Final Results from a Phase II Study. *Ann. Surg. Oncol.* **2024**, *31*, 4726–4734. [CrossRef]

*pharmaceutics*

MDPI

*Article*

# Biopharmaceutical Characterization and Stability of Nabumetone–Cyclodextrins Complexes Prepared by Grinding

**David Klarić [1], Željka Soldin [1], Anna Vincze [2,3], Rita Szolláth [2,3], György Tibor Balogh [2,3], Mario Jug [4,*] and Nives Galić [1,*]**

[1] Department of Chemistry, Faculty of Science, University of Zagreb, Horvatovac 102a, 10 000 Zagreb, Croatia; dklaric@chem.pmf.hr (D.K.); zeljka@chem.pmf.hr (Ž.S.)
[2] Department of Pharmaceutical Chemistry, Semmelweis University, Hőgyes Endre u. 9., H-1092 Budapest, Hungary; vincze.anna@semmelweis.hu (A.V.); szollath.rita.mariann@semmelweis.hu (R.S.); balogh.gyorgy.tibor@semmelweis.hu (G.T.B.)
[3] Center for Pharmacology and Drug Research & Development, Semmelweis University, Üllői u. 26. H-1092 Budapest, Hungary
[4] Department of Pharmaceutical Technology, Faculty of Pharmacy and Biochemistry, University of Zagreb, A. Kovačića 1, 10 000 Zagreb, Croatia
* Correspondence: mjug@pharma.hr (M.J.); ngalic@chem.pmf.hr (N.G.)

**Abstract: Background:** Nabumetone (NAB) is a poorly soluble nonsteroidal anti-inflammatory prodrug (BCS class II drug) whose solubility is significantly improved by complexation with cyclodextrins (CDs). **Methods**: The solid complexes, in a 1:1 molar ratio, were prepared by mechanochemical activation by grinding, using β-cyclodextrin (β-CD) and its derivatives, hydroxypropyl- and sulfobutylether-β-cyclodextrin (HP-β-CD and SBE-β-CD). The complexation was confirmed by differential scanning calorimetry (DSC), powder X-ray diffraction (PXRD), and attenuated total reflectance Fourier-transformed infrared spectroscopy (ATR–FTIR). Obtained products were further characterized regarding their solubility, in vitro dissolution, permeability and chemical stability. **Results**: Co-grinding with HP-β-CD and SBE-β-CD yielded products that showed in vitro dissolution profiles in hydrochloric acid medium (pH 1.2) that were substantially different from that of pure NAB, yielding dissolution efficiency enhancements of $34.86 \pm 1.64$ and $58.30 \pm 0.28$ times, respectively, for the optimized products. Their in vitro dissolution and gastrointestinal permeability were also studied in a low-volume environment at pH 6.8, corresponding to the intestinal environment. Both β-CD derivatives increased NAB dissolution rate and NAB mass transport across the biomimetic membrane. The effect of β-CD derivatives on NAB chemical stability was studied under the stress conditions by the developed and validated UHPLC–DAD–HRMS method. In acidic conditions, pure and complexed NAB was prone to hydrolytic degradation, yielding one degradation product—pharmacologically inactive NAB metabolite. However, under the oxidative conditions at elevated temperatures, 10 NAB degradation products were identified from co-ground samples. All systems were stable during photo- and long-term stability studies. **Conclusions**: NAB complexes with HP-β-CD and SBE-β-CD are promising candidates for pharmaceutical product development.

**Keywords:** nabumetone; cyclodextrins; mechanochemistry; solid-state characterization; in vitro permeability; in vitro dissolution; degradants; chemical stability

## 1. Introduction

Developing a new drug formulation is a demanding and complex procedure which needs a detailed characterization of the system both in solution and in the solid state. Cyclodextrins (CDs), a versatile family of cyclic oligosaccharides with a unique structure, have gathered significant interest as excipients due to their potential to form inclusion complexes [1]. These complexes can significantly enhance the solubility, chemical stability, and bioavailability of various drugs [2–4]. The biocompatibility, good tolerability, non-immunogenicity, and functional versatility make CDs a valuable asset in pharmaceutical formulations, particularly for newly emerging drug candidates with increasing molecular mass, lipophilicity, and reduced water solubility [5]. They also offer a solution for reformulating existing drugs with limited aqueous solubility, avoiding potentially irritant excipients like cosolvents and surfactants, resulting in formulations with enhanced tolerability and patient acceptance [6,7]. Numerous pharmaceutical products based on CDs have been subjected to clinical trials or have already reached the global market [2].

Very recently, within the ongoing project on drug–CDs complexes with enhanced properties, we have presented the results of a comprehensive investigation of nabumetone/CDs inclusion complexes in solution [8]. Since β-cyclodextrin (β-CD) and its derivatives increased nabumetone (NAB) solubility due to the formation of 1:1 inclusion complexes, in the continuation of our study on improving the solubility of poorly soluble drugs [9,10], in this work, the preparation and characterization of NAB complexes in the solid state is presented.

Solid drug/CD complexes, the starting material for dosage form development, may be prepared from solution through crystallization, spray-drying, and lyophilization; in the semisolid state by kneading; and in the solid state [11]. Considering the rising importance of green chemistry approaches, solid-state methods are of great interest, as they eliminate problems related to the low solubility and chemical instability of drugs in solution, as well as the potential toxic effect of residual solvents. In this light, mechanochemical activation by grinding appears as a fast, highly efficient, solvent-free, sustainable approach [12,13]. Furthermore, the grinding process may raise unconventional supramolecular interactions that lead to novel molecular arrangements not observed in solution, providing significant advantages in the formulation development [14].

Considering all the above, we applied mechanochemical activation by grinding to prepare solid CD complexes of NAB, a poorly soluble nonsteroidal anti-inflammatory prodrug (Figure 1). NAB exhibits a pharmacological effect via the metabolite 6-methoxy-2-naphthylacetic acid and is administered orally to treat patients with osteoarthritis and rheumatoid arthritis, showing comparable efficiency and better gastrointestinal tolerability than other nonsteroid anti-inflammatory drugs [15,16]. While the interactions of CDs and NAB have been extensively studied in solution [8,17–19], the systematic screening of preparation methods for NAB/CDs complexes in the solid state represents a novel and intriguing area of research. Previous studies have focused on methods like co-evaporation, kneading, and coprecipitation [20], which are suitable for laboratory-scale preparation but have limited potential for industrial application. In this study, a series of products were prepared by grinding in a high-energy vibrational mill that employed different CD derivatives and processing parameters to develop a product suitable for further formulation development. With that aim, we have screened the efficiency of nabumetone co-grinding with β-cyclodextrin (β-CD) as well as hydroxypropyl- and sulfobutylether-β-cyclodextrin (HP-β-CD and SBE-β-CD, respectively) by changing the grinding time and the grinding frequency. Complexes were prepared at an equimolar drug-to-cyclodextrin ratio, considering the results of a previous study performed by our group [8]. Differential scanning calorimetry (DSC), powder X-ray diffraction (PXRD), and attenuated total reflectance Fourier-transformed infrared spectroscopy (ATR–FTIR) were used to monitor the solid-state interactions in the products prepared. Obtained products were further characterized regarding their solubility, in vitro dissolution in the simulated gastric medium, and in vitro permeability, and flux was analyzed using a MicroFLUX device equipped with an artificial biomimetic membrane. To assess the stability profile of the cyclodextrin complexes obtained, forced degradation studies, employing oxidative, acidic, and basic conditions, were performed. The structures of degradants were proposed based on the results obtained using ultra-high-performance liquid chromatography coupled with high-resolution mass spectrometry (UHPLC–HRMS). This enabled the performance of the photostability and the long-term stability studies according to the ICH guidelines that, combined with other results, enabled the critical evaluation and selection of the complexes that were suitable for further formulation development.

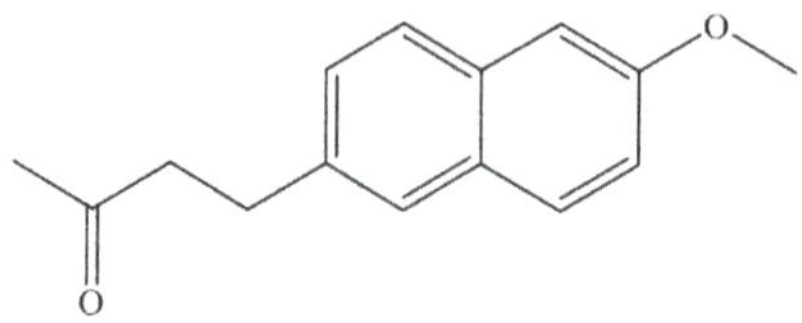

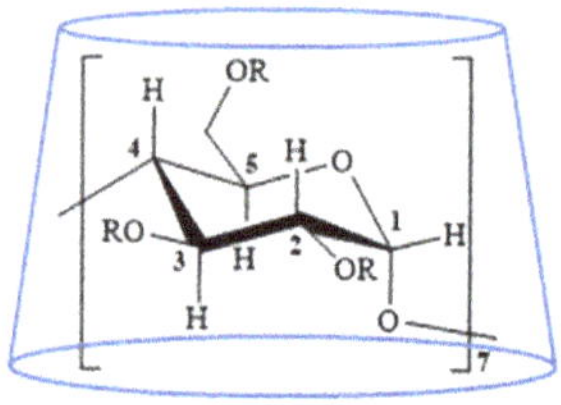


**β-CD**: R = $H_{21}$

**HP-β-CD**: R = $H_{21-n}$ or $(–CH_2CH(OH)CH_3)_n$, n = 2–8

**SBE-β-CD**: R = $H_{21-n}$ or $(–(CH_2)_4SO_3Na)_n$, n = 3–7

**Figure 1.** Structural formulas of nabumetone (NAB), β-cyclodextrin (β-CD), and their derivatives.

## 2. Material and Methods

### *2.1. Materials*

Nabumetone (NAB) was purchased from Cayman Chemical (Ann Arbor, MI, USA). β-cyclodextrin (β-CD), 2-hydroxypropyl-β-cyclodextrin (HP-β-CD, with an average degree of substitution, DS = 4.5), and sulfobutylether sodium salt β-cyclodextrin (SBE-β-CD, DS = 6.5) were obtained from CycloLab (Budapest, Hungary). Methanol and formic acid, LC–MS grade, were purchased from Carlo Erba (Milano, Italy). Ultrapure water was obtained from a Mili-Q Advantage A10 purification system (Merck, Darmstadt, Germany). All other chemicals were of p.a. grade and used as received.

Hydrochloric acid medium (pH 1.2) and hydrochloric medium (pH = 1.2) containing 2% (*w*/*V*) sodium lauryl sulfate were prepared according to European Pharmacopoeia [21].

Analytical-grade solvents (hexane, dodecane, chloroform), L-α-phosphatidylcholine, cholesterol, and all chemicals used for the buffer preparation were purchased from Merck KGaA (Darmstadt, Germany). Phosphate-buffered saline solution (PBS solution; 0.01 M, pH 6.8 and pH 7.4) was prepared by mixing 0.01 M monosodium phosphate solution (0.01 M $NaH_2PO_4$, 0.0027 M KCl, 0.138 M NaCl) and 0.01 M disodium phosphate solution together (0.01 M $Na_2HPO_4$, 0.0027 M KCl, 0.138 M NaCl), adjusting the pH with HCl. The phospholipid solution needed for flux measurements was prepared by dissolving 16 mg phosphatidylcholine and 4 mg cholesterol in 600 μL solvent mixture (70:25:5 *V/V* hexane:dodecane:chloroform).

### *2.2. Complex Preparation in the Solid State*

#### 2.2.1. Complex Preparation by Grinding

Cyclodextrin complexes of NAB were prepared by neat-grinding (NG) in a high-energy vibrational ball mill (Mixer Mill MM 500 control, Retch, GmbH, Germany), employing β-CD, HP-β-CD, and SBE-β-CD in equimolar ratios to the drug, in line with previous results [8]. Then, 6 g sample batches were prepared using 50 mL grinding jars coated with $ZrO_2$, equipped with 15 5 mm and 15 10 mm grinding balls made of the same material. The grinding was performed at a controlled temperature of 20 °C, applying the different grinding periods of up to 120 min in cycles comprising 1 min grinding at 5 Hz to homogenize the product followed by 15 min grinding at a frequency of 20 or 30 Hz to achieve complexation. The drug alone was also subjected to the same procedure at 20 Hz to evaluate the effect of mechanochemical activation on the physicochemical properties of the drug. The obtained products were transferred to the airtight glass containers and stored in a desiccator at room temperature until further analysis.

2.2.2. Complex Preparation by Co-Evaporation

Cyclodextrin complexes of NAB were also prepared by co-evaporation, according to the previously described method [20]. Briefly, 0.05 g of NAB was dissolved in 20 mL of concentrated ethanol, while an equimolar amount of CD in question was dissolved in the same volume of purified water. Then, both solutions were mixed, and the solvent was removed using an IKA KS 4000i control thermostated orbital shaker (IKA-Werke GmbH & Co., Staufen, Germany) operating at 50 °C with gentle mixing at 100 rpm. The drug alone was also subjected to the same procedure by omitting CDs from the preparation to evaluate the effect of co-evaporation on the physicochemical properties of the drug. The obtained products were transferred to the airtight glass containers and stored in a desiccator at room temperature until further analysis.

### 2.3. Solid State Analysis

Differential scanning calorimetry (DSC) was performed on a Perkin-Elmer Diamond differential scanning calorimeter (PerkinElmer, Inc., Waltham, MA, USA) calibrated with indium (99.98% purity; melting point 156.61 °C and fusion enthalpy of 28.71 J/g). The samples were accurately weighted into aluminum pans (1–3 mg, Mettler M3 Microbalance, Germany), sealed with pierced lids, and scanned under the inert atmosphere (nitrogen purge of 25 mL/min), employing a heating rate of 10 °C/min over the temperature range of 25–120 °C. The relative degree of drug crystallinity (*RDC*) in the samples was calculated according to Equation (1):

$$RDC = \frac{\Delta H_{sample}}{\Delta H_{drug}} \times 100\% \tag{1}$$

where $\Delta H_{\text{sample}}$ and $\Delta H_{\text{drug}}$ are the fusion enthalpies of the NAB in the product (normalized to the drug content) and the pure drug, respectively. Measurements were carried out in triplicate, and the relative standard deviation of crystallinity data was <1.0%.

Powder X-ray diffractograms (PXRD) of the starting compounds and co-ground products were recorded using a Malvern Panalytical Aeris diffractometer with Bragg–Brentano geometry (Malvern Panalytical LTD, Malvern, UK) with a copper anode (CuKα, 1.5406 Å) as a radiation source, a Ni filter, and a PIXcel1D-Medipix3 detector at room temperature on a silicon support. The intensity of the diffracted radiation was recorded by continuous scan in the range of 2θ values from 5 to 50° employing the scanning speed of 0.022 °/s, where the counter remained at a single point for 18.87 s. The Kα1/Kα2 intensity ratio was 0.5, the working voltage of the tube was 40 kV, and the cathode was heated with a current of 15 mA.

Attenuated total reflection infrared spectra (ATR–FTIR) spectra of the samples were recorded in the wave number range 4000–400 $cm^{-1}$, with an optical resolution of 2 $cm^{-1}$, using a Bruker Vector 22 IR spectrometer (Bruker Optics GmbH, Ettlingen, Germany) equipped with a Pike MIRacle ATR mount with diamond/ZnSe surface. All measurements were performed at ambient conditions by averaging 32 independent scans. The obtained spectra were further processed using the Opus 6.0 computer program, which applied ATR and background correction. Finally, the spectra were smoothed with the Savitzky–Golay algorithm through 25 data points.

### 2.4. Solubility and In Vitro Dissolution Study at pH 1.2

The saturated solubility of NAB and prepared co-ground products with CDs was determined by adding 30 mg of the drug or the equivalent amount of co-ground CD complex to 15 mL of the medium, which included a hydrochloric acid medium (pH = 1.2), a hydrochloric medium (pH = 1.2) containing 2% (*w*/*V*) sodium lauryl sulfate, and a series of aqueous methanolic solutions (5–40%, *V*/*V*). The flasks were hermetically sealed and shaken at 120 rpm in an orbital shaker thermostated at 37 °C (IKA® KS 4000 i control,

IKA-Werke GmbH & Co. KG, Staufen, Germany). After 24 and 48 h, the sample aliquots were filtered using Cromafil®Xtra PES 20/25 membrane filter (Macherey-Nagel GmbH & Co. KG, Düren, Germany) and spectrophotometrically assayed at $\lambda$ = 230 nm (Agilent Carry 60 spectrophotometer Agilent Technologies, Inc. Santa Clara, CA, USA) to determine the amount of dissolved drug [22]. Preliminary studies demonstrated that NAB did not adsorb to the filters used to separate the undissolved solids. The experiment was performed in triplicate for each sample.

The in vitro dissolution of NAB from the prepared solid systems was investigated using the mini paddle setup of the Agilent 708-DS Dissolution Apparatus (Agilent Technologies, Inc., USA). The sample quantity containing 250 mg of NAB was added to 125 mL of the dissolution medium, thermostated at 37 °C, and stirred at 100 rpm. At preselected time intervals (2, 5, 10, 15, 20, 30, 45, and 60 min), 5 mL aliquots of the dissolution medium were sampled and immediately replaced with the same volume of fresh medium, thermostated at 37 °C, to provide a constant volume of the dissolution medium during the experiment. Collected aliquots were filtered through Cromafil®Xtra PES 20/25 membrane filter (Macherey-Nagel GmbH & Co. KG, Düren, Germany) with 0.20 µm pore size and spectrophotometrically assayed for drug content as described above. The test was performed in triplicate (CV < 5.0%) for each sample. A correction was applied for the cumulative dissolution caused by adding the fresh dissolution medium.

The obtained in vitro dissolution profiles were characterized by calculating the dissolution efficiency (*DE*) parameter according to Equation (2):

$$DE_{60\ min} = \frac{\int_0^t Qdt}{Q_{100\%} \times t} \times 100 \quad (2)$$

where $Q$ is the percentage of the dissolved drug and $t$ is the examined dissolution time [23]. Furthermore, a model-independent similarity factor $f_2$ was used to compare the in vitro dissolution profiles, calculated according to Equation (3):

$$f_2 = 50 \times log\left\{\left[1 + \frac{1}{n}\sum_{t=1}^{n}(R_t - T_t)^2\right]^{-0.5} \times 100\right\} \quad (3)$$

where $n$ is the number of time points and $R_t$ and $T_t$ are the dissolution value of the reference and test product, respectively, at time $t$ [24].

### 2.5. In Vitro Assessment of Dissolution–Absorption Processes in a Low-Volume Environment

#### 2.5.1. In Vitro Dissolution Study at pH 6.8

For the in vitro dissolution studies, 20 mg of the samples (NAB, NAB/HP-β-CD GR 30 Hz/90 min, NAB/SBE-β-CD GR 30 Hz/120 min) were placed into small vessels containing 20 mL PBS solutions (pH 6.8, modeling the intestinal fluid). Measurements were carried out in triplicate. The suspensions were stirred at 300 rpm for only the first 6 h; then, they were allowed to settle for the remaining time. UV spectra were recorded by immersing the UV probes of a Rainbow R6 dynamic dissolution monitor (pION Inc., Billerica, MA, USA) over 24 h. The thermodynamic solubility of each sample was determined as the equilibrium concentration reached in this time period.

#### 2.5.2. In Vitro Gastrointestinal Permeability and Flux Measurements

The flux of nabumetone in different formulations was measured using a MicroFLUX device (pION Inc., USA), consisting of two low-volume absorption chambers and a separating PVDF membrane disk (0.45 µm pore size, 1.54 cm$^2$). First, the membrane disk was wetted with 20 µL phospholipid solution to create a gastrointestinal biomimetic membrane. The donor chamber was filled with 20 mL PBS pH 6.8 solution. Meanwhile, the acceptor chamber was filled with the same amount of 1 mM SBE-β-CD solution (dissolved in PBS pH 7.4) to ensure sink conditions throughout the measurement. Then, a magnetic stirrer bar was placed in both chambers. At the start of the experiment, 20 mg of the sample (NAB,

NAB/HP-β-CD GR 30 Hz/90 min, NAB/SBE-β-CD GR 30 Hz/120 min) was added to the donor chambers, and the stirring was immediately started. All measurements were carried out in triplicate at 37 °C and 300 rpm stirring. The UV–Vis data of each chamber were recorded by immersing the UV probes of a Rainbow R6 dynamic dissolution monitor (pION Inc., USA) over a 4-hour period.

Flux was calculated using Equation (4):

$$J(t) = \frac{\Delta n}{\times \Delta t} \tag{4}$$

where $J$ is the flux $\left(\frac{\text{mol}}{\text{cm}^2}\cdot\text{s}\right)$, $n$ is the amount of drug crossing the membrane (mol), $A$ is the area of the membrane (1.54 $cm^2$), and $t$ is the time (s).

Permeability was calculated using Equation (5):

$$P_a = \frac{J(t)}{c_D(t)} \tag{5}$$

where $P_a$ is the apparent permeability (cm/s) and $c_D(t)$ is the donor concentration at 4 h (mol/$cm^3$).

#### 2.5.3. UV–Vis Spectroscopy

The concentrations of NAB in the in vitro solubility (pH 6.8) and flux measurements were determined using a Rainbow R6 dynamic dissolution monitor (pION Inc., USA). The six UV–Vis immersion probes were equipped with 10 mm pathlength tips. Spectra were recorded in the 220–500 nm wavelength range. Concentration was calculated using the AuPRO 7.1 software (pION Inc., USA) based on a calibration curve generated prior to the measurements.

### *2.6. Stability Testing of Prepared Cyclodextrin Complexes*

#### 2.6.1. Stress Conditions

A stock solution of NAB was prepared in MeOH, LC–MS grade (1 mg/mL), while those of the CD complexes were prepared in a 1:1 mixture of MeOH and $H_2O$ (1 mg/mL). Forced degradation was performed under the following conditions: pure water, 2 M HCl, 2 M NaOH, and 3% $H_2O_2$ at 80 °C for 10 h and, in the case of oxidative degradation, at room temperature for 7 days.

#### 2.6.2. Photostability Study

NAB and the complexes were sieved in glass petri dishes ($\phi$ = 50 mm) to produce a 1 mm thin layer. The control samples were prepared in the same way, but the petri dish was covered and wrapped with aluminum foil. All samples were put in stability chambers and exposed for 141.2 h to a daylight source (8.5 Klux) and 40 h to a UV source (5 W/$m^2$) to ensure that standard ICH Q1B photostability testing conditions were achieved, i.e., 1,200,000 lux h and 200 W H/$m^2$ [25].

#### 2.6.3. Long-Term Stability

NAB and co-ground NAB/CD solids (200 ± 50 mg) were added to Eppendorf tubes and placed in a stability chamber (Memmert ICH110L eco) at 25 °C and 60% relative humidity (RH). Samples were collected and analyzed after 0, 1, 2, 3, 6, and 9 months. Next, 5 mg of NAB (10 mg of the complex) was dissolved in 5 mL of MeOH in the 10 mL flask using an ultrasonic bath. Water was then added until the volume reached the mark. The mass of the samples was corrected for the moisture content determined by dynamic thermogravimetric measurement at 10 °C/min using Discovery TGA 550 (TA Instruments, New Castle, DE, USA). All samples were analyzed in triplicate.

### 2.7. Chromatographic and MS/MS Measurements

Stability-indicating UHPLC–DAD (Agilent 1290 infinity II) and UHPLC–HRMS (Agilent 6550 iFunnel Q-TOF) methods were developed and validated for the quantitative determination of NAB and its degradation products (Supporting Information, Tables S1 and S2). Chromatographic separation was achieved on Agilent ZORBAX RRHD Eclipse Plus C18 column (2.1 × 50 mm, 1.8 μm) in gradient mode using a mobile phase consisting of 0.1% formic acid in water (solvent A) and in methanol (solvent B), with the flow rate set to 0.20 mL/min. The injection volume was 1 μL. NAB was detected at 231 nm. MS/MS experiments were conducted in ion-positive mode using $N_2$ as a collision gas. All samples were filtered through a Chromafil O-20/15 MS filter before LC–DAD and LC–MS analyses. The NAB concentration in MeOH:$H_2O$ 1:1 working solutions amounted to 2 μg/mL.

### 2.8. Statistical Analysis

Data plotting and statistical analysis were carried out using GraphPad Prism 8.0.1. software. For evaluating significant differences, one-way ANOVA with Tukey's multiple comparisons post hoc test was used ($p < 0.05$).

## 3. Results and Discussion

### 3.1. Preparation and Solid-State Characterization of Cyclodextrin Complexes

As the employed complex preparation method has a crucial role in the structural features and performance of the cyclodextrin product obtained, the efficiency of co-grinding, as a solid-state-based approach, was compared to that of the co-evaporation, a solution-based method. DSC and XRPD were used to characterize the co-evaporated and the co-ground products. It was previously postulated that the combined use of the complementary analytical techniques is a powerful tool to examine drug/CD interactions in the solid state, to select the most effective preparation technique, and to optimize the processing conditions of the complex preparation. The interactions in the co-evaporated and co-ground products were further analyzed by ATR–FTIR [11].

The DSC thermogram of NAB presented a sharp exothermic peak with an onset temperature of 80.9 °C and a fusion enthalpy of 139.0 J/g (Figure 2), corresponding to the melting of crystalline polymorphic form I of the drug [26,27]. This result was confirmed by XRPD analysis (Figure 2), which presented a diffractogram with numerous sharp peaks at 2θ values of 7.96, 8.60, 17.18, 17.75, 18.07, 18.48, 19.83, 21.51, 24.40, 26.94, and 27.31°, which are typical for the NAB's polymorphic form I [27,28]. The grinding of pure NAB did not significantly change its physicochemical properties. Although a slight reduction of drug residual crystallinity was observed (Table S3), the drug remained in the same polymorphic form. Namely, two polymorphic forms are described for NAB [26–29]. Polymorph II is a metastable form that transforms into the more stable form I upon slight mechanical contact. Form I is characterized by the onset of melting at a temperature of around 80 °C. In comparison, form II is characterized by melting at a temperature of around 65 °C [26,28]. Furthermore, these two forms can also be distinguished based on XRPD diffractograms, whereby form II is characterized by typical peaks at 6.50, 9.77, 13.04, and 19.61°, which were not observed in the diffractograms of ground NAB (Figure 2). During the grinding, the mechanical energy may be transferred to the treated material by impact or shearing, depending on the number and diameter of the grinding balls. In general, when milling is performed using a large number of smaller balls, as was the case in our experiments, the main mechanism of the energy transfer is the shearing. The transferred energy first reduces particle size to a critical threshold. Further energy input causes the amorphization of the treated material, increasing the molecular mobility and reactivity of the sample [30,31]. However, this state is unstable, and the mechanochemically activated system tends to stabilize, which, in the case of NAB, leads to the formation of the most stable polymorphic form I. At the same time, only a small fraction of the sample remains in the amorphous form, as suggested by the *RDC* values presented in Table S3. Furthermore, the co-evaporation procedure also had only a minor impact on the crystallinity of the drug, showing a similar reduction in *RDC* as observed for the ground NAB. The drug retained the most stable crystalline form in this sample, presenting a DSC curve and XRPD diffractogram typical for the polymorphic form I of NAB (Figure 2).

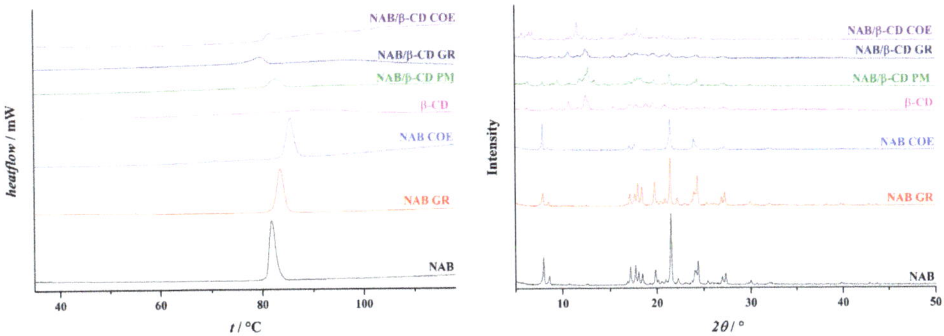


**Figure 2.** DSC thermograms (**left**) and XRPD diffractograms (**right**) of starting compounds (NAB and β-CD), ground and co-evaporated drug (NAB GR and NAB COE), physical mixture (NAB/β-CD PM), and complexes obtained by co-grinding (NAB/β-CD GR) and co-evaporation (NAB/β-CD COE). The results for the systems prepared with HP-β-CD and SBE-β-CD are presented in Supporting Information (Figures S1 and S2, respectively).

When the grinding was performed in the presence of cyclodextrins, a different degree of drug amorphization was observed, depending on the cyclodextrin type and the applied processing parameters (Table S3). The lowest degree of amorphization was obtained for the co-ground NAB with β-CD, presenting an *RDC* of 67.8%. Furthermore, in the case of NAB complexes with β-CD, co-evaporation appears as a more efficient technique, yielding a product with an *RDC* value of 26.6%. Grinding with HP-β-CD and SBE-β-CD was more efficient in establishing the solid-state interaction among the treated compounds, depending highly on the applied grinding frequency. After 120 min of grinding at 20 Hz, the *RDC* for the NAB/HP-β-CD was 75.1%, while processing for the same period but at 30 Hz resulted in a completely amorphous product, as shown by DSC and XRPD analysis (Figure 2). However, the consistency of such product was changed, and it remained compacted on the walls of the grinding jars, which caused the product to be difficult to collect. Therefore, the grinding time was intentionally reduced to 90 min, giving a powdered product with an *RDC* value of 49.2%. For comparison, the *RDC* in the NAB/HP-β-CD sample prepared by co-evaporation was 96.9%, clearly underlying the superior efficiency of the co-griding process in establishing efficient solid-state interactions among the drug and cyclodextrin used. Similar behavior was observed when grinding was performed with SBE-β-CD: processing at the lower grinding frequency (i.e., 20 Hz) for 120 min yielded a product where *RDC* was 84.3%, while increasing the grinding frequency for the same grinding period resulted in a product with *RDC* of 59.7%. On the contrary, the co-evaporation of NAB with SBE-β-CD resulted in a product with an *RDC* of 66.7% (Table S3). Furthermore, in all products with cyclodextrins, regardless of the preparation method employed, the residual drug fraction did not change the polymorphic form, presenting the most stable form—form I—as evident from DSC and XRPD results (Figure 2).

The starting components, their physical mixtures, and solid complexes prepared by grinding were further analyzed by ATR–FTIR spectroscopy. The ATR spectra are given in Figures S3–S5, while the assignation of vibrational bands is in Tables S4–S6. As can be seen, the ATR spectra of the physical NAB/β-CD mixture corresponded to the sum of the spectra of individual components. However, in the ATR spectra of the NAB/β-CD complex prepared by grinding, the shift of characteristic NAB bands, which were previously assigned by P. Govindasamy and S. Gunasekaran [32], to higher wavenumbers was observed, namely, from 1705 to 1706 cm$^{-1}$ ($\nu$(C=O)) and from 1633 and 1228 to 1635 and

1230 cm$^{-1}$ ($\nu$(CC) and $\tau$(HCOC), respectively). In addition, a decrease in band intensities was also observed, indicating the formation of inclusion complexes in the solid state [11,33].

By inspecting the ATR spectra obtained for complexes with CD derivatives (Figures S4 and S5), the similarity with the above-mentioned system can be easily observed. The spectra of physical mixtures are the superposition of those of pure components, while, in the ATR spectra of complexes, the shift and diminishing of NAB vibrational bands intensities were noticed.

The FTIR analyses of complexes prepared by the co-evaporation method reveals the fact that the preparation of the NAB-HP-β-CD complex by grinding was more efficient (Figures S6–S8).

During the grinding, the solid-state interactions between NAB and the cyclodextrin employed are mediated by an amorphous solid phase, allowing greater molecular mobility and the establishment of inclusion and non-inclusion interactions between the compounds [30]. As parent β-CD presents a very strong crystal lattice due to intramolecular hydrogen bonding among the adjacent glucopyranose units' C2 and C3 hydrogen groups, its potential for amorphization is significantly reduced. Because of that, solid-state interaction in the NAB/β-CD sample during the grinding is restricted, resulting in a product with a high fraction of *RDC*. A careful observation of Figure 2 reveals that most residual diffraction peaks in the NAB/β-CD GR sample are typical of β-CD. The weaker potential of β-CD to form effective solid-state interactions with the drug during co-grinding has also been observed with other drugs, while amorphous CD derivatives appear more effective [12,34–36]. In line with this, a relatively high *RDC* observed in the case of NAB/SBE-β-CD was somewhat surprising (Table S3). However, even if the product contains a significant fraction of residual crystalline drug, it could be readily converted into an inclusion complex upon dissolution in water, as demonstrated by Jablan et al. [35].

### *3.2. Solubility and In Vitro Dissolution Properties of the Co-Ground Complexes*

In vitro dissolution tests are crucial in drug dosage form development, quality control, and regulatory approval [37]. They are widely used to mimic and predict the in vivo performance of oral dosage forms in the gastrointestinal tract [38]. Media selection is critical when designing in vitro dissolution methods. Selected media should simulate human gastrointestinal fluid to provide an in vitro–in vivo correlation, enabling the development of clinically relevant dissolution methods. At the same time, the selected medium should be as simple as possible to avoid possible analytical interferences [39]. The US Pharmacopeia prescribes a 2% aqueous sodium lauryl sulfate (SLS) solution as a dissolution medium for NAB tablets [40]. Such a medium has been successfully applied to test the dissolution of micronized nabumetone prepared by a rapid expansion supercritical solution process [22]. To provide more relevant conditions to those encountered in the stomach, we have opted to modify this procedure using a hydrochloric acid medium prepared according to the prescription in monograph 5.17.1. Recommendation on dissolution testing of the European Pharmacopoeia [21], with or without 2% SLS. To assess the suitability of such media, we first tested the solubility of NAB and prepared co-ground products with cyclodextrins in such media. The obtained results are presented in Figure 3.

The solubility of tested samples in a hydrochloric acid medium clearly demonstrates the benefits obtained by the cyclodextrin complexation of NAB by grinding, increasing NAB solubility from 14.6 times in the case of β-CD complex up to 26.2 times for SBE-β-CD complexes. These results align with those observed by the phase solubility studies reported in our previous publication [8]. However, when a hydrochloric medium containing 2% (*w*/*V*) SLS was employed, the increase in NAB solubility brought up by cyclodextrin complexation was absent, probably due to the competition of SLS for inclusion complexation with CDs, thus displacing the drug from the complex [41]. In this light, the SLS-containing medium does not seem appropriate for the in vitro dissolution testing of CD complexes of NAB. Furthermore, the addition of an organic solvent like methanol was also considered; however, as organic solvent content in the dissolution medium is restricted to below 5%

($V/V$), such an approach did not yield any substantial increase in NAB solubility. Therefore, we have performed the in vitro dissolution studies in non-sink conditions using a hydrochloric acid medium without surfactants, employing conditions reflecting drug dose intake (i.e., 500 mg of NAB) with a glass of water (i.e., 250 mL). The performance of the experiments in such conditions enabled the assessment of cyclodextrin's performance in the worst-case scenario that may occur during the drug dissolution upon oral administration in vivo. The observed in vitro dissolution profiles of NAB and co-ground CD complexes in such conditions are presented in Figure 4.

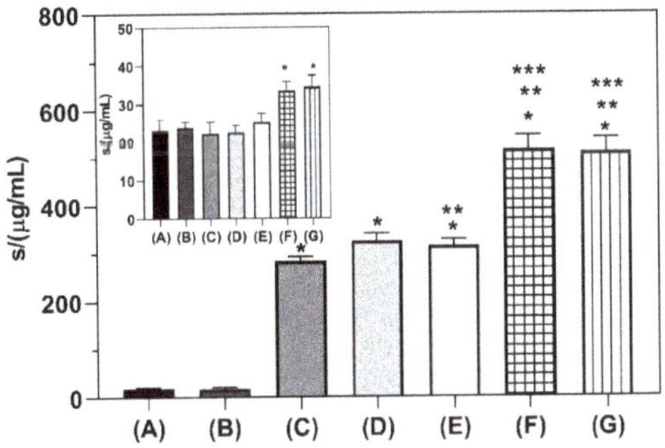


**Figure 3.** Saturation solubility of NAB and co-ground CD complexes in a hydrochloric acid medium pH 1.2 and a hydrochloric acid medium pH 1.2 with 2% ($w/V$) sodium lauryl sulfate (insert) at 37 °C. One asterisk (*) denotes a statistically significant difference ($p < 0.05$) compared to pure NAB, two asterisks (**) denote a statistically significant difference ($p < 0.05$) compared to β-CD complex, and three asterisks (***) denote a statistically significant difference ($p < 0.05$) compared to HP-β-CD complex. Sample codes: NAB (A), NAB GR (B), NAB/β-CD GR (C), NAB/HP-β-CD GR 20 Hz/120 min (D), NAB/HP-β-CD GR 30 Hz/90 min (E), NAB/SBE-β-CD GR 20 Hz/120 min (F), and NAB/SBE-β-CD GR 30 Hz/120 min (G).

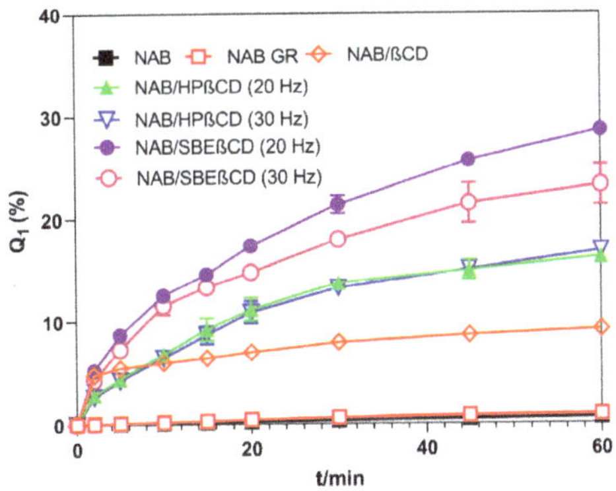


**Figure 4.** In vitro dissolution profiles of NAB and its co-ground products with CDs in hydrochloric acid medium at 37 °C.

The dissolution efficiency ($DE$) parameter, defined as the ratio of the area under the dissolution curve up to a testing time point to the area of the rectangle that describes 100% dissolution up to the same time point, was employed to characterize the obtained dissolution profiles. This enabled the calculation of the dissolution enhancement factor, defined as the ratio between the $DE$ of the co-ground sample and the $DE$ of the pure drug. The values obtained are presented in Table 1.

**Table 1.** Processing parameters, dissolution efficiency, and dissolution enhancement factor for the prepared co-ground samples.

| Sample | Cyclodextrin | Grinding Frequency (Hz) | Grinding Time (min) | Dissolution Efficiency (%) | Dissolution Enhancement Factor |
|---|---|---|---|---|---|
| NAB | - | - | - | 0.17 ± 0.03 | - |
| NAB GR | - | 20 | 120 | 0.26 ± 0.03 | 1.53 ± 0.19 |
| NAB/β-CD GR | β-CD | 20 | 120 | 3.70 ± 0.23 | 21.94 ± 1.35 |
| NAB/HP-β-CD GR 20 Hz | HP-β-CD | 20 | 120 | 5.87 ± 0.28 | 34.86 ± 1.64 |
| NAB/HP-β-CD GR 30 Hz | HP-β-CD | 30 | 90 | 5.81 ± 0.04 | 34.49 ± 0.26 |
| NAB/SBE-β-CD GR 20 Hz | SBE-β-CD | 20 | 120 | 9.83 ± 0.05 | 58.30 ± 0.28 |
| NAB/SBE-β-CD GR 30 Hz | SBE-β-CD | 30 | 120 | 8.30 ± 0.41 | 49.25 ± 2.45 |

To further evaluate the efficiency of co-ground products with CDs in enhancing the dissolution of NAB, the similarity factor $f_2$ was calculated using a model-independent mathematical method. Several FDA and EMA guidelines adopted the $f_2$ comparison as a criterion to estimate the similarity between two in vitro dissolution profiles. The two drug products are considered similar when the $f_2$ value falls between 50 and 100, where an $f_2$ of 100 signifies that the two profiles are identical, while an average variation of 10% at all determined time points leads to an $f_2$ value of 50 [24].

Pure NAB's in vitro dissolution profile is characterized by low dissolution efficiency due to its poor solubility in an aqueous medium (Table 1). The ground NAB sample presented almost the same dissolution profile ($f_2$ = 99.62 ± 0.23) and only an insignificant increase in dissolution efficiency ($p > 0.05$), in line with the lack of significant drug amorphization obtained by grinding. Co-grinding with CDs significantly increased the dissolution efficiency of the drug, depending on the employed CD derivative and applied grinding conditions. However, in the case of the NAB/β-CD sample, the observed dissolution enhancement did not lead to a substantially different dissolution profile, presenting an $f_2$ of 58.32 ± 1.15 compared to pure NAB. Only grinding with HP-β-CD and SBE-β-CD yielded products that showed dissolution profiles that were substantially different from that of pure NAB ($f_2$ values were 48.61 ± 0.76, 48.74 ± 0.16, 37.13 ± 0.05, and 40.87 ± 0.87 for HP-β-CD and SBE-β-CD complexes ground at 20 and 30 Hz, respectively). Interestingly, complexes prepared with the HP-β-CD at different grinding frequencies presented identical in vitro dissolution profiles, irrespective of the different amorphization degrees of the drugs obtained (Table 1, $f_2$ = 93.90 ± 3.38). In the case of co-ground complexes with SBE-β-CD, an anomalous behavior was observed, where the product prepared by grinding at 20 Hz (characterized by a lower degree of nabumetone amorphization) presented a higher dissolution enhancement index than that obtained at 30 Hz, which contained a higher fraction of the amorphous drug (Table 1). Such unusual behavior may be attributed to more pronounced product compaction, as discussed earlier.

### 3.3. *In Vitro Dissolution and Gastrointestinal Permeability Studies in a Low-Volume Environment*

An in vitro assessment of dissolution–absorption processes was performed using a device consisting of a low-volume absorption chamber separated from a low-volume donor chamber with a biomimetic gastrointestinal tract permeation membrane. This device is proposed as a valuable tool for understanding the complex interplay between solubility, permeability, and dissolution rate in vitro, enabling the prediction of in vivo outcomes [42].

#### 3.3.1. In Vitro Dissolution Study at pH 6.8

As Figure 5 shows, the cyclodextrins-containing nabumetone samples presented a greater dissolution rate than the API alone, as equilibrium was reached within 9 min and 50 min for NAB+HP-β-CD and NAB+SBE-β-CD, respectively. Meanwhile, NAB reached equilibrium only after 1.5 h. The equilibrium concentrations at 24 h were the following: 21.02 μg/mL for NAB, 35.53 μg/mL for NAB+HP-β-CD, and 43.41 μg/mL for NAB+SBE-β-CD. The different solubilities with respect to that observed in the hydrochloric medium may be attributed to a different ionic composition of the media [43]. Regardless, SBE-β-CD was shown to be the most effective solubilizing agent, allowing the highest concentration of nabumetone in the aqueous medium.

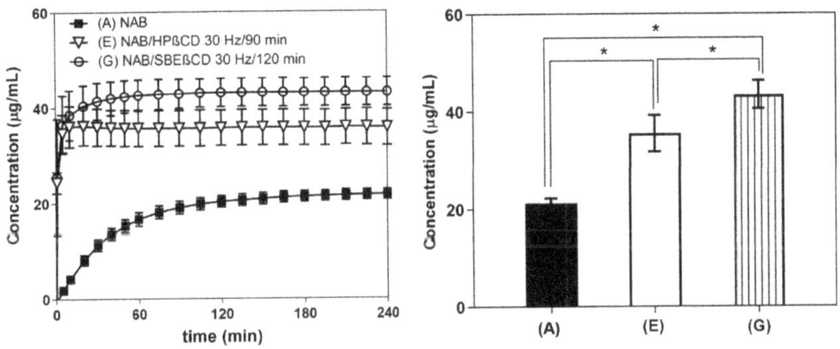


**Figure 5.** The 4-hour dissolution profiles of NAB (A), NAB/HP-β-CD 30 Hz/90 min (E), and NAB/SBE-β-CD 30 Hz/120 min (G) in PBS, pH 6.8, at 37 °C (**left**) and the thermodynamic solubility of the samples at 24 h (37 °C, PBS pH 6.8) (**right**). Significant differences are indicated with an asterisk: * $p < 0.05$ (n = 3, one-way ANOVA, Tukey's multiple comparisons test).

3.3.2. In Vitro Gastrointestinal Flux and Permeability Measurements

The fluxes of dissolved NAB across the biomimetic membrane are presented in Figure 6, clearly presenting the enhanced mass transport observed in the case of co-ground CD products. The higher solubility of NAB/HP-β-CD and NAB/SBE-β-CD created a higher local concentration of the drug available for the permeation, thus increasing the drug thermodynamic activity at the membrane, resulting in higher flux values [44]. This is significant, as it may enable faster achievement and higher levels of maximum drug plasma concentration, thus leading to a faster onset of drug action, as observed in the case of the CD complexes of piroxicam [45]. However, the apparent permeability coefficients for co-ground products with HP-β-CD and SBE-β-CD appeared lower than that of the pure drug. It should be noted that this result is only a consequence of higher drug concentrations in the donor compartment, as observed by in vitro dissolution studies (Figure 5). In line with this, the observed flux values appear more relevant in predicting the effect of CDs on the intestinal absorption of the drug from the tested formulations.

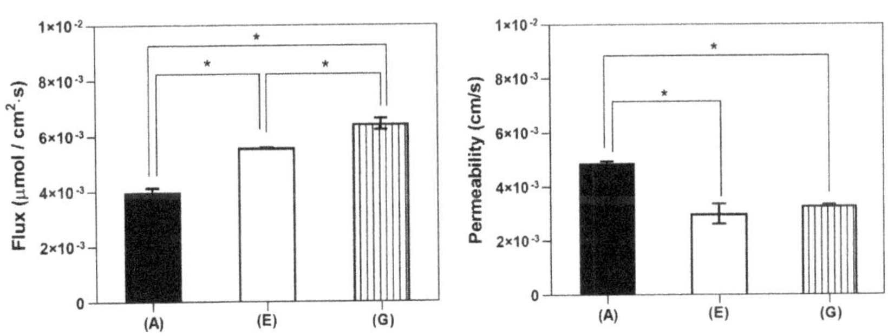


**Figure 6.** In vitro gastrointestinal flux (**left**) and permeability (**right**) of NAB (A), NAB/HP-β-CD 30 Hz/90 min (E), and NAB/SBE-β-CD 30 Hz/120 min (G). Significant differences are indicated with an asterisk: * $p < 0.05$ (n = 3, one-way ANOVA, Tukey's multiple comparisons test).

### 3.4. *Effect of Cyclodextrins on NAB Chemical and Photochemical Stability*

The stability of active pharmaceutical ingredients and their formulations is a critical parameter that ensures their safety and efficacy. Previously, it was shown that β-CDs can influence the chemical stability of a drug by increasing or even decreasing its stability [4,9,46]. Therefore, in the continuation of our study, based on the in vitro dissolution results, the stability of pure and co-ground NAB, CDs, and NAB complexes with HP-β-CD and SBE-β-CD was investigated. Before analysis, to be able to characterize and identify NAB degradation products [47], the stability-indication UHPLC–DAD–MS method for the quantitative determination of NAB in the presence of its degradation products was developed and validated (Tables S1 and S2). For that purpose, stress tests were performed in hydrolytic (acidic, neutral, and basic) and oxidative conditions both at room temperature and 80 °C.

At first, the analysis of pure NAB was performed. The total ion current chromatogram (TIC) of NAB and its MS spectrum are shown in Figures S9 and S10. The base peak (*m/z* 171) corresponds to the NAB in-source fragment ion, previously described by Valero and Costa [48] and by Wolff et al. [49], while peaks at *m/z* 229 and 251 to $[NAB+H]^+$ and $[NAB+Na]^+$ ions, respectively. All data are given in Table S7.

Nabumetone was prone to hydrolytic degradation only in acidic conditions, both alone and in systems with HP-β-CD and SBE-β-CD (Figure S11), yielding one degradation product (DP 1), which was noticed at the retention time of 10.9 min. The observed accurate *m/z* value of the singly protonated ion of DP 1 was 215.1062 (Figure 7). Structural characterization was based on the results of HRMS and MS/MS analysis (Table S8). This compound, 4-(6-hydroxy-2-naphthtyl)-2-butanone, was previously recognized as one of the pharmacologically inactive NAB metabolites [50,51].

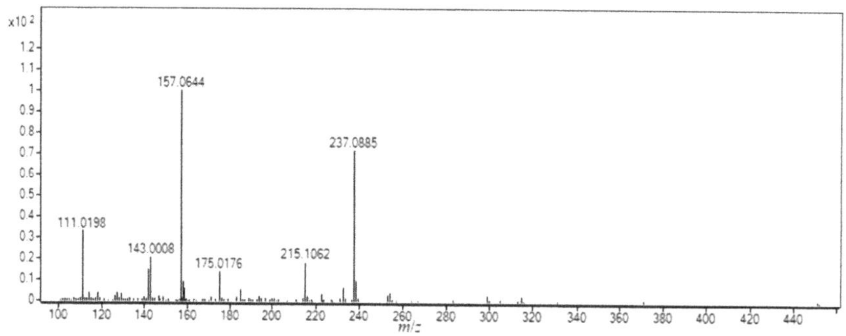


**Figure 7.** HRMS spectrum of degradation product DP 1 ($t_R$ = 10.9 min) formed during the acidic hydrolytic degradation.

The hydroxypropylated derivative of β-CD was also prone to hydrolytic degradation, yielding various differently substituted isomeric hydroxypropylated linear maltooligomers (Figure S12). The exact identification of degradation products is technically impossible, as HP-β-CD is a mixture of hundreds of thousands of isomeric species [52]. No degradation products were observed under neutral and basic hydrolytic conditions, which is in accordance with literature data on β-CD stability in neutral and basic media [53].

Nabumetone was not susceptible to oxidative degradation both at room temperature and at elevated temperatures. However, the presence of HP-β-CD and SBE-β-CD in their co-ground samples led to the formation of several degradation products only at elevated temperatures. The total ion chromatograms are given in Figure S13. Ten degradation products were identified in total as a result of the extensive HRMS and MS/MS analyses of protonated molecular ions (Tables S9–S18). The hydroxylation of the naphthalene moiety of NAB was the most pronounced degradation process. Such extensive hydroxylation can only be induced by hydroxy radicals. Indeed, hydrogen peroxide contains a very weak O–O bond, which can easily cleave to form hydroxyl radicals (•OH), a reactive oxidative reagent [54]. Likely, the presence of HP-β-CD and SBE-β-CD promote the •OH formation, making the hydroxylation of naphthalene moiety the dominating process at elevated temperature.

The proposed structures of NAB degradation products obtained during forced degradation studies are shown in Figure 8. It should be emphasized that the structures are proposed based on HRMS spectra and MS/MS data. The unambiguous determination of the structures will be confirmed by the isolation of degradation products and their analysis by NMR spectroscopy, which is the subject of upcoming investigations.

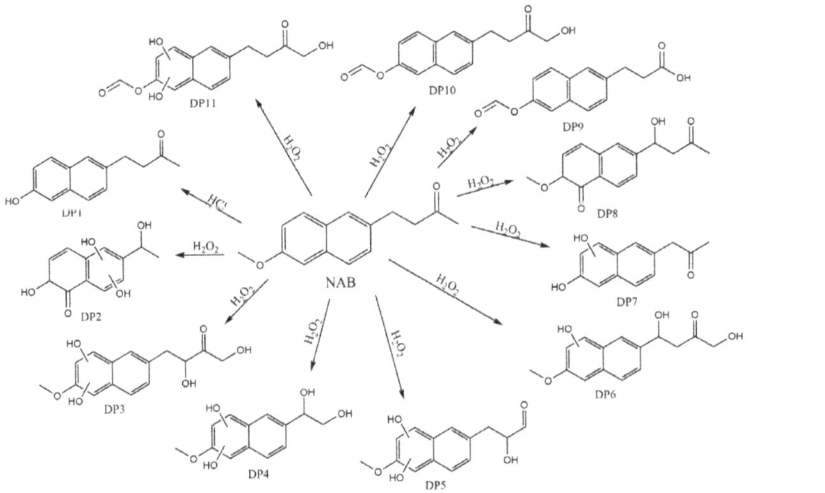


**Figure 8.** Proposed degradation products of NAB in hydrolytic (HCl) and oxidative conditions ($H_2O_2$). Experimental conditions: 2M HCl; 3% $H_2O_2$ at 80 °C.

Nabumetone, both alone and in systems with HP-β-CD and SBE-β-CD, was not prone to photodegradation. In all cases, the NAB content in samples subjected to photostability studies was within the specification of 98.5–102.6 of the control samples (Figure S14). To obtain deeper knowledge about possible minor degradation products formed during these studies, we performed a UHPLC–HRMS analysis. No degradation products were observed in any of the samples. The total ion chromatograms are given in the supporting information (Figure S15).

All co-ground systems showed satisfying chemical stability during the long-term stability studies. Both pure NAB and co-ground NAB were not prone to degradation. The recovered NAB content at the end of the 9-month testing was 93.5–100.5 of the initial content in all cases (Figure S16). No degradation products were observed in any of the samples during the UHPLC–HRMS analysis as well. The total ion chromatograms are given in the supporting information (Figure S17).

## 4. Conclusions

Grinding in high-energy vibrational mills is a sustainable, solvent-free, and eco-friendly approach for developing CD complexes of poorly soluble drugs like NAB. Processing NAB with CDs yielded powdered products, where the level of the drug amorphization depended on the CD derivative used and the grinding conditions applied. This rapid, one-step technological approach enables the easy control of the process by optimizing grinding time and frequency. Co-ground complexes with SBE-β-CD and HP-β-CD showed the most pronounced in vitro drug dissolution enhancement in both gastric and intestinal media. Enhanced dissolution has led to increased drug flux across the biomimetic membranes, indicating the possibility of achieving a faster onset of drug action upon oral administration of such co-ground complexes, which still needs to be verified in vivo.

Although forced degradation studies revealed various degradants originating from the drug and the CDs used, the co-ground NAB complexes with SBE-β-CD and HP-β-CD showed acceptable photo- and long-term stability, indicating their suitability for further pharmaceutical product development.

**Supplementary Materials:** The following supporting information can be downloaded at: https://www.mdpi.com/article/10.3390/pharmaceutics16121493/s1, The SI material published online alongside the article concerns the details for UHPLC and MS analyses (Tables S1 and S2); characterization of NAB complexes in the solid state by DSC and PXRD (Figures S1 and S2, Table S3); ATR–FTIR analysis of the complexes (Figures S3–S8 and Tables S4–S6); chemical stability (Figures S9–S13 and Tables S7–S18); photochemical stability (Figure S14 and S15); and long-term stability (Figures S16 and S17).

**Author Contributions:** Conceptualization G.T.B., M.J. and N.G.; Formal analysis, D.K., Ž.S., A.V. and R.S.; Investigation, D.K., Ž.S., A.V. and R.S.; Methodology, A.V. and R.S.; Supervision, G.T.B., M.J. and N.G; Validation, D.K.; Visualization, Ž.S., M.J. and N.G.; Resources, G.T.B. and N.G.; Funding Acquisition, N.G.; Project Administration, N.G.; Writing—original draft, M.J. and N.G.; Writing—review and editing, M.J. and N.G. All authors have read and agreed to the published version of the manuscript.

**Funding:** The research was funded by the Croatian Science Foundation (project IP-2022-10-6033) and supported by the European Regional Development Fund (infrastructural projects CIuK, KK.01.1.1.02.0016, and FarmInova, KK.01.1.1.02.0021).

**Institutional Review Board Statement:** Not applicable.

**Informed Consent Statement:** Not applicable.

**Data Availability Statement:** The original contributions presented in the study are included in the article/Supplementary Material; further inquiries can be directed to the corresponding author.

**Acknowledgments:** We are grateful to Vivien Bárdos for her assistance with the in vitro dissolution and permeability measurements. D. Klarić acknowledges the CEEPUS program for awarding him a scholarship within the RO-0010-19-2425 Network.

**Conflicts of Interest:** The authors declare no conflicts of interest.

## References

1. Jansook, P.; Ogawa, N.; Loftsson, T. Cyclodextrins: Structure, Physicochemical Properties and Pharmaceutical Applications. *Int. J. Pharm.* **2018**, *535*, 272–284. [CrossRef] [PubMed]
2. Kali, G.; Haddadzadegan, S.; Bernkop-Schnürch, A. Cyclodextrins and Derivatives in Drug Delivery: New Developments, Relevant Clinical Trials, and Advanced Products. *Carbohydr. Polym.* **2024**, *324*, 121500. [CrossRef] [PubMed]
3. Riccio, V.B.F.; Meneguin, A.B.; Baveloni, F.G.; de Antoni, A.J.; Robusti, L.M.G.; Gremião, M.P.D.; Ferrari, P.C.; Chorilli, M. Biopharmaceutical and Nanotoxicological Aspects of Cyclodextrins for Non-Invasive Topical Treatments: A Critical Review. *J. Appl. Toxicol.* **2023**, *43*, 1410–1420. [CrossRef]
4. Aiassa, V.; Garnero, C.; Zoppi, A.; Longhi, M.R. Cyclodextrins and Their Derivatives as Drug Stability Modifiers. *Pharmaceuticals* **2023**, *16*, 1074. [CrossRef]
5. Kovacs, T.; Nagy, P.; Panyi, G.; Szente, L.; Varga, Z.; Zakany, F. Cyclodextrins: Only Pharmaceutical Excipients or Full-Fledged Drug Candidates? *Pharmaceutics* **2022**, *14*, 2559. [CrossRef]
6. Ferreira, L.; Campos, J.; Veiga, F.; Cardoso, C.; Paiva-Santos, A.C. Cyclodextrin-Based Delivery Systems in Parenteral Formulations: A Critical Update Review. *Eur. J. Pharm. Biopharm.* **2022**, *178*, 35–52. [CrossRef] [PubMed]
7. Jacob, S.; Nair, A.B. Cyclodextrin Complexes: Perspective from Drug Delivery and Formulation. *Drug Dev. Res.* **2018**, *79*, 201–217. [CrossRef]
8. Klarić, D.; Kelrajter, M.; Čikoš, A.; Budimir, A.; Galić, N. Inclusion Complexes of Nabumetone with β-Cyclodextrins: Spectroscopic, Spectrometric and Calorimetric Studies in Solution. *J. Mol. Liq.* **2024**, *397*, 124152. [CrossRef]
9. Špehar, T.K.; Pocrnić, M.; Klarić, D.; Bertoša, B.; Čikoš, A.; Jug, M.; Padovan, J.; Dragojević, S.; Galić, N. Investigation of Praziquantel/Cyclodextrin Inclusion Complexation by NMR and LC-HRMS/MS: Mechanism, Solubility, Chemical Stability, and Degradation Products. *Mol. Pharm.* **2021**, *18*, 4210–4223. [CrossRef]
10. Pocrnić, M.; Hoelm, M.; Ignaczak, A.; Čikoš, A.; Budimir, A.; Tomišić, V.; Galić, N. Inclusion Complexes of Loratadine with β-Cyclodextrin and Its Derivatives in Solution. Integrated Spectroscopic, Thermodynamic and Computational Studies. *J. Mol. Liq.* **2024**, *410*, 125515. [CrossRef]
11. Mura, P. Analytical Techniques for Characterization of Cyclodextrin Complexes in the Solid State: A Review. *J. Pharm. Biomed. Anal.* **2015**, *113*, 226–238. [CrossRef] [PubMed]
12. Jug, M.; Mura, P.A. Grinding as Solvent-Free Green Chemistry Approach for Cyclodextrin Inclusion Complex Preparation in the Solid State. *Pharmaceutics* **2018**, *10*, 189. [CrossRef] [PubMed]

13. Nicoletti, C.D.; de Sá Haddad Queiroz, M.; de Souza Lima, C.G.; de Carvalho da Silva, F.; Futuro, D.O.; Ferreira, V.F. An Improved Method for the Preparation of β-Lapachone:2-Hydroxypropyl-β-Cyclodextrin Inclusion Complexes. *J. Drug Deliv. Sci. Technol.* **2020**, *58*, 101777. [CrossRef]
14. Cabrera-Quiñones, N.C.; López-Méndez, L.J.; Guadarrama, P. Inclusion and Non-Inclusion Complexes between Curcumin and β-Cyclodextrin with High-Curcumin Loading and Enhanced Aqueous Solubility Obtained by Mechanochemistry. *ChemistrySelect* **2023**, *8*, e202303254. [CrossRef]
15. Bannwarth, B. Safety of the Nonselective NSAID Nabumetone: Focus on Gastrointestinal Tolerability. *Drug Saf.* **2008**, *31*, 485–503. [CrossRef]
16. Hedner, T.; Samulesson, O.; Währborg, P.; Wadenvik, H.; Ung, K.A.; Ekbom, A. Nabumetone: Therapeutic Use and Safety Profile in the Management of Osteoarthritis and Rheumatoid Arthritis. *Drugs* **2004**, *64*, 2315–2343. [CrossRef]
17. Bensouilah, N.; Boutemeur-Kheddis, B.; Bensouilah, H.; Meddour, I.; Abdaoui, M. Host-Guest Complex of Nabumetone: β-Cyclodextrin: Quantum Chemical Study and QTAIM Analysis. *J. Incl. Phenom. Macrocycl. Chem.* **2017**, *87*, 191–206. [CrossRef]
18. Al-Rawashdeh, N.A.F. Interactions of Nabumetone with γ-Cyclodextrin Studied by Fluorescence Measurements. *J. Incl. Phenom. Macrocycl. Chem.* **2005**, *51*, 27–32. [CrossRef]
19. Valero, M.; Tejedor, J.; Rodríguez, L.J. Encapsulation of Nabumetone by Means of Drug: (β-Cyclodextrin)2:Polyvinylpyrrolidone Ternary Complex Formation. *J. Lumin.* **2007**, *126*, 297–302. [CrossRef]
20. Goyenechea, N.; Sánchez, M.; Vélaz, I.; Martín, C.; Martínez-Ohárriz, C.; Zornoza, A. Interactions of Nabumetone with Cyclodextrins in Solution and in the Solid State. *J. Incl. Phenom. Macrocycl. Chem.* **2002**, *44*, 283–288. [CrossRef]
21. 5.17.1. Recommendations on Dissolution Testing. In *European Pharmacopeia*; EDQM Council of Europe: Strasbourg, France, 2024.
22. Su, C.S.; Tang, M.; Chen, Y.P. Micronization of Nabumetone Using the Rapid Expansion of Supercritical Solution (RESS) Process. *J. Supercrit. Fluids* **2009**, *50*, 69–76. [CrossRef]
23. Anderson, N.H.; Bauer, M.; Boussac, N.; Khan-Malek, R.; Munden, P.; Sardaro, M. An Evaluation of Fit Factors and Dissolution Efficiency for the Comparison of in Vitro Dissolution Profiles. *J. Pharm. Biomed. Anal.* **1998**, *17*, 811–822. [CrossRef] [PubMed]
24. Xie, F.; Ji, S.; Cheng, Z. In Vitro Dissolution Similarity Factor (F2) and in Vivo Bioequivalence Criteria, How and When Do They Match? Using a BCS Class II Drug as a Simulation Example. *Eur. J. Pharm. Sci.* **2015**, *66*, 163–172. [CrossRef]
25. ICH Q1B, Stability Testing: Photostability Testing of New Drug Substances and Products. Available online: https://www.ema.europa.eu/en/documents/scientific-guideline/ich-q-1-b-photostability-testing-new-active-substances-and-medicinal-products-step-5_en.pdf (accessed on 7 October 2024).
26. Price, C.P.; Grzesiak, A.L.; Lang, M.; Matzger, A.J. Polymorphism of Nabumetone. *Cryst. Growth Des.* **2002**, *2*, 501–503. [CrossRef]
27. Türk, M.; Bolten, D. Polymorphic Properties of Micronized Mefenamic Acid, Nabumetone, Paracetamol and Tolbutamide Produced by Rapid Expansion of Supercritical Solutions (RESS). *J. Supercrit. Fluids* **2016**, *116*, 239–250. [CrossRef]
28. Chyall, L.J.; Tower, J.M.; Coates, D.A.; Houston, T.L.; Childs, S.L. Polymorph Generation in Capillary Spaces: The Preparation and Structural Analysis of a Metastable Polymorph of Nabumetone. *Cryst. Growth Des.* **2002**, *2*, 505–510. [CrossRef]
29. Suresh, K.; Ashe, J.S.; Matzger, A.J. Far-Infrared Spectroscopy as a Probe for Polymorph Discrimination. *J. Pharm. Sci.* **2019**, *108*, 1915–1920. [CrossRef]
30. Tan, D.; Loots, L.; Friščić, T. Towards Medicinal Mechanochemistry: Evolution of Milling from Pharmaceutical Solid Form Screening to the Synthesis of Active Pharmaceutical Ingredients (APIs). *Chem. Commun.* **2016**, *52*, 7760–7781. [CrossRef]
31. Julien, P.A.; Friščić, T. Methods for Monitoring Milling Reactions and Mechanistic Studies of Mechanochemistry: A Primer. *Cryst. Growth Des.* **2022**, *22*, 5726–5754. [CrossRef]
32. Govindasamy, P.; Gunasekaran, S. Experimental and Theoretical Studies of (FT-IR, FT-Raman, UV–Visible and DFT) 4-(6-Methoxynaphthalen-2-Yl) Butan-2-One. *Spectrochim. Acta A Mol. Biomol. Spectrosc.* **2015**, *149*, 800–811. [CrossRef]
33. Cannavà, C.; Crupi, V.; Ficarra, P.; Guardo, M.; Majolino, D.; Stancanelli, R.; Venuti, V. Physicochemical Characterization of Coumestrol/β-Cyclodextrins Inclusion Complexes by UV–Vis and FTIR-ATR Spectroscopies. *Vib. Spectrosc.* **2008**, *48*, 172–178. [CrossRef]
34. Mennini, N.; Bragagni, M.; Maestrelli, F.; Mura, P. Physico-Chemical Characterization in Solution and in the Solid State of Clonazepam Complexes with Native and Chemically-Modified Cyclodextrins. *J. Pharm. Biomed. Anal.* **2014**, *89*, 142–149. [CrossRef] [PubMed]
35. Jablan, J.; Bačić, I.; Kujundžić, N.; Jug, M. Zaleplon Co-Ground Complexes with Natural and Polymeric β-Cyclodextrin. *J. Incl. Phenom. Macrocycl. Chem.* **2013**, *76*, 353–362. [CrossRef]
36. Cugovčan, M.; Jablan, J.; Lovrić, J.; Cinčić, D.; Galić, N.; Jug, M. Biopharmaceutical Characterization of Praziquantel Cocrystals and Cyclodextrin Complexes Prepared by Grinding. *J. Pharm. Biomed. Anal.* **2017**, *137*, 42–53. [CrossRef]
37. Jug, M.; Hafner, A.; Lovrić, J.; Kregar, M.L.; Pepić, I.; Vanić, Ž.; Cetina-Čižmek, B.; Filipović-Grčić, J. An Overview of in Vitro Dissolution/Release Methods for Novel Mucosal Drug Delivery Systems. *J. Pharm. Biomed. Anal.* **2018**, *147*, 350–366. [CrossRef] [PubMed]
38. Lex, T.R.; Rodriguez, J.D.; Zhang, L.; Jiang, W.; Gao, Z. Development of In Vitro Dissolution Testing Methods to Simulate Fed Conditions for Immediate Release Solid Oral Dosage Forms. *AAPS J.* **2022**, *24*, 40. [CrossRef]
39. Grignard, E.; Taylor, R.; McAllister, M.; Box, K.; Fotaki, N. Considerations for the Development of in Vitro Dissolution Tests to Reduce or Replace Preclinical Oral Absorption Studies. *Eur. J. Pharm. Sci.* **2017**, *99*, 193–201. [CrossRef]

40. USP. Monographs, Nabumetone Tablets. In *United States Pharmacopeia*; The United State Pharmacopoeial Convention: Rockville, MD, USA, 2024.
41. Hao, L.S.; Wang, H.X.; Wang, Y.S.; Meng, Y.Q.; Nan, Y.Q. Inclusion Complexation of Surfactant with β-Cyclodextrin and Its Effect on the Mixed Micellization of Cationic/Anionic Surfactants. *Colloids. Surf. A Physicochem. Eng. Asp.* **2023**, *668*, 131437. [CrossRef]
42. Kádár, S.; Kennedy, A.; Lee, S.; Ruiz, R.; Farkas, A.; Tőzsér, P.; Csicsák, D.; Tóth, G.; Sinkó, B.; Borbás, E. Bioequivalence Prediction with Small-Scale Biphasic Dissolution and Simultaneous Dissolution-Permeation Apparatus—An Aripiprazole Case Study. *Eur. J. Pharm. Sci.* **2024**, *198*, 106782. [CrossRef]
43. Karkossa, F.; Klein, S. Assessing the Influence of Media Composition and Ionic Strength on Drug Release from Commercial Immediate-Release and Enteric-Coated Aspirin Tablets. *J. Pharm. Pharmacol.* **2017**, *69*, 1327–1340. [CrossRef]
44. Sripetch, S.; Prajapati, M.; Loftsson, T. Cyclodextrins and Drug Membrane Permeation: Thermodynamic Considerations. *J. Pharm Sci.* **2022**, *111*, 2571–2580. [CrossRef]
45. Scarpignato, C. Piroxicam-ß-Cyclodextrin: A GI Safer Piroxicam. *Curr. Med. Chem.* **2013**, *20*, 2415–2437. [CrossRef] [PubMed]
46. Popielec, A.; Loftsson, T. Effects of Cyclodextrins on the Chemical Stability of Drugs. *Int. J. Pharm.* **2017**, *531*, 532–542. [CrossRef] [PubMed]
47. Narayanam, M.; Handa, T.; Sharma, P.; Jhajra, S.; Muthe, P.K.; Dappili, P.K.; Shah, R.P.; Singh, S. Critical Practical Aspects in the Application of Liquid Chromatography–Mass Spectrometric Studies for the Characterization of Impurities and Degradation Products. *J. Pharm. Biomed. Anal.* **2014**, *87*, 191–217. [CrossRef] [PubMed]
48. Valero, M.; Costa, S.M.B. Photodegradation of Nabumetone in Aqueous Solutions. *J. Photochem. Photobiol. A. Chem.* **2003**, *157*, 93–101. [CrossRef]
49. Wolff, J.C.; Hawtin, P.N.; Monté, S.; Balogh, M.; Jones, T. The Use of Particle Beam Mass Spectrometry for the Measurement of Impurities in a Nabumetone Drug Substance, Not Easily Amenable to Atmospheric Pressure Ionisation Techniques. *Rapid. Commun. Mass. Spectrom.* **2001**, *15*, 265–272. [CrossRef]
50. Nobilis, M.; Mikušek, J.; Szotáková, B.; Jirásko, R.; Holčapek, M.; Chamseddin, C.; Jira, T.; Kučera, R.; Kuneš, J.; Pour, M. Analytical Power of LLE–HPLC–PDA–MS/MS in Drug Metabolism Studies: Identification of New Nabumetone Metabolites. *J. Pharm. Biomed. Anal.* **2013**, *80*, 164–172. [CrossRef]
51. Nobilis, M.; Kopecký, J.; Květina, J.; Svoboda, Z.; Pour, M.; Kuneš, J.; Holčapek, M.; Kolářová, L. Comparative Biotransformation and Disposition Studies of Nabumetone in Humans and Minipigs Using High-Performance Liquid Chromatography with Ultraviolet, Fluorescence and Mass Spectrometric Detection. *J. Pharm. Biomed. Anal.* **2003**, *32*, 641–656. [CrossRef] [PubMed]
52. Szente, L.; Szemán, J.; Sohajda, T. Analytical Characterization of Cyclodextrins: History, Official Methods and Recommended New Techniques. *J. Pharm. Biomed. Anal.* **2016**, *130*, 347–365. [CrossRef]
53. Saokham, P.; Muankaew, C.; Jansook, P.; Loftsson, T. Solubility of Cyclodextrins and Drug/Cyclodextrin Complexes. *Molecules* **2018**, *23*, 1161. [CrossRef]
54. Gabrić, A.; Hodnik, Ž.; Pajk, S. Oxidation of Drugs during Drug Product Development: Problems and Solutions. *Pharmaceutics* **2022**, *14*, 325. [CrossRef] [PubMed]

MDPI AG
Grosspeteranlage 5
4052 Basel
Switzerland
Tel.: +41 61 683 77 34

*Pharmaceutics* Editorial Office
E-mail: pharmaceutics@mdpi.com
www.mdpi.com/journal/pharmaceutics

www.ingramcontent.com/pod-product-compliance
Lightning Source LLC
Chambersburg PA
CBHW061446210926
51850CB00008B/1630
*9783725874729*